Common Childhood Diseases - Diagnosis, Prevention and Management

Edited by Enkhsaikhan Purevjav, Stephanie A. Storgion and Timothy Dean Minniear

Published in London, United Kingdom

Common Childhood Diseases - Diagnosis, Prevention and Management
http://dx.doi.org/10.5772/intechopen.1002574
Edited by Enkhsaikhan Purevjav, Stephanie A. Storgion and Timothy Dean Minniear

Contributors
Alessandro Maraschi, Asiya Uzun, Buyan-Ochir Orgil, Dalal R. Fatani, Derryl Miller, Dharanya Srinivasan, Enkhsaikhan Purevjav, Enkhzul Batsaikhan, Erica Cristina Vallocchia, Gantuul Narmandakh, Hala A. Helmi, Hind M. Alkatan, Kalaiarasi Raja, Kunal Bhakhri, Mirjam Močnik, Munirah Aldofyan, Nataša Marčun Varda, Nawaf AlAnazi, Neely Alberson, Rahaf Altwijri, Rakan Alsaad, Sarah AlMukhaylid, Sevgi Gözdaşoğlu, Timothy D. Minniear, Zafar Iqbal

First published in London, United Kingdom, 2024 by IntechOpen
IntechOpen is the global imprint of INTECHOPEN LIMITED, registered in England and Wales, registration number: 11086078, 167-169 Great Portland Street, London, W1W 5PF, United Kingdom

For EU product safety concerns: IN TECH d.o.o., Prolaz Marije Krucifikse Kozulić 3, 51000 Rijeka, Croatia, info@intechopen.com or visit our website at intechopen.com.

British Library Cataloguing-in-Publication Data
A catalogue record for this book is available from the British Library

Common Childhood Diseases - Diagnosis, Prevention and Management
Edited by Enkhsaikhan Purevjav, Stephanie A. Storgion and Timothy Dean Minniear
p. cm.
Print ISBN 978-0-85466-776-5
Online ISBN 978-0-85466-775-8
eBook (PDF) ISBN 978-0-85466-777-2

Meet the editors

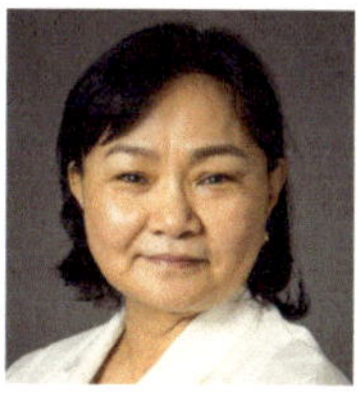

Dr. Enkhsaikhan Purevjav earned her MD from the Leningrad State Pediatric Medical Institute (LSPMI), Russia, in 1989. She completed a clinical residency in pediatrics at the Mongolian National Medical University, a fellowship in pediatric cardiology and electrophysiology at LSPMI, and a Ph.D. program in medical genetics and molecular biology at the Shimane Medical University, Japan, in 2003. Dr. Purevjav worked at Baylor College of Medicine, Texas Children's Hospital, and Cincinnati Children's Hospital Medical Center, USA. She is a Professor of Pediatrics at the University of Tennessee Health Science Center, USA, where she continues to study the genetics of cardiovascular diseases, focusing on pediatric cardiomyopathies, arrhythmias, and heart failure.

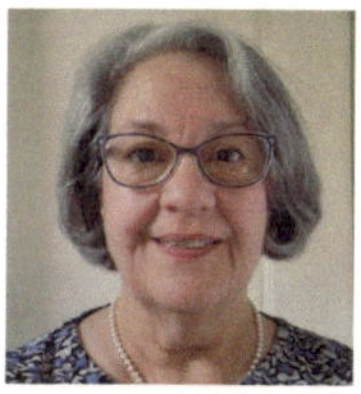

Dr. Stephanie Storgion has been at the University of Tennessee Health Science Center, USA, since 1987. She is a tenured professor in the College of Medicine in the Department of Pediatrics, Division of Pediatric Critical Care Medicine. She is also the Director of the Pediatric Critical Care Medicine fellowship and has served as Medical Director of the Pediatric Intensive Care Unit (PICU), Pediatric Neuro ICU, and the Intermediate Care Unit over the years. In addition to her work in pediatric critical care, she has been a professor and chair of the Department of Physician Assistant Studies since 2016. Dr. Storgion's research and medical interests include medical education, neurocritical care, trauma, and the management of chronically critically ill children.

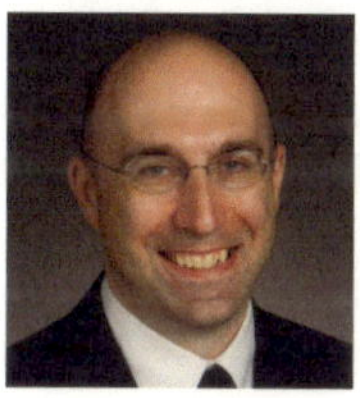

Dr. Timothy D. Minniear is an Assistant Professor of Pediatrics at the University of Tennessee Health Science Center (UTHSC), USA. Dr. Minniear earned his MD at Wayne State University School of Medicine, USA, in 2003. He completed a pediatric residency at UTHSC and a pediatric infectious diseases fellowship in the combined St. Jude Children's Research Hospital (SJCRH)/UTHSC program with an interest in and focus on children with acquired immunodeficiencies. He has worked in Lilongwe and Zomba, Malawi, as part of the Baylor Pediatric AIDS Initiative, as a Medical Officer at the U.S. Centers for Disease Control and Prevention, and as faculty at SJCRH. Currently, Dr. Minniear is the Clinical Director of Pediatric Transplant Infectious Diseases at Le Bonheur Children's Hospital and UTHSC and Associate Program Director for the SJCRH/UTHSC

Contents

Preface

The fact that nearly 32 million American children miss school yearly due to an illness demonstrates how vulnerable children are to disease. During the past centuries, substantial progress has been achieved in reducing childhood morbidity and mortality. According to the World Health Organization (WHO), the total number of deaths in children under the age of 5 worldwide has declined from 12.8 million in 1990 to 5 million in 2021. However, infectious diseases, including acute respiratory infections, diarrhea, malaria, birth complications, trauma, and congenital anomalies remain the leading causes of death for children. Furthermore, humankind is facing extreme climate change and pollution, poverty, migration crises, dangerous political conflicts, unsafe social and commercial networking, harmful lifestyles and diets, and the consequences of the COVID-19 pandemic. These threats change the landscape of human disorders, particularly for our children, the most vulnerable population. The diseases and devastating conditions of childhood, such as cancer, developmental and autism spectrum disorders, asthma and allergies, diabetes and obesity, trauma, and genetic anomalies, are on the rise.

Therefore, we have invited physicians and pediatric professionals around the world to present common diseases of childhood they currently encounter in their pediatric practice. This collection covers broad but important topics of childhood health including communicable and non-communicable disorders. The chapters in this book provide useful information on routine and emergency medical care for selected disorders of children with a discussion of current advancements and discoveries in prevention, diagnostics, and therapies. We are deeply grateful to the authors for providing broad information from their respective medical practice and expertise. We hope this book will be a valuable resource for physicians, nurses, researchers, patients, their families, and caregivers, as well as for the public.

Enkhsaikhan Purevjav, MD, Ph.D., FAHA
The Heart Institute,
Department of Pediatrics,
University of Tennessee Health Science Center,
Memphis, TN, USA

Stephanie A. Storgion and Timothy D. Minniear
University of Tennessee Health Science Center,
Memphis, TN, USA

Section 1

Common Rheumatic Disorders in Children

Chapter 1

Rheumatic Fever and Rheumatic Heart Disease in Children and Adolescents

Buyan-Ochir Orgil, Gantuul Narmandakh, Enkhzul Batsaikhan, Neely Alberson, Timothy D. Minniear and Enkhsaikhan Purevjav

Abstract

Acute rheumatic fever (ARF) is an inflammatory disease that produces cardiac, joint, neurological, and dermatological manifestations. It is caused by an abnormal immune response to Group A streptococcus (GAS) infection, most commonly after tonsillopharyngitis. ARF can affect anyone but commonly occurs in children. Severe or recurrent disease can cause rheumatic heart disease (RHD), which results in severe morbidity and mortality. Management of ARF includes eradicating GAS colonization, controlling symptoms, and secondary prophylaxis. Although the prevalence of ARF was high across the globe in the 1900s, its incidence has declined dramatically in industrialized countries after the development of antibiotics, accessible healthcare, and improved housing conditions and hygiene. However, this disease continues to affect people in developing nations. Improved international awareness of ARF and RHD is required for its control. This chapter will focus on the epidemiology, etiology, and pathogenesis of ARF and RHD along with a thorough description of clinical manifestations with their underlying mechanism. Diagnostic criteria, differentials, management, and prevention are also described in this chapter.

Keywords: rheumatic fever, rheumatic heart disease, *Streptococcus pyogenes*, toxin, valve disease

1. Introduction

Rheumatic heart disease (RHD) is a chronic and progressive systemic condition, a critical form of acquired heart disease caused by acute rheumatic fever (ARF) affecting children and adolescents and requiring specific targeted management [1]. Highly prevalent across the world in the 1900s, the worldwide burden of RHD on the healthcare system declined during the late twentieth century with the near elimination of ARF and a significant reduction in RHD rates in high-income countries such as the United States [2]. However, high rates of both ARF and RHD persist, and these diseases remain important causes of disability and cardiovascular mortality in some developing low- and middle-income countries, especially Oceania, South Asia, and central sub-Saharan Africa [3]. There are still more than 40 million people living with these diseases, over 15 million of which have evidence of RHD, and nearly 250,000 young people die from RHD each year worldwide [4]. Economic, healthcare, and social factors such as poverty, overcrowding, poor sanitation, low education level, improper disease prophylaxis, and limited medical care are associated with poor outcomes of this multi-system disease [5, 6].

Cardiac involvement with irreversible valve and cardiac muscle damage in RHD is the critical sequelae of ARF, which is a complication of upper respiratory tract infections with Group A *Streptococcus* (GAS). Due to an abnormal autoimmune response to GAS infection, this disease affects different organ systems in the body, including the heart, musculoskeletal system, skin, and neurological system [7]. Despite the complete reversibility of most symptoms, cardiac valve damage is irreversible and leads to life-long disability and death. This chapter will focus on different clinical aspects of GAS-associated rheumatic disease with a focus on ARF and RHD in children and young adults. In addition, the importance of primary prevention and secondary prophylaxis with multi-directional health management for these preventable conditions is described.

2. Epidemiology

The overall burden of diseases has decreased considerably over the last century, and these achievements are the results of improved housing conditions, reduced overcrowding, the development of antibiotic treatments, effective primary prevention and secondary prophylaxis, and accessible healthcare [2]. Moreover, the severity of rheumatic fever and disability-adjusted life years and death rates of subsequent RHD decreased markedly across the globe from 1990 to 2019 [8]. Incidence rates lower in developed countries compared to developing countries. For example, Germany has the lowest RHD deaths of 0.15 per 100,000 population among children 5–9 years of age compared to approximately 8 per 100,000 population [3]. Significant public health concerns yet persist around the world, particularly in developing countries with low economic, social, and health resources where persistent infections with GAS are more prevalent.

According to the 2019 global burden of disease findings, the age-standardized incidence and prevalence of RHD were 37.4 (28.6–46.7) and 513.7 (405.0–636.3) per 100,000 population, indicating the increase in RHD incidence and prevalence rates by 14.4 and 13.8%, respectively, compared to 1990 [8]. However, rates of disability-adjusted life years and mortality decreased globally by 53.1 and 56.9%, respectively, compared to 1990.

Approximately 3–5% of patients with pharyngeal infections caused by GAS develop secondary ARF because of the absence of antibiotic therapy or ineffective treatment [9, 10]. There are significant variances in the incidence of invasive GAS infection between geographic regions as well as resurgences within the same countries in different years likely related to changes in circulating GAS strains and/or host susceptibility [11–13]. Overall, the incidence of GAS pharyngitis infections was similar between nations (12.8–14 per 100 years), the GAS incidence was higher in socio-economic and healthcare-disadvantaged groups of both developing and developed countries [14]. These data are important as the GAS infection-induced ARF typically occurs in children who are 5–15 years of age, but the symptoms of RHD usually manifest in their young adulthood, while nearly 15–20% of all patients with RHD develop heart failure later during their lifespan [15].

3. Etiology

Streptococcus pyogenes is the GAS most commonly responsible for pharyngeal (tonsillitis and pharyngitis) and skin (impetigo, erysipelas, and cellulitis) infections. This group of bacteria also causes toxin-mediated diseases such as scarlet fever, streptococcal toxic shock syndrome, and necrotizing fasciitis [16]. Rheumatic fever is a cascade of inflammatory responses to GAS infection caused by an immune-mediated reaction against the patient's own tissues, potentially resulting in serious long-term complications. ARF occurs 2–3 weeks after GAS infection and is more related to upper respiratory tract infections. Some studies suggested that skin infections have also caused ARF among certain genetically susceptible populations [17, 18]. With the proper and prompt treatment of acute GAS infection, it is possible to prevent the development of ARF and consequent RHD. People with subclinical infections or those who are underserved to receive proper health care are at increased risk of developing ARF [19]. One or more episodes of rheumatic fever cause inflammation and damage of the heart valves by mechanisms which will be explained in the following sections.

4. Pathogenesis

The pathophysiology of ARF is multifactorial with the involvement of organism factors, host susceptibility factors, and factors of an individual's immune response.

4.1 Organism factors: Group A streptococcus

Group A streptococci are Gram-positive spherical or coccus [derived from the Greek word kokkos (berry)] shaped bacteria encapsulated in the outer membrane consisting of hyaluronic acids [20]. On its membrane surface, GAS expresses M-proteins that serve as the main virulence factor for the development of rheumatic heart disease [21]. M- and M-like proteins are molecules that contain conserved signal peptides on both N-terminal and C-terminal ends. These peptides can produce over 200 different types of M-proteins, providing a hypervariability of the N-terminal, while the C-terminal remains highly conserved [22]. This structure prevents phagocytosis of bacteria, making GAS one of the most prevalent pathogens and giving it the ability to persist in infected tissues [23]. The M-proteins are encoded by *emm* genes, which are labeled by chromosomal patterns A, B, C, D, and E, each of which is divided into serotypes. Studies have shown that gene patterns A, B, and C are associated with both pharyngitis and rheumatic fever [24]. Moreover, the >200 different serotypes based on the M-typing and GAS surface fibril markers (M1, M3, M6, M14, etc.), an individual may become infected by more than one serotype of GAS during the lifetime [25]. Recent association studies documented changes in the distribution of M serotypes in different geographic regions over time. Shulman et al. demonstrated a temporal association between ARF prevalence and GAS serotypes in the USA, which reflects the near-disappearance of ARF and reduction in detected rheumatogenic M serotypes [26].

4.2 Host susceptibility factors

Although ARF is associated with GAS infections, genetically determined factors of an individual's susceptibility to GAS also have been shown to play an important role in the development of ARF [27, 28]. Studies have demonstrated multiple genes involved in host susceptibility to ARF, such as genes encoding human leukocyte antigens, B-cell alloantigens, and cytokines [29]. Genetic variations in TNF-α (tumor necrosis factor α), human leukocyte antigen (HLA) DQA1-DQB1, and HLA class II alleles have been shown to be associated with RHD [30, 31]. The key mechanisms of RHD in an individual's susceptibility and pathogenesis have been linked to higher affinity DQA1-DQB1 alpha/beta dimers to M5 and M6 serotypes in the 2-risk HLA-DQA1*0101_DQB1*0503 and HLA-DQA1*0103_DQB1*0601 haplotypes than the HLA_DQA1*0301-DQB1*0402 determined as the protective haplotype [31]. Moreover, studies have shown a high heritability pattern based on the concordance risk for ARF identified in 44% of monozygotic twins, while 12% risk was shown in dizygotic twins [32], underscoring the importance of large whole genome studies to discover the genetic susceptibility factors in human populations.

4.3 Host immune response

After GAS enters the body, the immune system responds to the invading organism including the production of antibodies. Proteins on the surface of GAS share similar or "similar enough" epitopes with human proteins. This similarity produces an autoimmune reaction, resulting in the rheumatic manifestations [33]. This immunological cross-reactivity between the bacterial antigen and the host tissue is known as "molecular mimicry" [34, 35]. Three types of molecular mimicry have been identified: (1) identical amino acid sequences shared between different proteins in the tissue and the bacterium; (2) similar antibody sequences within protein structures such as the streptococcal M-protein and the host body's proteins such as myosin, keratin, tropomyosin, vimentin, and laminin; and (3) diverse molecules such as DNA, carbohydrates, and proteins that share identical epitopes in their molecular structure [36]. Once autoantibodies form, they activate other immune processes such as lymphoproliferation and infiltrate the valve through the endocardial surface causing autoinflammatory damage [37]. Cross-reaction with myosin leads to myositis and valvulitis, whereas cross-reaction with keratin causes erythema marginatum, the dermatologic manifestation that occurs in ARF.

The development of valvular disease occurs when autoantibodies cross-react with the endothelial cells of valves, leading to activation of vascular cell adhesion protein 1 (VCAM1) on the endothelial surface [38]. This triggers cytotoxic T cells to infiltrate through the endothelium and further recruitment of T cells and macrophages leading to inflammation and valve injury. As a result of T-cell- and macrophage-mediated inflammation, granulomas form underneath the endocardium around or at the valve. These lesions are called the Aschoff bodies, which are commonly seen in patients with ARF and RHD [30].

In addition to valvular disease, rheumatic fever causes Sydenham chorea or rheumatic chorea, a disorder characterized by rapid and uncoordinated jerking movements in patients after GAS pharyngitis. This is likely due to molecular mimicry between the Group A carbohydrate epitope called N-acetyl-β-D-glucosamine (NABG) of GAS and an antigen in the basal ganglia of brain cells [39], causing autoinflammatory damage in the dorsal corpus striatum, caudate nucleus, and putamen. This inflammation leads to imbalanced functions between the intrastriatal cholinergic, dopaminergic, and inhibitory gamma-aminobutyric acid (GABA) systems, clinically manifesting as chorea [30, 40].

5. Clinical manifestations

Clinical features of ARF typically present 2–3 weeks after the precipitating GAS infections. Most patients report a preceding GAS pharyngitis as the most common diagnosis [41]. However, almost one-third of patients never recall any previous infections. While these subclinical cases can be confirmed by streptococcal antibody testing. The clinical manifestations of ARF range widely, from an asymptomatic subclinical disease to more serious, life-threatening disease like acute fulminant pancarditis. Some patients do not have symptoms until they develop RHD after several decades.

The most common presenting symptoms of ARF are fever (>90% of patients) and arthritis (75% of patients) followed by carditis (>50% of patients). Chorea presents differently among various populations depending on age and sex and can occur in up to 30% of patients with ARF. Chorea is much less frequent today, and the symptoms are less severe than in the past. Erythema marginatum and subcutaneous nodules are infrequent manifestations, occurring in less than 10% of patients [30]. In addition to specific symptoms, other constitutional symptoms such as fever, chills, fatigue as well as an increase in C-reactive protein (CRP) and erythrocyte sedimentation rate (ESR) are almost universal. Joint pain in the absence of arthritis is among the minor manifestations.

5.1 Involvement of joints

The cross-reactive immune response leads to immune complex formation and causes transient migratory polyarthritis. Joint involvement is a major and minor manifestation, depending on its features. Frequently, multiple joints are involved, either occurring at the same time or separately, giving rise to the description of "migratory polyarthritis" [42–44]. Arthritis occurs in approximately 75% of patients with ARF and usually is one of the earliest signs of ARF. Inflammation of joints (arthritis) typically affects the larger joints such as the knees, ankles, hips, elbows, and wrists, and is asymmetric. Smaller joints of the hands and feet and the axial skeleton are rarely involved. Rheumatic joints are usually hot, red, swollen, and extremely tender, requiring analgesics. Inflammatory signs in one joint can be resolved within a few days, with the entire arthritis course resolving after 1 month without treatment [45].

One unique feature of ARF arthritis is its quick response to aspirin and other nonsteroidal anti-inflammatory drugs (NSAIDs). A profound response to even a small dose of salicylates is highly suggestive of rheumatic fever, and if joint symptoms persist 1–2 days after salicylate administration, a different diagnosis should be suspected. For this reason, aspirin and other NSAIDs or steroidal medications should be withheld in patients with monoarthritis and fever, who are highly suspicious of ARF. This strategy assists in observing the migratory nature of the arthritis which will aid in differential diagnosis. Alternative medications such as acetaminophen or codeine should be used to manage the pain.

5.2 Heart involvement

Rheumatic carditis and consequent RHD are the most serious manifestations of ARF and are the main cause of disability and mortality. It occurs in 50% of patients with ARF. Rheumatic inflammation may involve the endocardium, pericardium, and myocardium, and involvement of all layers of heart ventricular walls leads to pancarditis. Endocarditis and valvulitis are universal findings in rheumatic carditis, while pericardium and myocardium are affected variably [30]. Isolated pericarditis or myocarditis is unlikely to be rheumatic in origin. Most rheumatic carditis cases involve either only the mitral valve or combined damage involving aortic or tricuspid valves, while isolated cases of aortic or right-sided valvular involvement are rare. Both single and recurrent attacks of ARF can cause severe and long-term valvular damage. Pathologically, lesions characteristic of RHD called Aschoff nodules result from inflammation in the heart muscle and can be found in valves and small blood vessels of the myocardium and endocardium. They are rarely found in the pericardium of patients with RHD [30, 46].

5.2.1 Valvulitis

The majority of valvulitis cases involve the mitral valve, which is affected in 50–60% of cases. Mitral valve damage leads to mitral regurgitation, which can be observed in both the acute and convalescent stages. On clinical examination, mitral regurgitation produces a holosystolic murmur that is heard best at the apex and radiates to the left axilla [47]. If the mitral regurgitation is more severe, cardiomegaly and congestive heart failure may develop. In this case, patients may present with dyspnea, hepatomegaly, and lower extremity edema due to congestive heart failure. Several years or even decades later, mainly due to recurrent episodes, ARF patients may develop leaflet thickening and scarring, calcification, and valvular stenosis. This may require invasive procedures such as interventional catheterization and valve replacement surgery to repair.

Up to 20% of patients with ARF valvulitis present with aortic valve involvement. Aortic valvular damage usually manifests as aortic regurgitation, which display a decrescendo early-diastolic murmur heard as a blowing whisper at the base of the heart. The tricuspid valve is the least affected—accounting for 10% of rheumatic valvulitis cases—and presents with tricuspid regurgitation [18]. Like the development of mitral valvular stenosis, aortic and tricuspid stenosis also develop several years or even decades after initial rheumatic damage of the corresponding valve.

5.2.2 Carditis

Clinical carditis has been defined as the presence of an audible murmur consistent with the affected valvular regurgitation and is considered universally a major manifestation in all populations. However, with the more widespread use of echocardiography for diagnostic purposes, recent studies have emphasized the use of echocardiography in confirming the presence of carditis. Moreover, the term "subclinical carditis" has been incorporated as a major manifestation into guidelines, including those followed in Australia and New Zealand, and the revised 2015 Jones Criteria are shown in **Table 1**. Subclinical carditis is defined as mitral or aortic valvulitis seen on echocardiography and Doppler studies (**Tables 2** and **3**), but the signs of ARF are not present on physical examination as an auscultatory finding. Myocardial involvement

Criteria	Patient population	Manifestations
Major	Low risk*	• Carditis† (clinical and/or subclinical) • Arthritis (polyarthritis only) • Chorea • Erythema marginatum • Subcutaneous nodules
	Moderate and high risk	• Carditis (clinical and/or subclinical) • Arthritis (including polyarthritis, monoarthritis or polyarthralgia) • Chorea • Erythema marginatum • Subcutaneous nodules
Minor	Low risk	• Polyarthralgia • Fever (≥38.5°C) • ESR ≥60 mm in the first hour and/or CRP of ≥3.0 mg/dL • Prolonged PR interval, after accounting for age variability (unless carditis is a major criterion)
	Moderate and high risk	• Monoarthralgia • Fever (≥38°C) • ESR ≥30 mm/h and/or CRP of ≥3.0 mg/dL • Prolonged PR interval, after accounting for age variability (unless carditis is a major criterion)
For all patient populations with evidence of preceding Group A Streptococcus infection (except chorea and indolent carditis) Diagnosis of initial ARF: two major or one major plus two minor manifestations. Diagnosis of recurrent ARF: either two major or one major and two minor or three minor manifestations.		

**Low-risk populations with annual ARF incidence of ≤2 per 100,000 school-aged children or all-age RHD prevalence of ≤1 per 1000 people per year.*
*†Subclinical carditis indicates echocardiographic valvulitis (see **Tables** 2 and 3).*

Table 1.
2015 revised Jones criteria for the diagnosis of acute rheumatic fever.

in ARF may also affect the electrical conduction system, resulting in first-degree atrioventricular (AV) block on ECG tracing with a prolongation of PR interval and rare higher-degree heart blocks [46]. Particularly in the early stages of the AFR course, mitral or aortic valve morphology may be normal on echocardiograms, while Doppler may show regurgitation, as defined in **Table 2**. These findings can also be seen in chronic RHD.

5.3 Dermatologic manifestations

Dermatologic manifestations of acute rheumatic fever include subcutaneous nodules and erythema marginatum. Both these signs are included in the revised Jones criteria as a major manifestation. Occurring in less than 10% of patients with ARF, subcutaneous nodules are small (0.5–2 cm in diameter), firm, painless, mobile lumps that are found on extensor surfaces of joints, mostly the knees, elbow, and wrists.

Pathological mitral regurgitation (all 4 criteria met)
• Seen in at least two views
• Jet length ≥ 2 cm in at least one view
• Peak velocity > 3 m/s
• Pansystolic jet in at least one envelope
Pathological aortic regurgitation (all 4 criteria met)
• Seen in at least two views
• Jet length ≥ 1 cm in at least one view
• Peak velocity > 3 m/s
• Pan diastolic jet in at least one envelope
This table was adapted from the Scientific Statement From the AHA. Gewitz et al. [48].

Table 2.
Doppler findings in rheumatic valvulitis.

Acute mitral valve changes
• Annular dilation
• Chordal elongation
• Chordal rupture resulting in flail leaflet with severe mitral regurgitation
• Anterior (or less commonly posterior) leaflet tip prolapse
• Beading/nodularity of leaflet tips
Chronic mitral valve changes not seen in acute carditis
• Leaflet thickening
• Chordal thickening and fusion
• Restricted leaflet motion
• Calcification
Aortic valve changes in either acute or chronic carditis
• Irregular or focal leaflet thickening
• Coaptation defect
• Restricted leaflet motion
• Leaflet prolapse
This table was adapted from the Scientific Statement From the AHA. Gewitz [48].

Table 3.
Morphological findings on echocardiogram in rheumatic valvulitis.

Nodules can rarely be seen in the occiput and along the spinous processes. They are usually seen in patients with severe rheumatic carditis. The subcutaneous nodules most likely form due to delayed hypersensitivity against GAS antigens. They present a few days to 3 weeks after GAS infection and can last a few days to 3 weeks. The formation of these nodules shares a similar mechanism with Aschoff body formations, which are granulomatous lesions that are seen in heart valves [30, 46].

Seen in less than 10% of ARF patients, erythema marginatum is a highly characteristic lesion. These lesions generally appear as a bright pink annular or serpiginous, nonpruritic rash with raised edges and a central clearing found mostly on the trunk and extremities. Lesions of erythema marginatum do not appear on the face. Warming up the skin may accentuate the rash, and it blanches with pressure [49]. The mechanism behind this rash is likely due to the antibodies against Group A carbohydrate that cross-react with the keratin of the skin [30].

5.4 Sydenham chorea

Sydenham chorea is one of the major manifestations of acute rheumatic fever and reflects neurological involvement. Studies have shown that antibodies to the NABG peptide of GAS cross-react with the basal ganglia of the brain cells [50] and cause a release of excess dopamine from neuronal cells in culture [51] producing the choreiform movement [30].

Sydenham chorea occurs in 10–30% of ARF cases. When it occurs, it usually presents in the absence of other symptoms [skin, heart, or joint), probably, due to a more prolonged latent period, typically, requiring 1–8 months after GAS infection [18]. When Sydenham chorea first presents, the anti-streptococcal antibodies may have already declined to normal levels. Therefore, diagnosis is predominantly based on clinical signs. Signs of chorea in ARF present as purposeless, uncontrollable, irregular, and jerking movements of the face and extremities. They usually occur on one side of the body, worsen with stress, and disappear during sleep. Tics and facial grimaces are characteristic. Chorea is often associated with emotional lability and behavioral symptoms such as anxiety, obsessive-compulsive disorder, agitation, and anxiety. A clinical sign characteristic of Sydenham Chorea is the "milkmaid's grip" where the patient is unable to maintain the grip due to irregular contractions of the hand muscles while squeezing the examiner's fingers. Chorea almost always resolves completely, usually within 6 weeks.

6. Diagnosis and evaluation

The diagnosis of ARF is established according to the revised Jones Criteria, originally established by T. Duckett Jones in 1944. Since then, the Jones Criteria underwent multiple modifications and updates, and the most recent revision summarized in **Table 1** was published by the AHA in 2015 [48]. There are five major and four minor criteria. The diagnosis of an initial ARF is determined if a patient fulfills two major manifestations or one major plus two minor manifestations. For recurrent ARF, the patient should have two major manifestations or one major and two minor or three minor to qualify for a diagnosis. Even when the patient fulfills these criteria, evidence of preceding GAS infection must be confirmed. A positive throat culture for GAS or a positive rapid GAS carbohydrate antigen testing in suspected patients serves as evidence for active or prior infection [52]. However, at the time of symptom presentation, these tests are usually negative. Thus, serology tests should be used for confirmation only. Increased or rising anti-streptolysin O (ASO) and antideoxyribonuclease B (ADB) antibody titers on serology serve as evidence of preceding infection as well [52].

There are some circumstances in which the diagnosis of ARF can be made without following the Jones Criteria and evidence of GAS infection. These include patients who present with chorea or indolent carditis because these manifestations may come to medical attention months after the inciting streptococcal infection. Most cases of ARF present with fever. In the past, the cutoff value for fever was 39°C. However, recent studies showed that lowering this threshold increased the sensitivity of detecting ARF cases [53], thus the revised Jones Criteria has set the number to ≥38.0°C in moderate- and high-risk populations, and ≥ 38.5°C in low-risk populations.

7. Differential diagnosis

Rheumatic fever shares signs and symptoms with many other infectious and non-infectious diseases. During the differential diagnostics of ARF, we should consider each of the major manifestations. **Table 4** shows a list of differential diagnoses.

When a child or adult presents with arthritis, we should consider connective tissue and autoimmune diseases such as rheumatoid arthritis, idiopathic juvenile arthritis, and systemic lupus erythematosus. Poststreptococcal syndromes are often confused with rheumatic fever. These include poststreptococcal reactive arthritis (PSRA) which has a shorter latent period presenting within 1 week of GAS infection with symmetrical involvement of the small joint and responds slower to salicylate medications than ARF arthritis. A prospective study conducted in the Netherlands has shown that PSRA was not associated with long-term heart involvement [54]. Other arthritis of different etiologies such as septic arthritis (including gonococcal), serum sickness, sickle cell disease, cancer, Lyme disease, and reactive arthritis present secondary to gastrointestinal infections (e.g., Shigella, Salmonella, Yersinia) should also be considered in the differential diagnosis [48, 49].

When using echocardiogram analysis in patients with subclinical carditis, valvular changes that resemble ARF should be carefully investigated. Because systemic blood pressure affects the echocardiographic gradient measurements, it is important to measure the blood pressure values while performing echocardiograms and when possible, do serial echocardiograms in the same patient to ensure diagnostic accuracy [48].

Arthritis	Carditis	Chorea
• Connective tissue and other autoimmune disease (rheumatoid arthritis, juvenile idiopathic arthritis) • Poststreptococcal reactive arthritis • Septic arthritis (including gonococcal) • Viral arthropathy • Reactive arthropathy • Lyme disease • Sickle cell anemia • Gout and pseudogout	• Physiological mitral regurgitation • Mitral valve prolapse • Myxomatous mitral valve • Fibroelastoma • Innocent murmurs • Congenital valve disease • Infective endocarditis • Myocarditis (viral or idiopathic) • Cardiomyopathy • Kawasaki disease	• Pediatric autoimmune neuropsychiatric disorders associated with streptococcal infections (PANDAS) • Drug intoxication • Wilson disease • Huntington disease • Tic disorder • Cerebral palsy • Intracranial tumor • Encephalitis

Table 4.
Criteria of differential diagnosis of acute rheumatic fever.

8. Treatment

The treatment of ARF is multimodal and involves GAS eradication therapy, symptomatic therapy of acute manifestations such as arthritis and fever, and management of carditis and chorea if present. It is important to commence secondary prophylaxis against future GAS infection to prevent ARF recurrences and progression of valvular damage and to provide education to patients on their diagnosis. Once diagnosed with ARF, all patients should be hospitalized and monitored closely to ensure that necessary tests and care are performed and, if necessary, repeated to evaluate treatment response and monitor the disease course.

8.1 Group A streptococcus eradication therapy

All patients diagnosed with GAS infection should receive antibiotic therapy to eradicate GAS. This serves as the primary prevention for acute rheumatic fever. All patients with ARF should be initiated on antibiotic treatment regardless of negative throat cultures to eradicate GAS carriage, prevent ARF recurrences in the future, and reduce the risk of developing RHD [52].

The antibiotic therapy of choice for GAS eradication is penicillin. Penicillin is a very effective and inexpensive drug with a narrow spectrum of activity. It can be administered orally or intramuscularly, depending on whether the patient will adhere to the oral regimen and on the risks of rheumatic fever in the population. Amoxicillin has a slightly broader spectrum compared to penicillin, but some physicians prefer it for its once-daily administration [55, 56].

If allergic to penicillin, cephalosporins, macrolides, or oral clindamycin are given. Some penicillin-allergic patients are also allergic to cephalosporin; thus, cephalosporins should not be used in patients who have had a severe anaphylactic reaction to penicillin [57]. Checking the QT interval before commencing macrolides is advised as they may cause QT interval prolongation in a dose-dependent manner. **Table 5** summarizes the antimicrobial agents and their dosages for the treatment of GAS pharyngitis.

8.2 Management of arthritis

Anti-inflammatory agents may be used for treating arthritis, arthralgia, and fever after the diagnosis is confirmed. Premature treatment with anti-inflammatory medications may hinder the characteristic development of migratory polyarthritis in patients who initially presented only with arthritis. Thus, confirming the diagnosis of acute rheumatic fever before initiating these medications is important. In the meantime, acetaminophen may be used for pain management. Historically, aspirin with a dose of 100 mg/kg/day in divided doses has been the mainstay of treatment of ARF arthritis based on previous literature [58–60]. Aspirin required frequent measurements of serum salicylate levels and increased the risk of liver toxicity and Reye syndrome [18]. Subsequent studies have shown that the use of NSAIDs, particularly naproxen, was effective, easier to use, and had lower adverse effects compared to aspirin [61–63]. Naproxen is given in a dose of 5–10 mg/kg every 12 hours with a maximum daily dose of 1000 mg until symptoms resolve. Gastrointestinal toxicity risk is increased during NSAID therapy. Therefore, patients are often concurrently prescribed proton pump inhibitors. For pediatric patients, gastrointestinal

Agent	Dose
Penicillins	
Penicillin V	• If ≤27 kg (60 lb): 250 mg two to three times daily PO for 10 days • If >27 kg (60 lb): adolescents, and adults: 500 mg two to three times daily PO for 10 days
Amoxicillin	50 mg/kg once daily PO for 10 days
Benzathine penicillin G	• If ≤27 kg (60 lb): 600,000 units IM as a single dose • If >27 kg (60 lb): 1200,000 units IM as a single dose
If allergic to penicillin	
Narrow-spectrum cephalosporins (cephalexin, cefadroxil)*	Variable
Clindamycin	• 20 mg/kg/day divided into three doses PO for 10 days (maximum 300 mg per dose)
Azithromycin	• 12 mg/kg once daily PO for five days (maximum 500 mg per dose)
Clarithromycin	• 7.5 mg/kg/day twice daily for 10 days (maximum 250 mg per dose)

*PO, by mouth; IM, intramuscularly. *Some penicillin-allergic patients are also allergic to cephalosporin; thus, cephalosporin should not be used in patients who have anaphylactic reactions to penicillin.*

Table 5.
Primary prevention of ARF (treatment of GAS pharyngitis).

prophylaxis is often not necessary unless there is a history of previous gastrointestinal bleeding or GERD. Recurrence of arthritis after discontinuation or dose reduction of anti-inflammatory medications is called a "rebound phenomenon" of ARF. It is not a recurrence of rheumatic fever, while a prolonged course of treatment is required.

8.3 Management of cardiac involvement

Patients with signs of carditis/valvulitis and heart failure should be assessed with echocardiography. Corticosteroids are widely used in severe acute carditis. Corticosteroid pulse therapy may be effective in managing patients with severe rheumatic carditis [64], however, there is not enough evidence that corticosteroids prevent or reduce valvular damage at a 12-month follow-up [65, 66]. Intravenous immunoglobulin therapy also did not show any benefit according to a randomized controlled trial [67].

In patients who develop congestive heart failure, diuretics, fluid retention, and bed rest are the mainstay of treatment. Angiotensin-converting enzyme (ACE) inhibitors may be used in patients with aortic regurgitation and left ventricular dysfunction to reduce the afterload [68]. There are limited experiences with beta-blockers used for the treatment of heart failure due to ARF, and their use is not recommended [69].

Immediate cardiac surgery is indicated in patients with severe mitral valve regurgitation due to chordae tendinae rupture and subsequent pulmonary edema [70]. In general, surgery is deferred until the acute inflammation has subsided. In pediatric and young adult patients, mitral valve repair rather than valve replacement is advised as a general rule [30].

8.4 Management of chorea

Sydenham chorea usually occurs as an isolated finding after the acute phase of rheumatic fever has resolved. It is often self-limited and benign and resolves within weeks to months even with no medication, while severe cases of chorea have shown improvement in symptoms following corticosteroids [71, 72]. Milder cases can be managed by rest and a calm environment to minimize overstimulation [73]. In patients with severe chorea, sedatives may be helpful. Commonly used medications are valproic acid and carbamazepine. Recent studies demonstrated the possibility of levetiracetam use due to its effectiveness and safety profile [74, 75]. However, additional evidence from clinical trials is needed to support this effect.

9. Preventive measures

9.1 Primary prevention

The current strategy for primary prevention aims to prevent the development of ARF after Group A streptococcal tonsillopharyngitis by administering a single dose of intramuscular benzathine penicillin G or oral administration of penicillin or amoxicillin for 10 days (**Table 5**). Treating GAS tonsillopharyngitis will eradicate the bacteria before the bacterial toxins can trigger the autoimmune reaction responsible for the ARF mechanism. The ideal primary prevention would be vaccination against GAS, but no vaccine has been developed to date. Efforts to develop a vaccine against GAS are ongoing.

9.2 Secondary prophylaxis

The risk of recurrent attack of rheumatic fever after GAS infection is dramatically higher in individuals with a history of ARF compared to the general population. Subsequent ARF attacks can cause cardiac involvement in individuals who did not have carditis in the previous attack or worsen the severity of rheumatic heart disease in those who had already developed carditis from the previous attack. For this reason, patients with a history of RHD should receive secondary antibiotic prophylaxis against GAS infection.

The best regimen for secondary prophylaxis of RHD is intramuscular benzathine penicillin G injections of 600,000 U every 4 weeks (or 1,200,000 U for those >27 kg). It can be given every 3 weeks if the patient is at high risk. Oral penicillin V (250 mg per dose) can also be used, but requires twice daily dosing, and is associated with low adherence and increased recurrence. Patients allergic to penicillin can be given sulfadiazine with a recommended dose of 0.5 g once daily (1 g once daily for patients weighing >27 kg). If a patient is allergic to both penicillin and sulfisoxazole, an oral macrolide can be given [52].

The duration of prophylaxis can depend on several factors. Individuals with multiple previous attacks and those who are more susceptible to GAS pharyngitis are at increased risk of recurrent GAS infection, requiring continuous antimicrobial

Category	Duration after last attack
Rheumatic fever with carditis and residual heart disease (persistent valvular disease*)	• 20 mg/kg/day divided in three doses PO for 10 days (maximum 300 mg per dose)
Rheumatic fever with carditis but no residual heart disease (no valvular disease*)	• 12 mg/kg once daily PO for 5 days (maximum 500 mg per dose)
Rheumatic fever without carditis	• 7.5 mg/kg/day twice daily for 10 days (maximum 250 mg per dose)

Adapted from Ref. [52].
**Clinical or echocardiographic evidence.*

Table 6.
American Heart Association recommendations for the duration of secondary rheumatic fever prophylaxis.

prophylaxis. Patients with persistent valvular damage should receive prophylaxis for 10 years after the last ARF episode or until 40 years of age, whichever is longer [52]. After that, GAS infection risk should be re-evaluated, and lifelong prophylaxis should be considered for high-risk individuals. For patients with a history of ARF but with no carditis, secondary prophylaxis is continued until the patient reaches 21 years of age or for 5 years since the last attack, whichever is longer. **Table 6** summarizes the secondary prophylaxis indications and duration [52].

10. Complications

The main complication of ARF is RHD, which occurs 10–20 years after the initial rheumatic fever attack. It typically occurs after severe ARF or due to recurrent attacks and usually develops during adulthood, and leads to heart failure, pulmonary hypertension, arrhythmia, embolic strokes, and sudden cardiac death [18, 76]. Cardiomyopathy and heart failure can also occur even during the acute phase of rheumatic fever. ARF arthritis generally does not lead to long-term osteoarticular sequelae. In rare cases, Sydenham chorea is associated with increased psychiatric symptoms in some patients.

11. Prognosis

If untreated, most cases of ARF last 3 months on average. If treated, ARF patients are usually discharged within 1–2 weeks. However, it takes at least 1 month for the inflammatory markers to normalize. Therefore, an echocardiogram should be performed after 1 month in cases of rheumatic carditis to evaluate progressive changes. Carditis resolves without sequelae in 70% of patients.

12. Patient education

Both ARF and RHD are a significant cause of morbidity and mortality due to acquired valvular heart disease, especially in developing countries. Educating the patient is vital for the successful management of ARF. It is important to provide full and adequate information about the patient's ongoing disease and possible consequences. Educating pediatric patients and their parents about antibiotic prophylaxis, reasons to seek medical evaluation, and encouraging continuous adherence to treatment is very important.

13. Conclusion

Acute rheumatic fever and rheumatic heart disease are among the most common acquired valvular heart diseases in children and young people worldwide. Although ARF can lead to serious cardiovascular sequelae, it can be effectively prevented and managed with antibiotics. Although this disease is no longer prevalent in developed countries, it remains to be a global challenge. Therefore, healthcare providers should be equipped with the knowledge and skills to diagnose and treat ARF and implement primary and secondary preventive measures.

Conflict of interest

The authors declare no conflict of interest.

Author details

Buyan-Ochir Orgil[1,2], Gantuul Narmandakh[3], Enkhzul Batsaikhan[4], Neely Alberson[1,2], Timothy D. Minniear[2,5]* and Enkhsaikhan Purevjav[1,2]*

1 The Heart Institute, Department of Pediatrics, University of Tennessee Health Science Center, Memphis, TN, USA

2 Children's Foundation Research Institute, Le Bonheur Children's Hospital, Memphis, TN, USA

3 Department of Cardiology, Third State Central Hospital, Ulaanbaatar, Mongolia

4 Department of Pharmacology, Addiction Science, and Toxicology, University of Tennessee Health Science Center, Memphis, TN, USA

5 Division of Pediatric Infectious Diseases, Department of Pediatrics, University of Tennessee Health Science Center, Memphis, TN, USA

*Address all correspondence to: tminniea@uthsc.edu and epurevja@uthsc.edu

References

[1] Bocchi EA, Guimaraes G, Tarasoutshi F, Spina G, Mangini S, Bacal F. Cardiomyopathy, adult valve disease and heart failure in South America. Heart. 2009;**95**(3):181-189. Epub 2008/11/04. DOI: 10.1136/hrt.2008.151225

[2] Gordis L. The virtual disappearance of rheumatic fever in the United States: Lessons in the rise and fall of disease. T. Duckett Jones memorial lecture. Circulation. 1985;**72**(6):1155-1162. . Epub 1985/12/01. DOI: 10.1161/01.cir.72.6.1155

[3] Watkins DA, Johnson CO, Colquhoun SM, Karthikeyan G, Beaton A, Bukhman G, et al. Global, regional, and National Burden of rheumatic heart disease, 1990-2015. The New England Journal of Medicine. 2017;**377**(8):713-722. Epub 2017/08/24. DOI: 10.1056/NEJMoa1603693

[4] Seckeler MD, Hoke TR. The worldwide epidemiology of acute rheumatic fever and rheumatic heart disease. Clinical Epidemiology. 2011;**3**:67-84. Epub 2011/03/10. DOI: 10.2147/CLEP.S12977

[5] Longo-Mbenza B, Bayekula M, Ngiyulu R, Kintoki VE, Bikangi NF, Seghers KV, et al. Survey of rheumatic heart disease in school children of Kinshasa town. International Journal of Cardiology. 1998;**63**(3):287-294. Epub 1998/05/13. DOI: 10.1016/s0167-5273(97)00311-2

[6] Meira ZM, Goulart EM, Colosimo EA, Mota CC. Long term follow up of rheumatic fever and predictors of severe rheumatic valvar disease in Brazilian children and adolescents. Heart. 2005;**91**(8):1019-1022. Epub 2005/07/16. DOI: 10.1136/hrt.2004.042762

[7] Marijon E, Mirabel M, Celermajer DS, Jouven X. Rheumatic heart disease. Lancet. 2012;**379**(9819):953-964. Epub 2012/03/13. DOI: 10.1016/S0140-6736(11)61171-9

[8] Ghamari SH, Abbasi-Kangevari M, Saeedi Moghaddam S, Aminorroaya A, Rezaei N, Shobeiri P, et al. Rheumatic heart disease is a neglected disease relative to its burden worldwide: Findings from global burden of disease 2019. Journal of the American Heart Association. 2022;**11**(13):e025284. Epub 2022/06/23. DOI: 10.1161/JAHA.122.025284

[9] Wannamaker LW. The chain that links the heart to the throat. Circulation. 1973;**48**(1):9-18. DOI: 10.1161/01.cir.48.1.9

[10] Breese BB. Beta-hemolytic streptococcus: Its bacteriologic culture and character. American Journal of Diseases of Children. 1978;**132**(5):502-508. DOI: 10.1001/archpedi.1978.02120300062013

[11] You Y, Davies MR, Protani M, McIntyre L, Walker MJ, Zhang J. Scarlet fever epidemic in China caused by streptococcus pyogenes serotype M12: Epidemiologic and molecular analysis. eBioMedicine. 2018;**28**:128-135. Epub 2018/01/18. DOI: 10.1016/j.ebiom.2018.01.010

[12] Mosites E, Frick A, Gounder P, Castrodale L, Li Y, Rudolph K, et al. Outbreak of invasive infections from subtype emm26.3 group a streptococcus among homeless adults-Anchorage, Alaska, 2016-2017. Clinical Infectious Diseases. 2018;**66**(7):1068-1074. Epub 2017/10/27. DOI: 10.1093/cid/cix921

[13] Kaplan EL, Wotton JT, Johnson DR. Dynamic epidemiology of group a streptococcal serotypes associated with pharyngitis. Lancet. 2001;**358**(9290):1334-1337. Epub 2001/10/31. DOI: 10.1016/S0140-6736(01)06415-7

[14] Pearce S, Bowen AC, Engel ME, de la Lande M, Barth DD. The incidence of sore throat and group a streptococcal pharyngitis in children at high risk of developing acute rheumatic fever: A systematic review and meta-analysis. PLoS One. 2020;**15**(11):e0242107. Epub 2020/11/19. DOI: 10.1371/journal.pone.0242107

[15] Auala T, Zavale BG, Mbakwem AC, Mocumbi AO. Acute rheumatic fever and rheumatic heart disease: Highlighting the role of group a streptococcus in the global burden of cardiovascular disease. Pathogens. 21 Apr 2022;**11**(5):496. Epub 2022/05/29. DOI: 10.3390/pathogens11050496

[16] Walker MJ, Barnett TC, McArthur JD, Cole JN, Gillen CM, Henningham A, et al. Disease manifestations and pathogenic mechanisms of group a streptococcus. Clinical Microbiology Reviews. 2014;**27**(2):264-301. DOI: 10.1128/CMR.00101-13

[17] McDonald M, Currie BJ, Carapetis JR. Acute rheumatic fever: A chink in the chain that links the heart to the throat? The Lancet Infectious Diseases. 2004;**4**(4):240-245. Epub 2004/03/31. DOI: 10.1016/S1473-3099(04)00975-2

[18] Chowdhury MDS, Koziatek CA, Rajnik M. Acute Rheumatic Fever. Treasure Island (FL) with ineligible companies. Disclosure: Christian Koziatek declares no relevant financial relationships with ineligible companies. Disclosure: Michael Rajnik declares no relevant financial relationships with ineligible companies: StatPearls; 2024

[19] McDonald MI, Towers RJ, Andrews RM, Benger N, Currie BJ, Carapetis JR. Low rates of streptococcal pharyngitis and high rates of pyoderma in Australian aboriginal communities where acute rheumatic fever is hyperendemic. Clinical Infectious Diseases. 2006;**43**(6):683-689. Epub 2006/08/17. DOI: 10.1086/506938

[20] Zapun A, Vernet T, Pinho MG. The different shapes of cocci. FEMS Microbiology Reviews. 2008;**32**(2):345-360. Epub 2008/02/13. DOI: 10.1111/j.1574-6976.2007.00098.x

[21] Sharma AK, Dhasmana N, Dubey N, Kumar N, Gangwal A, Gupta M, et al. Bacterial virulence factors: Secreted for survival. Indian Journal of Microbiology. 2017;**57**(1):1-10. Epub 2017/02/06. DOI: 10.1007/s12088-016-0625-1

[22] Perez-Casal J, Caparon MG, Scott JR. Introduction of the emm6 gene into an emm-deleted strain of streptococcus pyogenes restores its ability to resist phagocytosis. Research in Microbiology. 1992;**143**(6):549-558. DOI: 10.1016/0923-2508(92)90112-2

[23] Iyer V, Sagar V, Toor D, Lyngdoh V, Nongrum G, Kapoor M, et al. Group a streptococcus infections: Their mechanisms, epidemiology, and current scope of vaccines. Cureus. 2022;**14**(12):e33146. Epub 20221230. DOI: 10.7759/cureus.33146

[24] Bessen DE, Sotir CM, Readdy TL, Hollingshead SK. Genetic correlates of throat and skin isolates of group A streptococci. The Journal of Infectious Diseases. 1996;**173**(4):896-900. DOI: 10.1093/infdis/173.4.896

[25] Lancefield RC. Current knowledge of type-specific M antigens of group A

streptococci. Journal of Immunology. 1962;**89**:307-313

[26] Shulman ST, Stollerman G, Beall B, Dale JB, Tanz RR. Temporal changes in streptococcal M protein types and the near-disappearance of acute rheumatic fever in the United States. Clinical Infectious Diseases. 2006;**42**(4):441-447. Epub 2006/01/20. DOI: 10.1086/499812

[27] Wilson MG, Schweitzer M. Pattern of hereditary susceptibility in rheumatic fever. Circulation. 1954;**10**(5):699-704. DOI: 10.1161/01.cir.10.5.699

[28] Abdallah AM, Abu-Madi M. The genetic control of the rheumatic heart: Closing the genotype-phenotype gap. Frontiers in Medicine (Lausanne). 2021;**8**:611036. Epub 20210324. DOI: 10.3389/fmed.2021.611036

[29] Bryant PA, Robins-Browne R, Carapetis JR, Curtis N. Some of the people, some of the time. Circulation. 2009;**119**(5):742-753. DOI: 10.1161/CIRCULATIONAHA.108.792135

[30] Carapetis JR, Beaton A, Cunningham MW, Guilherme L, Karthikeyan G, Mayosi BM, et al. Acute rheumatic fever and rheumatic heart disease. Nature Reviews. Disease Primers. 2016;**2**:15084. Epub 2016/05/18. DOI: 10.1038/nrdp.2015.84

[31] Gray LA, D'Antoine HA, Tong SYC, McKinnon M, Bessarab D, Brown N, et al. Genome-wide analysis of genetic risk factors for rheumatic heart disease in aboriginal Australians provides support for pathogenic molecular mimicry. The Journal of Infectious Diseases. 2017;**216**(11):1460-1470. Epub 2017/10/14. DOI: 10.1093/infdis/jix497

[32] Engel ME, Stander R, Vogel J, Adeyemo AA, Mayosi BM. Genetic susceptibility to acute rheumatic fever: A systematic review and meta-analysis of twin studies. PLoS One. 2011;**6**(9):e25326. Epub 20110930. DOI: 10.1371/journal.pone.0025326

[33] Zen M, Gatto M, Domeneghetti M, Palma L, Borella E, Iaccarino L, et al. Clinical guidelines and definitions of autoinflammatory diseases: Contrasts and comparisons with autoimmunity-a comprehensive review. Clinical Reviews in Allergy and Immunology. 2013;**45**(2):227-235. Epub 2013/01/17. DOI: 10.1007/s12016-013-8355-1

[34] Krisher K, Cunningham MW. Myosin: A link between streptococci and heart. Science. 1985;**227**(4685):413-415. DOI: 10.1126/science.2578225

[35] Cunningham MW. Pathogenesis of group A streptococcal infections. Clinical Microbiology Reviews. 2000;**13**(3):470-511. DOI: 10.1128/CMR.13.3.470

[36] Cunningham MW. Molecular mimicry, autoimmunity, and infection: The cross-reactive antigens of group a streptococci and their sequelae. Microbiology Spectrum. Spectr7:10.1128/microbiolspec.gpp3-0045-2018

[37] Quinn A, Kosanke S, Fischetti VA, Factor SM, Cunningham MW. Induction of autoimmune valvular heart disease by recombinant streptococcal m protein. Infection and Immunity. 2001;**69**(6):4072-4078. DOI: 10.1128/IAI.69.6.4072-4078.2001

[38] Passos LSA, Nunes MCP, Aikawa E. Rheumatic heart valve disease pathophysiology and underlying mechanisms. Frontiers in Cardiovascular Medicine. 2020;**7**:612716. Epub 2021/02/05. DOI: 10.3389/fcvm.2020.612716

[39] Dash D, Pandey S. Movement disorders associated with neuronal antibodies. Acta Neurologica

Scandinavica. 2019;**139**(2):106-117. Epub 2018/10/20. DOI: 10.1111/ane.13039

[40] Teixeira AL, Vasconcelos LP, Nunes M, Singer H. Sydenham's chorea: From pathophysiology to therapeutics. Expert Review of Neurotherapeutics. 2021;**21**(8):913-922. Epub 2021/08/07. DOI: 10.1080/14737175.2021.1965883

[41] Gordis L. Effectiveness of comprehensive-care programs in preventing rheumatic fever. The New England Journal of Medicine. 1973;**289**(7):331-335. DOI: 10.1056/NEJM197308162890701

[42] Congeni B, Rizzo C, Congeni J, Sreenivasan VV. Outbreak of acute rheumatic fever in Northeast Ohio. The Journal of Pediatrics. 1987;**111**(2):176-179. DOI: 10.1016/s0022-3476(87)80063-x

[43] Jansen TL, Janssen M, de Jong AJ, Jeurissen ME. Post-streptococcal reactive arthritis: A clinical and serological description, revealing its distinction from acute rheumatic fever. Journal of Internal Medicine. 1999;**245**(3):261-267. DOI: 10.1046/j.1365-2796.1999.0438e.x

[44] Jaggi P. Rheumatic fever and postgroup-a streptococcal arthritis. The Pediatric Infectious Disease Journal. 2011;**30**(5):424-425. DOI: 10.1097/INF.0b013e318217ca5a

[45] Sika-Paotonu D, Beaton A, Raghu A, Steer A, Carapetis J. Acute rheumatic fever and rheumatic heart disease. In: Ferretti JJ, Stevens DL, Fischetti VA, editors. *Streptococcus pyogenes*: Basic Biology to Clinical Manifestations. Oklahoma City (OK): University of Oklahoma Health Sciences Center; 2016

[46] Singhi AK, Bobhate P, Kappanayil M. Acute rheumatic fever. Circulation. 2010;**121**(7):946-947. DOI: 10.1161/CIR.0b013e3181d30e96

[47] Dass C, Kanmanthareddy A. Rheumatic Heart Disease. Treasure Island (FL): StatPearls; 2024

[48] Gewitz MH, Baltimore RS, Tani LY, Sable CA, Shulman ST, Carapetis J, et al. Revision of the Jones criteria for the diagnosis of acute rheumatic fever in the era of Doppler echocardiography. Circulation. 2015;**131**(20):1806-1818. DOI: 10.1161/CIR.0000000000000205

[49] Kliegman R, Nelson WE. Nelson Textbook of Pediatrics. 19th ed. Philadelphia, PA: Elsevier/Saunders; 2011. 923 p

[50] Kirvan CA, Swedo SE, Heuser JS, Cunningham MW. Mimicry and autoantibody-mediated neuronal cell signaling in Sydenham chorea. Nature Medicine. 2003;**9**(7):914-920. DOI: 10.1038/nm892

[51] Husby G, van de Rijn I, Zabriskie JB, Abdin ZH, Williams RC Jr. Antibodies reacting with cytoplasm of subthalamic and caudate nuclei neurons in chorea and acute rheumatic fever. The Journal of Experimental Medicine. 1976;**144**(4):1094-1110. DOI: 10.1084/jem.144.4.1094

[52] Gerber MA, Baltimore RS, Eaton CB, Gewitz M, Rowley AH, Shulman ST, et al. Prevention of rheumatic fever and diagnosis and treatment of acute streptococcal pharyngitis: A scientific statement from the American Heart Association rheumatic fever, endocarditis, and Kawasaki disease Committee of the Council on cardiovascular disease in the young, the interdisciplinary council on functional genomics and translational biology, and the interdisciplinary council on quality of care and outcomes research: Endorsed

by the American Academy of Pediatrics. Circulation. 2009;**119**(11):1541-1551. Epub 20090226. DOI: 10.1161/CIRCULATIONAHA.109.191959

[53] Carapetis JR, Currie BJ. Rheumatic fever in a high incidence population: The importance of monoarthritis and low grade fever. Archives of Disease in Childhood. 2001;**85**(3):223-227. DOI: 10.1136/adc.85.3.223

[54] van Bemmel JM, Delgado V, Holman ER, Allaart CF, Huizinga TW, Bax JJ, et al. No increased risk of valvular heart disease in adult poststreptococcal reactive arthritis. Arthritis and Rheumatism. 2009;**60**(4):987-993. DOI: 10.1002/art.24401

[55] Lennon DR, Farrell E, Martin DR, Stewart JM. Once-daily amoxicillin versus twice-daily penicillin V in group a beta-haemolytic streptococcal pharyngitis. Archives of Disease in Childhood. 2008;**93**(6):474-478. Epub 20080312. DOI: 10.1136/adc.2006.113506

[56] Shvartzman P, Tabenkin H, Rosentzwaig A, Dolginov F. Treatment of streptococcal pharyngitis with amoxycillin once a day. BMJ. 1993;**306**(6886):1170-1172. DOI: 10.1136/bmj.306.6886.1170

[57] Shulman ST, Bisno AL, Clegg HW, Gerber MA, Kaplan EL, Lee G, et al. Clinical practice guideline for the diagnosis and management of group A streptococcal pharyngitis: 2012 update by the Infectious Diseases Society of America. Clinical Infectious Diseases. 2012;**55**(10):1279-1282. DOI: 10.1093/cid/cis847

[58] The Rheumatic Fever Working Party of the Medical Research Council of Great B, The Subcommittee of Principal Investigators of the American Council on Rheumatic F, Congenital Heart Disease AHA. TREATMENT of acute rheumatic fever in children a co-operative clinical trial of a.C.T.H., cortisone, and aspirin; a joint report by the rheumatic fever working party of the Medical Research Council of Great Britain and the subcommittee of principal investigators of the American council on rheumatic fever and congenital heart disease, American Heart Association. British Medical Journal. 1955;**1**(4913):555-574

[59] Illingworth RS, Lorber J, Holt KS, Rendle-Short J. Acute rheumatic fever in children; a comparison of six forms of treatment in 200 cases. Lancet. 1957;**273**(6997):653-659. DOI: 10.1016/s0140-6736(57)92104-9

[60] Kliegman R, Nelson WE. Nelson Textbook of Pediatrics. 19th ed. Philadelphia, PA: Elsevier/Saunders; 2011. p. lxvii, 2610 p

[61] Uziel Y, Hashkes PJ, Kassem E, Padeh S, Goldman R, Wolach B. The use of naproxen in the treatment of children with rheumatic fever. The Journal of Pediatrics. 2000;**137**(2):269-271. DOI: 10.1067/mpd.2000.107158

[62] Hashkes PJ, Tauber T, Somekh E, Brik R, Barash J, Mukamel M, et al. Naproxen as an alternative to aspirin for the treatment of arthritis of rheumatic fever: A randomized trial. The Journal of Pediatrics. 2003;**143**(3):399-401. DOI: 10.1067/s0022-3476(03)00388-3

[63] Cetin II, Ekici F, Kocabas A, Cevik BS, Eminoglu S, Azak E, et al. The efficacy and safety of naproxen in acute rheumatic fever: The comparative results of 11-year experience with acetylsalicylic acid and naproxen. The Turkish Journal of Pediatrics. 2016;**58**(5):473-479. DOI: 10.24953/turkjped.2016.05.003

[64] Torres RPA, Torres RFA, Torres RA, Torres RSLA. Pulse therapy combined with oral corticosteroids in the management of severe rheumatic carditis and rebound. Cardiology in the Young. 2018;**28**(2):309-314. Epub 2017/10/25. DOI: 10.1017/S1047951117002062

[65] Albert DA, Harel L, Karrison T. The treatment of rheumatic carditis: A review and meta-analysis. Medicine (Baltimore). 1995;**74**(1):1-12. DOI: 10.1097/00005792-199501000-00001

[66] Cilliers AM, Manyemba J, Saloojee H. Anti-inflammatory treatment for carditis in acute rheumatic fever. Cochrane Database of Systematic Reviews. Jun 2012;**13**;(6):CD003176. DOI: 10.1002/14651858.CD003176

[67] Voss LM, Wilson NJ, Neutze JM, Whitlock RM, Ameratunga RV, Cairns LM, et al. Intravenous immunoglobulin in acute rheumatic fever: A randomized controlled trial. Circulation. 2001;**103**(3):401-406. DOI: 10.1161/01.cir.103.3.401

[68] Thatai D, Turi ZG. Current guidelines for the treatment of patients with rheumatic fever. Drugs. 1999;**57**(4):545-555. DOI: 10.2165/00003495-199957040-00007

[69] Ralph AP, Noonan S, Wade V, Currie BJ. The 2020 Australian guideline for prevention, diagnosis and management of acute rheumatic fever and rheumatic heart disease. The Medical Journal of Australia. 2021;**214**(5):220-227. Epub 20201115. DOI: 10.5694/mja2.50851

[70] Anderson Y, Wilson N, Nicholson R, Finucane K. Fulminant mitral regurgitation due to ruptured chordae tendinae in acute rheumatic fever. Journal of Paediatrics and Child Health. 2008;**44**(3):134-137. Epub 20070914. DOI: 10.1111/j.1440-1754.2007.01214.x

[71] Cardoso F, Maia D, Cunningham MC, Valenca G. Treatment of Sydenham chorea with corticosteroids. Movement Disorders. 2003;**18**(11):1374-1377. DOI: 10.1002/mds.10521

[72] Fusco C, Spagnoli C. Corticosteroid treatment in Sydenham's chorea. European Journal of Paediatric Neurology. 2018;**22**(2):327-331. Epub 20171216. DOI: 10.1016/j.ejpn.2017.11.011

[73] Lessof MH, Bywaters EG. The duration of chorea. British Medical Journal. 1956;**1**(4982):1520-1523. DOI: 10.1136/bmj.1.4982.1520

[74] Direk M, Epcacan S, Epcacan Z, Yildirim DD, Okuyaz C. Efficacy of levetiracetam in the treatment of Sydenham chorea. Pediatrics International. 2020;**62**(11):1264-1268. Epub 20201105. DOI: 10.1111/ped.14318

[75] Douvoyiannis M, Fautsch KJ, Miles J. The role of levetiracetam and prednisolone in the treatment of Sydenham's chorea. Clinical Pediatrics (Phila). Oct 2024;**63**(9):1185-1188. DOI: 10.1177/00099228231222663. Epub 2024 Jan 10

[76] Marcus RH, Sareli P, Pocock WA, Barlow JB. The spectrum of severe rheumatic mitral valve disease in a developing country. Correlations among clinical presentation, surgical pathologic findings, and hemodynamic sequelae. Annals of Internal Medicine. 1994;**120**(3):177-183. DOI: 10.7326/0003-4819-120-3-199402010-00001

Section 2

Common Neurological Disorders in Children

Chapter 2

Childhood Epilepsies and When to Refer for Epilepsy Surgery Evaluation

Derryl Miller

Abstract

Many providers feel uncomfortable with the recognition of epileptic seizures, the diagnosis and classification of epilepsy syndromes, and initial treatments to offer to patients with epilepsy. Available therapies for children with epilepsy include medical management with antiseizure medications, trial of the ketogenic diet, and evaluation for epilepsy surgeries. This chapter will highlight the diagnostic criteria for epilepsy, common epilepsy syndromes according to the recent updated International League Against Epilepsy (ILAE) Classification, and when to refer to an epilepsy center for specialized treatments if not readily available such as the ketogenic diet, phase 1 presurgical evaluation, and epilepsy surgery. This chapter will also briefly highlight frequent comorbidities with epilepsy such as psychogenic nonepileptic seizures and attention deficit hyperactivity disorder and the challenges related to seizure mimics. This chapter will therefore highlight the diagnosis, workup, and management of both medically responsive epilepsy and drug resistant epilepsy (DRE) as well as its comorbidities. This chapter is a comprehensive review of the literature for the diagnosis and treatment of epilepsy and the author's experience of practice working at Riley Hospital for Children at Indiana University Health which is a National Association of Epilepsy Centers (NAEC) Level 4 Epilepsy Center.

Keywords: epilepsy, seizures, antiseizure medications, ketogenic diet, presurgical evaluation, epilepsy surgery, neuromodulation, magnetic resonance imaging, electroencephalogram, next generation sequencing

1. Introduction

Epilepsy is a syndrome of recurrent seizures with an operational definition of high risk of occurrence of seizures at or above 60% [1]. This risk of occurrence of seizures can be met several ways with the following: two unprovoked seizures which are 24 hours apart or one unprovoked seizure and a diagnostic workup placing the patient at high risk of occurrence of seizure with the Electroencephalogram (EEG), structural imaging with Magnetic Resonance Imaging (MRI) of the brain, or genetic testing [1]. Following the diagnosis of epilepsy, the clinician should initiate therapy to reduce the risk of continued seizures to prevent sudden unexplained death in epilepsy (SUDEP) [2, 3].

For most patients with epilepsy, the first two seizure medications with appropriate mechanisms for the treatment of their seizures result in seizure freedom if side effects are not encountered [4]. Despite the development of many available new antiseizure medications, rates of seizure freedom with medical management alone are not increased for those patients with drug resistant epilepsy (DRE) [5].

Given that rates of seizure freedom following the diagnosis of DRE are low with medical management alone, referral to a comprehensive epilepsy center which is capable of treatments such as the ketogenic diet, presurgical evaluation, and epilepsy surgeries such as resective, ablative, disconnective, and neuromodulation surgeries should be performed at the time of diagnosis of DRE [6].

1.1 Recognizing epileptic seizures

Epileptic seizures are paroxysmal events with discrete onset, offset, and often post ictal state [7]. The International League Against Epilepsy (ILAE), an international association of clinicians and scientists dedicated to evidence-based and efficacious practice of medicine for children and adults with epilepsy, recently released a position paper which describes epileptic seizures by semiology for identification of focal onset, generalized onset, or unknown onset [7]. Seizure classification begins with the history of the patient's description of their seizures along with visual analysis of the events by caregivers [7].

Seizures are broadly divided into generalized onset and focal onset referring to the early activation of networks in the brain, and within these two broad categories are subgroups of epileptic seizures which will be described [7].

Generalized onset seizures are subdivided into motor or nonmotor seizures with the motor features being tonic, atonic, tonic clonic, or myoclonic, while nonmotor seizures are classified as typical absence, atypical absence, absence with myoclonia or absence with eyelid myoclonia [7]. Focal onset seizures by contrast can be classified with hypermotor movements, automatic behavior, arrest of behavior, emotional response, sensory changes, or lateralized motor features such as tonic, atonic, tonic clonic, or myoclonic movements [7]. Focal onset seizures furthermore can be classified as retained awareness or impaired awareness to designate whether memory remains intact throughout the seizure or not [7]. Assessing awareness during a seizure requires delivery of a code word to determine if memory is intact throughout a seizure. At Riley Hospital for Children, code words are a color and an object such as "red truck" which, if remembered by the patient after the seizure is over, suggest focal retained awareness at the onset of the seizure symptoms. At times, seizures cannot be adequately classified as focal or generalized in onset based on the semiology alone and so are classified as unknown onset [7]. It is also possible for patients to have comorbid focal onset and generalized onset seizures [7].

One feature of seizure which highly supports focal onset by history is the patient self-reporting positive symptoms such as tastes, smells, déjà vu, visual phenomena, paresthesias, or strong emotional response which could all be auras [8]. Auras which do not progress to a secondarily generalized seizure with loss of awareness could be consistent with focal retained awareness seizures [8]. Focal retained awareness seizures can be challenging to diagnose other than by empiric treatment due to many patients with focal retained awareness seizures having negative EEG tracings during the ictus [9]. As the focal onset seizure spreads to involve both hemispheres, impacting the circuits of papez, the patient then loses awareness and an ictal pattern is seen in most cases [10, 11].

Table 1 describes the typical semiology, duration, and features of each subtype of seizure commonly experienced by the patient.

1.2 Provoked and unprovoked epileptic seizures

Epileptic seizures may be provoked or unprovoked [12–14]. A provoked epileptic seizure is a seizure with cause explaining its occurrence which is not intrinsic to the patient's brain [12, 13]. Provoked seizures have a broad differential including electrolyte abnormalities (hyponatremia, hypocalcemia, hypomagnesemia, hypoglycemia, and hyperglycemia), metabolic derangements such as hyperammonemia,

Seizure Type	Focal or Generalized Onset	Typical Duration	Semiology
Typical Absence (Petit Mal)	Generalized	5–10 seconds	Staring with behavior arrest, possibly eyelid fluttering, and loss of awareness without post ictal state
Atypical Absence	Generalized	20–60 seconds	Slowing of movement with staring and decreased responsiveness but often not clear behavior arrest
Focal Retained Awareness Seizure (Simple Partial)	Focal	60–120 seconds	Aura of tastes, smells, déjà vu, visual phenomena, paresthesia, or strong emotional response without loss of awareness
Focal Impaired Awareness Seizure (Complex Partial or Dyscognitive)	Focal	60–120 seconds	Aura of tastes, smells, déjà vu, visual phenomena, paresthesia, or strong emotional response progressing to loss of awareness and possibly secondary generalized tonic clonic seizure with post ictal state
Myoclonic Seizure	Focal or Generalized	< 1 second each	Twitching of the extremities with rapid and sudden movement which can cluster but typically are not rhythmic in a cluster
Clonic Seizure	Focal or Generalized	5–120 seconds	Rhythmic twitching of the extremities with rapid and sudden movement which clusters into rhythmic shaking
Generalized Tonic clonic Seizure (Grand Mal)	Generalized	60–120 seconds	Sudden loss of awareness with or without vocalization and stiffening of the extremities followed by rhythmic shaking and post ictal state and patients often fall
Tonic Seizure (Drop attack)	Focal or Generalized	3–10 seconds	Sudden stiffening of the extremities with or without loss of awareness and generally without post ictal state and patients often fall
Atonic Seizure (Drop attack)	Generalized	< 1–2 seconds	Sudden loss of tone with head drop and patients often will hit their head and fall without post ictal state
Infantile Epileptic Spasms Syndrome (Epileptic Spasms)	Focal or Generalized	< 3 seconds and cluster out of sleep	Stereotyped flexor or extensor clonic tonic stiffening events which each are each about 3 seconds and cluster out of sleep about every 10–15 seconds. These often disturb the patient and result in crying.

Table 1.
Seizure subtypes which are classified by onset (generalized or focal), duration in seconds, and expected semiology of each subtype.

hyperthermia seen commonly with febrile seizures between 6 months and 6 years of age, hypoxia, trauma with intracranial hemorrhage, and infectious causes such as meningitis/encephalitis [12, 13].

In the case of provoked seizures, the clinician should correct any offending provoking factor, though antiepileptics may raise the seizure threshold while the provoking factor is addressed. For example, electrolyte abnormalities which are detected should be corrected, lesions on head imaging requiring surgical management should be repaired/excised, intoxications with illicit substances should be detected and detoxified, and infectious causes ruled out with lumbar puncture or treated as appropriate [12, 13]. Patients with provoked seizures should still be treated with antiseizure medications while the provoking factor is addressed [12, 13]. Workup for provoked seizures which is generally performed in the emergency department following complete history and neurologic examination includes complete blood count (CBC), complete metabolic panel (CMP), Magnesium, and head imaging with either computed tomography (CT) or magnetic resonance imaging (MRI). Other workups to consider include Urine Drug Screen, Lactate, Pyruvate, Ammonia, Arterial Blood Gas (ABG), and lumbar puncture for total nucleated cell count, glucose, protein, and culture and stain [14].

Unprovoked seizures by contrast occur spontaneously in patients with epilepsy in the absence of provoking factors [14]. Multiple seizures which are unprovoked are highly suggestive of epilepsy as multiple unprovoked seizures constitutes high risk of recurrence of unprovoked seizures [1, 14]. Once a patient has multiple unprovoked seizures, the clinician should initiate treatment even prior to workup for the underlying cause.

1.3 Nonepileptic seizure mimics

Complicating the diagnosis of epilepsy are the many seizure mimics which include inattentiveness as is seen with attention deficit hyperactivity disorder (ADHD), sleep disturbances, autism spectrum disorder with poor social reciprocity, stereotypies, self-gratification behaviors, other subcortical movement disorders such as tic disorders, and psychogenic nonepileptic spells [15–17]. For this reason, if there is a low clinical suspicion of epileptic seizure, video EEG (VEEG) to spell capture events can be very helpful to rule out seizures, while routine EEG and head imaging are helpful for ruling in a diagnosis of epilepsy. In other words, the routine EEG and head imaging are sensitive for diagnosis of epilepsy, though they are not specific, while VEEG with characteristic events captured can both rule in and rule out epileptic seizures.

1.4 Diagnostic workup after suspected first unprovoked seizure

Diagnostic workup for epilepsy etiology in the outpatient setting after first time seizure includes imaging of the head with either CT or more ideally MRI of the brain to look for symptomatic lesions. Some of these lesions may be surgical such as hemorrhages which need to be evacuated in the case of accidental or nonaccidental trauma, supratentorial tumors, or infectious causes such as abscesses or empyema [1]. The EEG may be utilized to predict risk of occurrence of seizures as well by detecting interictal discharges or demonstrating seizure onset if seizures are captured [1, 18]. Genetic testing with chromosome microarray, epilepsy gene panels, or next generation sequencing testing, and metabolic testing can also be considered [19, 20].

Generally, the diagnosis of epilepsy is made following a first-time unprovoked seizure with rule out of provoking factors along with the detection of interictal discharges or ictal patterns on an EEG, the detection of a lesion on the imaging of the head which indicates continued risk of occurrence of seizures, or having known genetic predisposition from testing [1, 14].

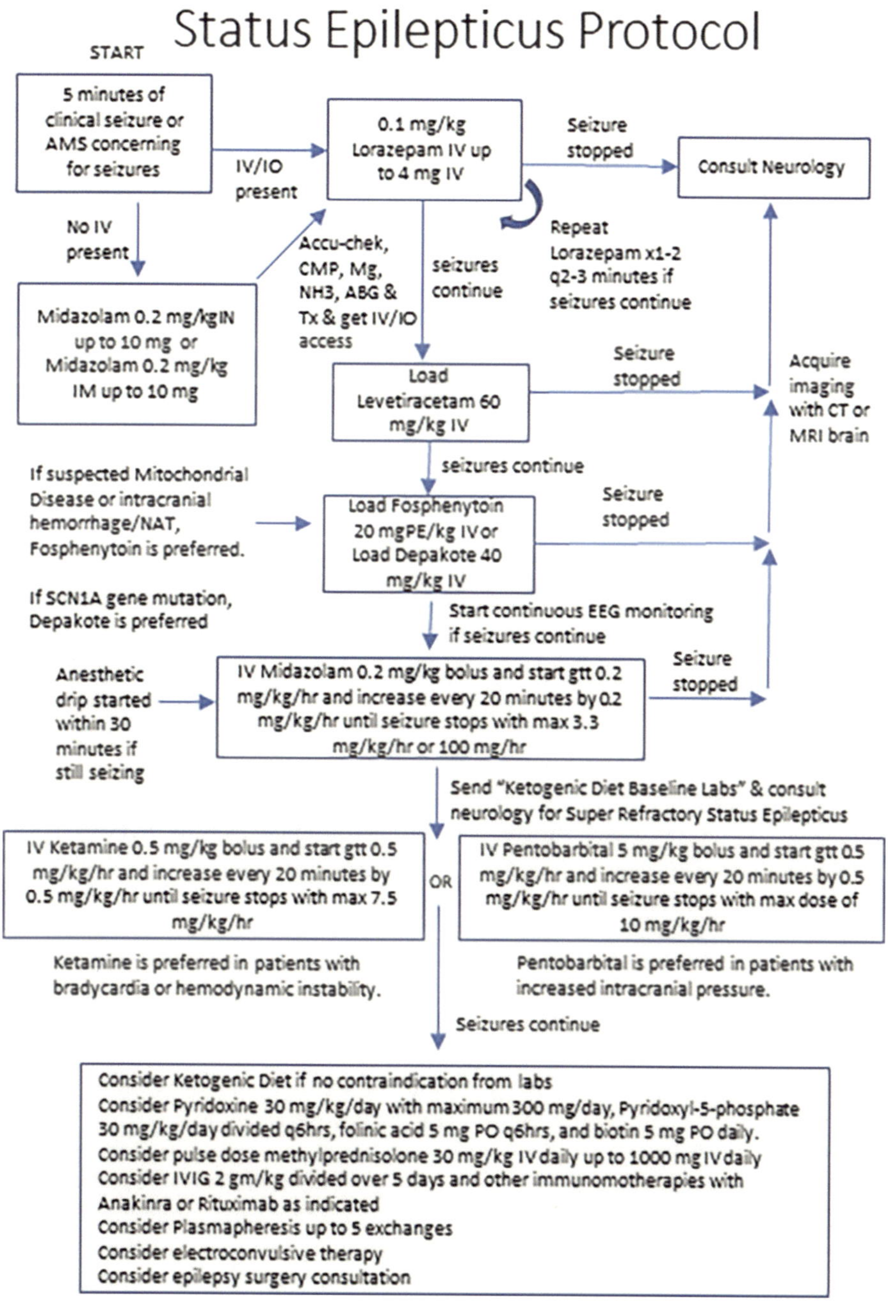

Figure 1.
Status epilepticus protocol for children beyond the neonatal period which begins at 5 minutes of clinical seizure and ends with cessation of status epilepticus. IM = intramuscular, IN = intranasal, IV = intravenous, IO = intraosseous, gtt = drip.

1.5 Protocol for status epilepticus

The first time provoked or unprovoked seizure in a patient may be consistent with status epilepticus if a seizure is longer than 5 minutes [1]. Status epilepticus as a first-time seizure is not equivalent to a diagnosis of epilepsy, though it is a medical emergency requiring urgent management with associated morbidity and mortality if not treated emergently [1, 14]. At Riley Hospital for Children, a status epilepticus protocol is utilized for the prompt and efficacious treatment of status epilepticus with concomitant diagnosis and management of the prolonged seizure (**Figure 1**).

Treatment of seizure per this protocol involves detecting and correcting provoking factors while initiating therapies for resolution of status epilepticus starting at 5 minutes [21]. Initiating treatment for status epilepticus at 5 minutes is indicated to reduce risk of physiologic loss of neurons which occurs if status is not treated quickly [21]. Refractory status epilepticus (RSE) occurs when the seizure does not stop with loads of seizure medication and super refractory status epilepticus (SRSE) is defined as continuous seizure despite initiation of anesthetic coma [21]. SRSE carries morbidity and mortality, so additional diagnostic testing to determine the underlying cause of SRSE should be conducted by the neurologist if seizures do not respond to anesthetic coma as expected.

The treatment of status epilepticus at Riley Hospital for Children in the neonatal period starts with loads of phenobarbital 20 mg/kg IV given twice followed by keppra 30 mg/kg IV given twice, while considering treatment of underlying metabolic epilepsy from inborn errors of metabolism with pyridoxine, pyridoxyl-5-phosphate, folinic acid, and biotin followed by midazolam anesthetic drip [22].

Neuronal loss and injury due to status epilepticus is seen as evidenced by cytotoxic edema seen on MRI of the brain following treatment of prolonged status epilepticus [21]. Status epilepticus should by promptly identified and the clinician should initiate an aggressive treatment protocol to avoid injury [21]. Thankfully, the majority of patients without a provoking cause of seizure which needs to be corrected do respond to appropriately dosed benzodiazepines and the first load of appropriately dosed antiseizure medications, making very prolonged status epilepticus rare if treated aggressively [21]. This protocol for treatment of status epilepticus is invaluable for the prompt treatment of status epilepticus. Involving the pediatric neurologist at the start or throughout this protocol is appropriate given that status epilepticus can cause permanent neurologic injury if not promptly treated.

2. Treatment of epileptic seizures with maintenance medications

Broadly, there are three common treatments for epileptic seizures, being antiseizure medications, the ketogenic diet, and epilepsy surgeries [4–6].

Of the available treatments, antiseizure medications are generally first line and easiest to attempt, with minimal effect on quality of life in many cases. At Riley Hospital for Children, antiseizure medications are dosed via the guidelines in **Table 2**.

Approximately 2/3 of patients with epilepsy will respond to medical management and become seizure free on an appropriate therapeutic dosing of antiseizure medications [23]. For those who are not seizure free with trial of 2 therapeutic trials of antiseizure medications for efficacy, the epileptologist should be involved for the workup and treatment of drug resistant epilepsy (DRE) as even newer medications

Generic Name (Brand Name)	Dosing	Forms	Levels	Seizure Types Treated
Brivaracetam (Briviact)	3–5 mg/kg/day	• Liquid • Tablet • Injection	0.2–2.0 mcg/mL	Broad Spectrum
Cannabidiol (Epidiolex)	2.5–20 mg/kg/day	• Liquid	300–450 ng/mL studies only	Broad Spectrum, Dravet Syndrome, Lennox Gastaut Syndrome
Carbamazepine (Tegretol, Epitol, Carbatrol, Tegretol XR)	10–20 mg/kg/day	• Liquid • Tablet • Chewable • XR capsule & tablet	4–12 mg/L of metabolite	Focal Seizures
Cenobamate (Xcopri)	1–7 mg/kg/day	• Tablet	>0.2 mcg/mL	Focal Seizures
Clobazam (Onfi)	0.3–1.3 mg/kg/day	• Liquid • Tablet	30–300 ng/mL	Broad Spectrum
Clonazepam (Klonopin)	0.01–0.05 mg/kg/day	• Tablet • Oral dissolving tablet	Not Established	Broad Spectrum
Ethosuximide (Zarontin)	10–60 mg/kg/day	• Liquid • Capsule	45–100 mcg/mL	Absence Seizures Only
Eslicarbazepine (Aptiom)	20–30 mg/kg/day	• Tablet	3–35 mg/L of metabolite	Focal Seizures
Felbamate (Felbatol)	15–45 mg/kg/day	• Liquid • Tablet	30–60 mg/L	Focal Seizures and Lennox Gastaut Syndrome
Fenfluramine (Fintepla)	0.1–0.35 mg/kg/day	• Liquid	<50 mcg/L in studies	Dravet Syndrome and Lennox Gastaut Syndrome
Gabapentin (Neurontin)	10–50 mg/kg/day	• Liquid • Tablet • Capsule	2–20 mg/L	Focal Seizures
Ganaxolone (Ztalmy)	63 mg/kg/day	• Liquid	500–900 ng/mL	CDKL5 deficiency disorder associated seizures
Lacosamide (Vimpat)	5–10 mg/kg/day	• Liquid • Tablet • Injection	5–10 mg/L	Focal Seizures
Lamotrigine (Lamictal)	1–5 mg/kg/day (On Depakote) 5–15 mg/kg/day (Not on Depakote)	• Tablet • Long acting tablet • Oral dissolving tablet • Chewable	3–14 mg/L	Broad Spectrum but may worsen Myoclonus

Generic Name (Brand Name)	Dosing	Forms	Levels	Seizure Types Treated
Levetiracetam (Keppra)	20–60 mg/kg/day	• Liquid • Tablet • Long acting tablet • Disperse tablet • Injection	12–46 mg/L	Broad Spectrum but generally ineffective for absence seizures
Pregabalin (Lyrica)	2.5–14 mg/kg/day	• Liquid • Capsule	2.8–8.3 mg/L	Focal Seizures
Oxcarbazepine (Trileptal)	20–40 mg/kg/day	• Liquid • Tablet • Long acting tablet	3–35 mg/L of metabolite	Focal Seizures
Perampanel (Fycompa)	8–12 mg/day	• Liquid • Tablet	180–610 ng/mL	Focal Seizures
Phenobarbital (Sezaby)	5–7 mg/kg/day	• Liquid • Tablet	15–40 mcg/mL	Broad Spectrum
Phenytoin (Dilantin)	5–7 mg/kg/day	• Liquid • Chewable tablet • Long acting capsule • Injection	10–20 mcg/mL	Broad Spectrum though avoided in Dravet Syndrome
Prednisolone (Rayos)	8 mg/kg/day with taper	• Liquid • Tablet • Oral dissolving tablet	Not established though can measure for compliance	Infantile Spasms
Primidone (Mysoline)	10–25 mg/kg/day	• Tablet	5–10 mg/L	Broad Spectrum
Rufinamide (Banzel)	45 mg/kg/day	• Liquid • Tablet	5–30 mcg/mL	Lennox Gastaut Syndrome
Stiripentol (Diacomit)	50 mg/kg/day	• Capsule • Powder Packet	4–22 mg/L	Dravet Syndrome
Tiagabine (Gabitril)	32 mg/day	• Tablet	0.02–0.2 mg/L	Focal Seizures
Topiramate (Topamax, Eprontia, Trokindi XR, Qudexy XR)	4–9 mg/kg/day	• Liquid, • Sprinkle Capsule • Tablet • Long acting tablet	5–20 mg/L	Broad Spectrum
Valproic Acid (Depakote, Valproate, Depakene)	15–60 mg/kg/day	• Liquid • Sprinkle Capsule • Delayed Release Tablet • Extended Release Tablet • Injectable	40–100 mcg/mL	Broad Spectrum

Generic Name (Brand Name)	Dosing	Forms	Levels	Seizure Types Treated
Vigabatrin (Sabril)	50–150 mg/kg/day	• Tablet • Packets of powder to mix with water	0.8–36 mg/L	Infantile Spasms
Zonisamide (Zonegran)	4–9 mg/kg/day	• Liquid • Capsules	10–40 mg/L	Broad Spectrum
Corticotropin injection (Acthar, ACTH Gel)	40–150 units/m^2/day	• Injectable Gel	Not established	Infantile Spasms
Diazepam (Valium)	0.1–1 mg/kg/day	• Liquid • Tablet	0.2–2.5 mcg/mL	Broad Spectrum

Table 2.
Guidelines for dosing of antiseizure medications in children utilized commonly at Riley Hospital for children including formulations of each medication, therapeutic levels of medications where appropriate, and seizure types treated.

which have been developed have not appreciably increased seizure freedom in children diagnosed with DRE [23–34].

The choice of initial antiseizure medications is based on the patient's epilepsy onset [35–38]. If a patient's epilepsy is determined to be focal, there are many choices for antiseizure medications for focal seizures and broad-spectrum agents both being efficacious [35–38]. If an epilepsy is determined to be generalized by interictal profile and semiology of seizures or unknown in onset, broad-spectrum antiseizure medications are preferentially utilized as narrow spectrum medications could worsen absence seizures and myoclonic seizures [36, 37]. Titration of monotherapy antiseizure medication to side effect or maximal therapeutic dose is generally recommended to demonstrate true medication failure before switching medications or before considering antiseizure medications in combination [39].

There are also dietary therapies with the ketogenic diet, modified Adkins diet, and low glycemic index diet [40], and many surgical options ranging from resection and ablation, disconnection such as corpus callosotomy or functional hemispherotomy, and neuromodulation techniques which are utilized in DRE which will be discussed later in this chapter [41–43].

2.1 Diagnosis and treatment of drug resistant epilepsy

Drug resistant epilepsy (DRE) is diagnosed following trials of two appropriate antiseizure medications failed for efficacy at high therapeutic doses for controlling seizures [4, 6, 18, 23, 41]. Medications can also be tried in synergistic combinations as these do exist; however, it is not necessary to prescribe medications in combination to diagnose DRE [39].

Once a child is diagnosed with DRE with focal onset, generalized onset, focal and generalized onset, or unknown onset, workup initiates to better understand the epilepsy etiology if it is incompletely understood as well as to determine if the patient would be a candidate for potentially curative epilepsy surgery [24–26]. The ILAE has further assembled a framework for the definition of epilepsy syndromes which are clinically similar though heterogeneous by etiology [44–49]. Within each epilepsy syndrome is a wide range of etiologies with tailored medications and dietary therapy in many cases, so workup for diagnosis of etiology will be important to the neurologist to determine the cause of the drug resistant epilepsy as structural, genetic, metabolic, infectious, autoimmune, or idiopathic [44]. Structural abnormalities causing epilepsy would include cortical dysplasia, periventricular nodular heterotopia, and neoplastic processes as etiologies [44]. Genetic epilepsy is caused by either single gene disorders or is polygenic [44]. Metabolic epilepsies include mitochondrial disorders, vitamin deficiencies, and metabolite storage disorders [44]. Infectious and autoimmune causes are often diagnosed by lumbar puncture showing inflammation of the cerebrospinal fluid [44]. Furthermore, many cases of epilepsy remain idiopathic despite thorough diagnostic workup [44].

A practical example of this approach is the treatment of infantile epileptic spasms syndrome (IESS) which can present as the complete triad of developmental regression, hypsarrhythmia on the EEG, and ictal spasms captured on EEG which was originally described as West Syndrome [50]. In the patient with IESS without known etiology, available therapies include adrenocorticotropic hormone (ACTH), Vigabatrin, and high dose prednisolone [51]. In the case of patients with infantile spasms with comorbid Tuberous Sclerosis as an etiology, Vigabatrin is superior therapy to the hormonal therapies for seizure freedom [50, 51]. For this reason, a thorough physical exam looking for stigmata of tuberous sclerosis such as shagreen patches, ash-leaf macules, angiokeratomas, and imaging studies to identify cortical tubers may prompt genetic testing for the genetic causes in TSC1 and TSC2 and identification of superior therapy with Vigabatrin [50–52].

Another example of a heterogeneous etiology which is medically refractory but often responsive to tailored therapy would be the identification of early infantile developmental epileptic encephalopathies (EIDEE) [46]. EIDEE presents with global developmental delay, tone abnormalities, and seizures under 3 months old, and genetic testing and metabolic testing are high yield, resulting in guidance of therapy [46]. Such genetic mutations include SCN8A or SCN2A which generally are gain of function mutations and so respond to sodium channel blockade [46]. For this reason, early onset seizures with associated developmental delay, dysmorphism, or consanguinity history suggests that genetic testing is high yield. Available genetic testing for patients with suspected genetic epilepsies include chromosome microarray (CMA) and next generation sequencing (NGS) testing such as genetic panels, whole exome sequencing (WES), and whole genome sequencing (WGS) [19, 20]. Of these tests, NGS testing while more expensive remains higher yield than CMA with the cost per diagnosis favoring NGS testing over CMA [20]. Additionally, professional opinion suggests that NGS is very high yield in patients with global developmental delay and epilepsy of any kind.

Following the diagnosis of drug resistant epilepsy, care should be directed to an epilepsy center with pediatric neurologists with epilepsy training to assess candidacy for epilepsy surgery or for continued management through medical and dietary means [4, 6, 18, 24–26].

2.2 Phase 1 presurgical evaluation for drug resistant epilepsy

If a phase 1 presurgical evaluation cannot be performed at your center, referral to an epilepsy center is appropriate once a patient is diagnosed with DRE whether or not the etiology of their epilepsy is known [23–26]. Phase 1 presurgical evaluation is noninvasive testing aimed at defining as precisely as possible a region of the brain called the epileptogenic zone, which is the smallest region of brain which if removed or destroyed would render the patient with DRE seizure free [18].

Phase 1 evaluation testing for DRE for epilepsy surgery generally includes high resolution MRI of the brain with 3 tesla or higher resolution if available and with thin coronal cuts to detect subtle mesial temporal lesions, prolonged video EEG monitoring with wean of antiseizure medications as needed to capture and lateralize/localize seizures with scalp electrodes, and neuropsyciatric testing if the patient may cooperate with this [26].

Discussion of these patients in multidisciplinary epilepsy committees with input from epileptologists, neurosurgeons, neuropsychologists, and neuroradiologists is critical to establish adequate concordance of the phase 1 presurgical data [25]. The committee will determine if surgery candidacy is clear, if additional phase 1 testing is required, if an invasive phase 2 monitoring will be needed, or if the patient is not a good candidate for resection or ablation [25].

If additional testing is needed to establish surgical candidacy in phase 1, interictal 18F-Fluorodeoxyglucose positron emission tomography computed tomography (FDG-PET/CT) can be utilized to determine regions of the brain where hypometabolism of glucose is noted [53]. Ictal and interictal blood flow studies with Technecium-99 m single-photon emission computed tomography (SPECT) are utilized to directly highlight the epileptogenic zone and can be co-registered with MRI of the brain for anatomic localization [54, 55]. If both interictal SPECT and ictal SPECT scans are acquired, a subtraction scan called Subtraction Ictal SPECT Coregistered to MRI (SISCOM) can be produced which highlights the epileptogenic zone with better delineation if the ictal SPECT is inconclusive [55]. In cases where nonradial dipoles are suspected, magnetoencephalography (MEG) can be utilized to anatomically localize interictal or ictal findings on the EEG by analyzing the magnetic fields detected around the head and solving the "inverse problem" to determine the most likely anatomic localization of the discharges [56].

Functional MRI of the brain, MEG, and Wada testing all are utilized to lateralize the patient's language and motor cortices to prevent injury to these eloquent regions when planning epilepsy surgery [25, 56, 57]. This evaluation is especially important in patients who are left-handed or who had injury to the suspected dominant hemisphere from stroke or other previous pathology as language lateralization is not clearly delineated in this group [58, 59]. The goal of phase 1 presurgical evaluation is definitive epilepsy surgery with ablation or resection which remain the most efficacious interventions, or lateralization or localization of the seizure focus such that a strong hypothesis for seizure localization/lateralization can prompt a phase 2 presurgical evaluation [26].

2.3 Phase 2 presurgical evaluation for drug resistant epilepsy

If lateralization is achieved but localization is unclear after comprehensive phase 1 presurgical evaluation, a decision is often made to explore the brain with phase 2 presurgical evaluation including grids, strips, depth electrodes, or stereo electroencephalography, with placement guided by the epileptologist and neurosurgeon to more accurately localize the patient's seizure onset zone for definitive surgical treatment [26]. At times during the phase 1 or phase 2 of testing for epilepsy surgery, the patient is determined not to be a candidate for resection or ablation surgery due to the epileptogenic zone being multifocal or generalized or involving eloquent cortices [18, 26]. Rather than performing disabling resective or ablative surgery in these cases, neuromodulation and dietary management are possible for these patients [40, 43]. Cortical mapping during phase 2 evaluation can be performed by the epileptologist by delivering small shocks to each contact which is implanted to determine the location of eloquent cortices at the bedside, which is an additional advantage of phase 2 monitoring [26].

2.4 Neuromodulation

There are currently multiple devices available for neuromodulating seizures which are either placed peripherally or centrally and are open loop or closed loop for reducing seizures [43, 60].

Vagus Nerve Stimulators (VNS) are commonly placed with the generator in the left chest and leads attached to the vagus nerve (CN10) at the neck which produces open loop stimulation with afferent nerves delivering signal through the brainstem and to the cortex which reduces seizures [43]. The more modern generators also have tachycardia detection for delivering shock during a rapid rise in heart rate and comes with a magnet which the family may swipe over the generator to send a larger impulse with the goal of stopping seizures when they occur [43]. VNS has furthermore been shown to reduce risk of SUDEP in cohorts with DRE over 3–10 years of monitoring [61].

Deep Brain Stimulation (DBS) is another open loop system stimulating various nuclei of the brain with the goal of reducing seizures [62]. The anterior nucleus of the thalamus DBS has reduced seizures in patients with frontotemporal epilepsy [62]. Anterior nucleus DBS also has been shown to reduce risk of SUDEP, though it involves intracranial surgery [63]. There is evidence for DBS placement in the centromedian parafascicular nuclei complex which may show efficacy for generalized or multifocal onset seizures, though this target is being studied [60].

Reactive neurostimulation (RNS) is also approved for the treatment of focal epilepsy and is a closed loop system [60, 64]. This device is implanted within the skull and with electrodes placed on the surface of the brain or depth electrodes, which are capable of recording seizures with electrocorticography and delivering current to stop seizures [60, 64]. Like VNS and DBS, there is evidence for reduction of seizures over time and reduction in SUDEP risk as well [60, 64]. RNS can be utilized to treat two foci of seizure onset once localized and can treat seizures arising from eloquent cortex which cannot be addressed with resection or ablative surgeries [64].

2.5 Corpus callosotomy

Corpus callosotomy (CC) is a disconnection procedure which divides the hemispheres of the brain by severing the commissural white matter tract between hemispheres [65]. CC is especially effective for seizures which are generalized and result in fall injuries, such as tonic and atonic seizures [65]. CC has been used to lateralize a seizure focus that appeared bilateral on scalp and intracranial monitoring for definitive epilepsy surgery when focal semiology was suspected [66].

2.6 Ketogenic diet

For patients with drug resistant epilepsy who are not candidates for definitive surgery or if the family prefers additional nonsurgical and nonmedical therapies for epilepsy, the ketogenic diet can be utilized for both generalized and focal onset seizures [40]. Through phase 1 presurgical evaluation, many patients with drug resistant epilepsy are determined not to be effective surgical candidates and have side effects from antiseizure medication polytherapy. Certain metabolic disorders such as patients with SLC2A1 gene mutation are also excellent candidates for the diet [40]. The ketogenic diet is a high fat and low carbohydrate diet aimed at adjusting the metabolism of the brain to reduce hyperexcitability of neurons and to reduce seizures [40]. Before starting the ketogenic diet, contraindications to its use should first be ruled out including fatty acid oxidation disorders, or other metabolic disorders which could potentially be worsened by the high fat diet [40].

At Riley Hospital for Children, baseline labs are performed with serum Complete Blood Count, Complete Metabolic Panel, Phosphorous, Magnesium, Lipid Panel, Vitamin D, Free and total carnitine, Prealbumin, Lactate, Ammonia, Uric acid, Zinc, Selenium, Amino Acid Profile, acylcarnitine analysis, and Ferritin along with urine Amino Acid Profile and Organic Acid Screen. If no contraindications to the diet are found, the ketogenic diet can be attempted with the help of a registered dietician generally titrating to a 4:1 ratio of fat to protein and carbohydrates [40].

Side effects of the ketogenic diet include weight loss, constipation, risk of kidney stones, risk of pancreatitis, and hyperlipidemia [40]. Additional considerations are that liquid medication often contains too many carbohydrates for use so families generally have to switch medications to tablet formulations [67].

3. Seizure safety and acute treatment

Even before epilepsy is diagnosed and treated, seizure precautions and first aid should be discussed with patients and families presenting for a first-time seizure, while performing diagnostic workup [68, 69]. Seizure first aid includes staying with the patient, rolling them on their side, and keeping the patient safe while timing the seizure [70]. For seizures over 5 minutes, various rescue medications are utilized which may be made available if prescribed by treating physicians, and activating emergency services is advised if a seizure is longer than 5 minutes, as this is consistent with status epilepticus which should be treated emergently (**Figure 1**). **Table 3** shows available seizure rescue medications.

Seizure precautions to prevent injuries during even brief seizures should be discussed with patients who have had even one seizure [68]. Precautions include

Medication	Sizes	Route of Administration	Dosing
Diazepam (Diastat)	2.5 mg, 10 mg, 20 mg	Rectal gel	2–5 years = 0.5 mg/kg/dose 6–11 years = 0.3 mg/kg/dose ≥12 years = 0.2 mg/kg/dose
Diazepam (Valtoco)	5 mg, 10 mg, 15 mg, 20 mg	Intranasal kit	6–11 years = 5 mg if 10–18 kg, 10 mg if 19–37 kg, 15 mg if 38–55 kg, and 20 mg if ≥56 kg ≥12 years = 5 mg if 14–27 kg, 10 mg if 28–50 kg, 15 mg if 51–75 kg, and 20 mg if ≥76 kg
Midazolam (Versed, Nayzilam)	5 mg	Intranasal kit	≥12 years = 5 mg intranasal and may repeat for 10 mg total

These are pre-dosed by the prescribing physician so can be utilized for seizure over 5 minutes or clusters of seizures over 5 minutes without return to baseline.

Table 3.
Available antiseizure medications for seizure first aid with bystanders.

swimming with only 1:1 adult supervision, avoiding baths while unattended, not climbing heights which are not enclosed, refraining from using hot objects, power tools, or other objects which may result in injury during a seizure, and generally considering the safety of an activity with the occurrence of a typical seizure [68].

Activities generally considered safe for children with epilepsy are sports without heavy contact, standing water, or heights. Photosensitive epilepsy can be ruled out by exposing the patient to various flash frequencies (1, 3, 6, 9, 12, 15, 20, and 30 Hz) while hooked to EEG. Children with epilepsy should be given autonomy to select safe activities with their peers to improve their quality of life [68–70].

4. Conclusions

For the primary care physician and other subspecialists providing care to patients with seizures, identification of epilepsy requires assessment of the complete history including number of suspected seizures that the patient has previously experienced along with the semiology of those events. If the patient has had two or more events consistent with epileptic seizures which are separated by time, the risk of recurrence is high enough to diagnose with epilepsy undetermined as to generalized or focal onset and start seizure medications, generally with broad spectrum agents as the first choice if the onset of seizures is unclear. Workup following a first-time unprovoked seizure includes an EEG and MRI of the brain with additional electrographic data or lesions contributing to the diagnosis of epilepsy after a single seizure. Drug resistant epilepsy (DRE) is diagnosed with failure of two appropriate antiseizure medications at therapeutic trials for efficacy. Patients with DRE are unlikely to achieve seizure freedom with antiseizure medications alone so should be referred to an epilepsy center for presurgical evaluation while additional medical management and the ketogenic diet can be considered. Seizure precautions and first aid education should be provided to all families with children who are diagnosed with epilepsy and for children with even one seizure to reduce risk of injuries with subsequent seizures. Rescue medication can be provided after a first unprovoked seizure in anticipation of the possibility of additional seizures.

Acknowledgements

This chapter was written without funding.

Conflict of interest

There are no conflicts of interest.

Thanks

I would like to thank my wife, Trisha Miller, who always supports me through my work and is the best spouse I could fathom. I would also like to thank all of my mentors at the Indiana University School of Medicine and Graduate Medical Education for my training and for preparing me to write this chapter.

DOI: http://dx.doi.org/10.5772/intechopen.1005271

Author details

Derryl Miller
Riley Hospital Dr., Indiana University School of Medicine, Indianapolis, IN, USA

*Address all correspondence to: miller89@iupui.edu

References

[1] Fisher RS, Acevedo C, Arzimanoglou A, Bogacz A, Cross H, Elger CE, et al. A practical clinical definition of epilepsy. Epilepsia. 2014;**55**(4):475-482. DOI: 10.1111/epi.12550

[2] Shankar R, Donner EJ, McLean B, Nashef L, Tomson T. Sudden unexpected death in epilepsy (SUDEP): What every neurologist should know. Epileptic Disorders. 2017;**19**(1):1-9. DOI: 10.1684/epd.2017.0891

[3] Maguire M, Jackson C, Marson A, Nevitt S. Treatments to prevent sudden unexplained death in epilepsy (SUDEP). The Cochrane Database of Systematic Reviews. 2020;**4**:CD011792. DOI: 10.1002/14651858.CD011792.pub3

[4] Kwan P, Arzimanoglou A, Berg AT, Brodie MJ, Hauser WA, Mathern G, et al. Definition of drug resistant epilepsy: Consensus proposal by the ad hoc task force of the ILAE commission on therapeutic strategies. Epilepsia. 2010;**51**(6):1069-1077. DOI: 10.1111/j.1528-1167.2009.02397.x

[5] Chen Z, Brodie MJ, Liew D, Kwan P. Treatment outcomes in patients with newly diagnosed epilepsy treated with established and new antiepileptic drugs: A 30-year longitudinal cohort study. JAMA Neurology. 2018;**75**(3):279-286. Erratum in: JAMA Neurol. 2018;75(3):384. DOI: 10.1001/jamaneurol.2017.3949

[6] Jehi L, Jette N, Kwon CS, Josephson CB, Burneo JG, Cendes F, et al. Timing of referral to evaluate for epilepsy surgery: Expert consensus recommendations from the surgical therapies commission of the international league against epilepsy. Epilepsia. 2022;**63**(10):2491-2506. DOI: 10.1111/epi.17350

[7] Fisher RS, Cross JH, French JA, Higurashi N, Hirsch E, Jansen FE, et al. Operational classification of seizure types by the international league against epilepsy: Position paper of the ILAE Commission for Classification and Terminology. Epilepsia. 2017;**58**(4):522-530. DOI: 10.1111/epi.13670

[8] Ighodaro ET, Maini K, Arya K, Sharma S. Focal Onet Seizure. In: Statpearls. Treasure Island (FL): StatPearls Publishing; 2024. Available from: https://www.ncbi.nlm.nih.gov/books/NBK500005/

[9] Devinsky O, Kelley K, Porter RJ, Theodore WH. Clinical and electroencephalographic features of simple partial seizures. Neurology. 1988;**38**(9):1347-1352. DOI: 10.1212/wnl.38.9.1347

[10] Bhattacharyya KB. James Wenceslaus Papez, his circuit, and emotion. Annals of Indian Academy of Neurology. 2017;**20**(3):207-210. DOI: 10.4103/aian.AIAN_487_16

[11] Kumar A, Sharma S. Focal Impaired Awareness Seizure. Treasure Island, FL: StatPearls Publishing; 2024. Available from: https://www.ncbi.nlm.nih.gov/books/NBK519030/

[12] Misra UK, Kalita J. Management of provoked seizure. Annals of Indian Academy of Neurology. 2011;**14**(1):2-8. DOI: 10.4103/0972-2327.78041

[13] Berg AT. Are febrile seizures provoked by a rapid rise in temperature? American Journal of Diseases of Children. 1993;**147**(10):1101-1103. DOI: 10.1001/archpedi.1993.02160340087020

[14] Gulati S, Kaushik JS. How I treat a first single seizure in a

child. Annals of Indian Academy of Neurology. 2016;**19**(1):29-36. DOI: 10.4103/0972-2327.173404

[15] Patel H, Blake H, Dunn D. Psychogenic nonepileptic seizures in children and adolescents. Indian Pediatrics. 2021;**58**(3):259-265. DOI: 10.1007/s13312-021-2167-9

[16] Seeber M, Cantonas LM, Hoevels M, Sesia T, Visser-Vandewalle V, Michel CM. Subcortical electrophysiological activity is detectable with high-density EEG source imaging. Nature Communications. 2019;**10**(1):753. DOI: 10.1038/s41467-019-08725-w

[17] Miller DJ, Komanapalli H, Dunn DW. Comorbidity of attention deficit hyperactivity disorder in a patient with epilepsy: Staring down the challenge of inattention versus nonconvulsive seizures. Epilepsy & Behavior Reports. 2024;**25**:100651. DOI: 10.1016/j.ebr.2024.100651

[18] Jehi L. The epileptogenic zone: Concept and definition. Epilepsy Currents. 2018;**18**(1):12-16. DOI: 10.5698/1535-7597.18.1.12

[19] Chang YT, Hong SY, Lin WD, Lin CH, Lin SS, Tsai FJ, et al. Genetic testing in children with developmental and epileptic encephalopathies: A review of advances in epilepsy genomics. Children (Basl). 2023;**10**(3):556. DOI: 10.3390/children10030556

[20] Sánchez Fernández I, Loddenkemper T, Gaínza-Lein M, Sheidley BR, Poduri A. Diagnostic yield of genetic tests in epilepsy: A meta-analysis and cost-effectiveness study. Neurology. 2019;**92**(5):e418-e428. DOI: 10.1212/WNL.0000000000006850

[21] Samanta D, Garrity L, Arya R. Refractory and super-refractory status epilepticus. Indian Pediatrics. 2020;**57**(3):239-253. DOI: 10.1007/s13312-020-1759-0

[22] Moeller AA, Stefanescu AR, Stefanescu BM, Golomb MR, Boyle FA, Buss WF, et al. A standardized, 3-tiered, seizure burden-based protocol for the treatment of neonatal seizures. Journal of Child Neurology. 2023;**38**(3-4):142-152. DOI: 10.1177/08830738231164704

[23] Moosa ANV. Antiepileptic drug treatment of epilepsy in children. Continuum (Mineap Minn). 2019;**25**(2 Epilepsy):381-407. DOI: 10.1212/CON.0000000000000712

[24] Mesraoua B, Brigo F, Lattanzi S, Abou-Khalil B, Al Hail H, Asadi-Pooya AA. Drug-resistant epilepsy: Definition, pathophysiology, and management. Journal of the Neurological Sciences. 2023;**452**:120766. DOI: 10.1016/j.jns.2023.120766

[25] Guery D, Rheims S. Clinical management of drug resistant epilepsy: A review on current strategies. Neuropsychiatric Disease and Treatment. 2021;**17**:2229-2242. DOI: 10.2147/NDT.S256699

[26] Baumgartner C, Koren JP, Britto-Arias M, Zoche L, Pirker S. Presurgical epilepsy evaluation and epilepsy surgery. F1000Res. 2019;**8**:F1000 Faculty Rev-1818. DOI: 10.12688/f1000research.17714.1

[27] Makridis KL, Bast T, Prager C, Kovacevic-Preradovic T, Bittigau P, Mayer T, et al. Real-world experience treating pediatric epilepsy patients with cenobamate. Frontiers in Neurology. 2022;**13**:950171. DOI: 10.3389/fneur.2022.950171

[28] Krasowski MD. Therapeutic drug monitoring of the newer anti-epilepsy

medications. Pharmaceuticals (Basel). 2010;**3**(6):1909-1935. DOI: 10.3390/ph30619109

[29] Shi LL, Dong J, Ni H, Geng J, Wu T. Felbamate as an add-on therapy for refractory partial epilepsy. Cochrane Database of Systematic Reviews. 2017;**7**(7):CD008295. DOI: 10.1002/14651858.CD008295.pub4

[30] Li Y, Dong N, Qin YX, Dai HR, Hu YH, Zhao YT, et al. Therapeutic drug monitoring of parampanel in children diagnosed with epilepsy: Focus on influencing factors on the plasma concentration-to-dose-ratio. Epilepsia Open. 2022;**7**(4):737-746. DOI: 10.1002/epi4.12653

[31] Bentué-Ferrer D, Verdier MC, Tribut O. Therapeutic drug monitoring of primidone and phenobarbital. Thérapie. 2012;**67**(4):381-390. French. DOI: 10.2515/therapie/2012036

[32] Singh RK, Singh R, Stewart A, Van Poppel K, Klinger S, Hulihan J, et al. Intravenous ganaxolone in pediatric super-refractory status epilepticus: A single hospital experience. Epilepsy & Behavior Reports. 2022;**20**:100567. DOI: 10.1016/j.ebr.2022.100567

[33] Vaitkevicius H, Ramsay RE, Swisher CB, Husain AM, Aimetti A, Gasior M. Intravenous ganaxolone for the treatment of refractory status epilepticus: Results from an open-label, dose-finding, phase 2 trial. Epilepsia. 2022;**63**(9):2381-2391. DOI: 10.1111/epi.17343

[34] Kanner AM, Ashman E, Gloss D, Harden C, Bourgeois B, Bautista FJ, et al. Practice guideline update summary: Efficacy and tolerability of the new antiepileptic drugs I: Treatment of new-onset epilepsy: Report of the guideline development, dissemination, and implementation Subcommittee of the American Academy of neurology and the American Epilepsy Society. Neurology. 2018;**91**(2):74-81. DOI: 10.1212/WNL.0000000000005755

[35] Gunasekera CL, Sirven JI, Feyissa AM. The evolution of antiseizure medication therapy selection in adults: Is artificial intelligence-assisted antiseizure medication selection ready for prime time? Journal of Central Nervous System Disease. 2023;**15**:1-13. DOI: 10.1177/11795735231209209

[36] Håkansson S, Wickström R, Zelano J. Selection and continuation of antiseizure medication in children with epilepsy in Sweden from 2007 to 2020. Pediatric Neurology. 2023;**144**:19-25. DOI: 10.1016/j.pediatrneurol.2023.03.016

[37] Glauser T, Ben-Menachem E, Bourgeois B, Cnaan A, Chadwick D, Guerreiro C, et al. ILAE treatment guidelines: Evidence-based analysis of antiepileptic drug efficacy and effectiveness as initial monotherapy for epileptic seizures and syndromes. Epilepsia. 2006;**47**(7):1094. DOI: 10.1111/j.1528-1167.2006.00585.x

[38] Arya R, Glauser TA. Pharmacotherapy of focal epilepsy in children: A systemic review of approved agents. CNS Drugs. 2013;**27**(4):273. DOI: 10.1007/s40263-013-0048-z

[39] Park KM, Kim SE, Lee BI. Antiepileptic drug therapy in patients with drug-resistant epilepsy. Journal of Epilepsy Research. 2019;**9**(1):14-26. DOI: 10.14581/jer.19002

[40] D'Andrea MI, Romão TT, Pires do Prado HJ, Krüger LT, MEP P, da Conceição PO. Ketogenic diet and epilepsy: What we know so far. Frontiers in Neuroscience. 2019;**13**:5. DOI: 10.3389/fnins.2019.00005

[41] Miller JW, Hakimian S. Surgical treatment of epilepsy. Continuum (Minneap Minn). 2013;**19**(3 Epilepsy):730-742. DOI: 10.1212/01.CON.0000431398.69594.97

[42] Hwang JK, Kim DS. From resection to disconnection for seizure control in pediatric epilepsy children. Journal of Korean Neurosurgical Association. 2019;**62**(3):336-343. DOI: 10.3340/jkns.2019.0031

[43] Ryvlin P, Rheims S, Hirsch LJ, Sokolov A, Jehi L. Neuromodulation in epilepsy: State-of-the-art approved therapies. Lancet Neurology. 2021;**20**(12):1038-1047. DOI: 10.1016/S1474-4422(21)00300-8. Erratum in: Lancet Neurol. 2021;20(12):e7

[44] Scheffer IE, Berkovic S, Capovilla G, Connolly MB, French J, Guilhoto L, et al. ILAE classification of the epilepsies: Position paper of the ILAE Commission for classification and terminology. Epilepsia. 2017;**58**(4):512-521. DOI: 10.1111/epi.13709

[45] Wirrell E, Tinuper P, Perucca E, Moshé SL. Introduction to the epilepsy syndrome papers. Epilepsia. 2022;**63**(6):1330-1332. DOI: 10.1111/epi.17262

[46] Zuberi SM, Wirrell E, Yozawitz E, Wilmshurst JM, Speccio N, Riney K, et al. ILAE classification and definition of epilepsy syndromes with onset in neonates and infants: Position statement by the ILAE task force on nosology and definitions. Epilepsia. 2022;**63**(6):1349-1397. DOI: 10.1111/epi.17239

[47] Speccio N, Wirrell EC, Scheffer IE, Nabbout R, Riney K, Samia P, et al. International league against epilepsy classification and definition of epilepsy syndromes with onset in childhood: Position paper by the ILAE task force on nosology and definitions. Epilepsia. 2022;**63**(6):1398-1442. DOI: 10.1111/epi.17241

[48] Riney K, Bogacz A, Somerville E, Hirsch E, Nabbout R, Scheffer IE, et al. International league against epilepsy classification and definition of epilepsy syndromes with onset at a variable age: Position statement by the ILAE task force on nosology and definitions. Epilepsia. 2022;**63**(6):1443-1474. DOI: 10.1111/epi.17240

[49] Hirsch E, French J, Scheffer IE, Bogacz A, Alsaadi T, Sperling MR, et al. ILAE definition of the idiopathic generalized epilepsy syndromes: Position statement by the ILAE task force on nosology and definitions. Epilepsia. 2022;**63**(6):1475-1499. DOI: 10.1111/epi.17236

[50] Nelson GR. Management of infantile spasms. Translational Pediatrics. 2015;**4**(4):260-270. DOI: 10.3978/j.issn.2224-4336.2015.09.01

[51] Go CY, Mackay MT, Weiss SK, Stephens D, Adams-Webber T, Ashwal S, et al. Child neurology society, American Academy of Neurology. Evidence-based guideline update: Medical treatment of infantile spasms. Report of the guideline development Subcommittee of the American Academy of neurology and the practice Committee of the Child Neurology Society. Neurology. 2012;**78**(24):1974-1980. DOI: 10.1212/WNL.0b013e318259e2cf

[52] Miller D, Felker M, Ciccarelli M. Transitioning ambulatory medicine from pediatrics to adult care for patients with epilepsy and intellectual disability. Journal of Pediatric Epilepsy. 2020;**9**(4):172-176. DOI: 10.1055/s-0040-1717135

[53] de Laat NN, Tolboom N, Leijten FSS. Optimal timing of interictal FDG-PET

for epilepsy surgery: A systemic review on time since last seizure. Epilepsia. 2022;7(3):512-517. DOI: 10.1002/epi4.12617

[54] Lee WW, K-SPECT Group. Clinical applications of technetium-99m quantitative single-photon emission computed tomography/computed tomography. Nuclear Medicine and Molecular Imaging. 2019;**53**(3):172-181. DOI: 10.1007/s13139-019-00588-9

[55] Yassin A, El-Salem K, Al-Mistarehi AH, Momani A, Zein Alaabdin AM, Shah P, et al. Use of innovative SPECT techniques in the presurgical evaluation of patients with nonlesional extratemporal drug-resistant epilepsy. Molecular Imaging. 2021;**2021**:6614356. DOI: 10.1155/2021/6614356

[56] Singh SP. Magnetoencephalography: Basic principles. Annals of Indian Academy of Neurology. 2014;**17**(Suppl. 1):S107-S112. DOI: 10.4103/0972-2327.128676

[57] Somers M, Negers SF, Diederen KM, Boks MP, Kahn RS, Sommer IE. The measurement of language lateralization with functional transcranial Doppler and functional MRI: A critical evaluation. Frontiers in Human Neuroscience. 2011;**5**:31. DOI: 10.3389/fnhum.2011.00031

[58] Pritchard VE, Malone SA, Burgoyne K, Heron-Delaney M, Bishop DVM, Hulme C. Stage 1 registered report: The relationship between handedness and language ability in children. Wellcome Open Research. 2019;**4**:30. DOI: 10.12688/wellcomeopenres.15077.1

[59] Rolinski R, You X, Gonzalez-Castillo J, Norato G, Reynolds RC, Inati SK, et al. Language lateralization from task-based and resting state functional MRI in patients with epilepsy. Human Brain Mapping. 2020;**41**(11):3133-3146. DOI: 10.1002/hbm.25003

[60] Simpson HD, Schulze-Bonhage A, Cascino GD, Fisher RS, Jobst BC, Sperling MR, et al. Practical considerations in epilepsy neurostimulation. Epilepsia. 2022;**63**(10):2445-2460. DOI: 10.1111/epi.17329

[61] Ryvlin P, So EL, Gordon CM, Hesdorffer DC, Sperling MR, Devinsky O, et al. Long-term surveillance of SUDEP in drug-resistant epilepsy patients treated with VNS therapy. Epilepsia. 2018;**59**(3):562-572. DOI: 10.1111/epi.14002

[62] Fisher R, Salanova V, Witt T, Worth R, Henry T, Gross R, et al. Electrical stimulation of the anterior nucleus of thalamus for treatment of refractory epilepsy. Epilepsia. 2010;**51**(5):899-908. DOI: 10.1111/j.1528-1167.2010.02536.x

[63] Salanova V, Sperling MR, Gross RE, Irwin CP, Vollhaber JA, Giftakis JE, et al. The SANTÉ study at 10 years of follow-up: Effectiveness, safety, and sudden unexpected death in epilepsy. Epilepsia. 2021;**62**(6):1306-1317. DOI: 10.1111/epi.16895

[64] Bergey GK, Morrell MJ, Mizahi EM, Goldman A, King-Stephens D, Nair D, et al. Long-term treatment with responsive brain stimulation in adults with refractory and partial seizures. Neurology. 2015;**84**(8):810-817. DOI: 10.1212/WNL.0000000000001280

[65] Luat AF, Asano E, Kumar A, Chugani HT, Sood S. Corpus Callosotomy for intractable epilepsy revisited: The Children's Hospital of Michigan Series. Journal of Child

Neurology. 2017;**32**(7):624-629. DOI: 10.1177/0883073817697847

[66] Truong VT, Tayah T, Bouthillier A, Nguyen DK. Anterior corpus callosotomy in multistep invasive monitoring and surgery for atonic seizures. Epilepsy & Behavior Case Reports. 2014;**2**:11-14. DOI: 10.1016/j.ebcr.2013.12.003

[67] Feldstein TJ. Carbohydrate and alcohol content of 200 oral liquid medications for use in patients receiving ketogenic diets. Pediatrics. 1996;**97**(4):506-511. DOI: 10.1542/peds.97.4.506

[68] Nguyen R, Téllez Zenteno JF. Injuries in epilepsy: A review of its prevalence, risk factors, type of injuries and prevention. Neurology International. 2009;**1**(1):e20. DOI: 10.4081/ni.2009.e20

[69] ILAE Commission Report. Restrictions for children with epilepsy. Commission of Pediatrics of the ILAE. International league against epilepsy. Epilepsia. 1997;**38**(9):1054-1056. DOI: 10.1111/j.1528-1157.1997.tb01493.x

[70] Rank WP. Seizure first aid for bystanders. Nursing. 2020;**50**(10):11-12. DOI: 10.1097/01.NURSE.0000697196.36554.fe

Chapter 3

Cerebral Palsy

Asiya Uzun

Abstract

Cerebral palsy is one of the most common neurodevelopmental and musculoskeletal problems in the world. Two or four out of 1000 births each year are born with this disease. Cerebral palsy, with its various etiologies impacting different areas of the brain, adds to a broad spectrum of clinical findings that may result in secondary problems like hip pain or dislocation, balance issues, hand dysfunction, joint deformities, and social challenges. Children with cerebral palsy have difficulties in providing trunk postural control and balance, which is critical for independence in daily living activities. Treatment requires a multidisciplinary approach, and the aim is for the child to continue daily life and education with maximum independence. With the development of technology, new technological methods are applied in the rehabilitation process and contribute to the improvement of activity and participation.

Keywords: cerebral palsy, childhood disability, rehabilitation, quality of life, education

1. Introduction

Cerebral palsy (CP) is a permanent childhood disease that affects the functionality, participation in social life, and independence of the person from the earliest periods. Health professionals make important contributions to increase the level of participation and independence of children in home, school, and social environments at every stage of their lives. Recent research results have shown that new technological treatment options also have important contributions in this field.

2. Definition

Cerebral palsy is a group of disorders that can be defined as an overarching term. It constitutes a persistent condition, albeit not inherently fixed, marked by deficits in both movement and/or posture as well as motor functionality. It results from a non-progressive response/impairment/abnormality that occurs in the developing/immature brain. These “five essential elements” provide a clear and concise definition of CP and reflect the main features of the definitions to date [1–4]. CP is a physical and developmental disability caused by disorders in the brain before or during birth. CP causes permanent impairments in movement and posture. Described in 1861, ideas and knowledge about CP have evolved over time. In 2006, an international panel reached a consensus definition of CP as a condition associated with non-progressive impairments. CP is a common developmental disorder encountered by many pediatric healthcare providers.

This update reviews current knowledge on the diagnostic methods, prevalence, risk factors, genetic research, and clinical management of CP. These data are evaluated with the aim of providing better healthcare for patients with CP and their families [3–5].

3. Prevalence of cerebral palsy

Epidemiological studies indicate that the prevalence of CP varies between 2 and 4 per 1000 live births. However, it is important to note that the data contain geographical differences and that there are different rates between countries [6, 7]. In a meta-analysis conducted by Oskoui et al., the total prevalence of CP worldwide was reported to be 2.11 per 1000 live births [8]. In a comprehensive study conducted to determine trends and current estimates regarding the regional and global prevalence of CP, 27 countries and 41 regions from five continents were included in the study. The study concluded that the prevalence rate for CP of prenatal and perinatal origin in high-income countries was 1.5 per 1000 live births, and when postneonatal CP was included, this rate was 1.6. In contrast, the prevalence of CP in low- and middle-income countries was reported to be significantly higher at 3.4 per 1000 live births. It has been reported that the prevalence trends in low- and middle-income countries cannot be measured at the moment. However, it is evident that prevalence tends to decrease in high-income countries [9].

4. Etiology

Cerebral palsy is a condition with various etiologies, resulting in a variety of clinical manifestations due to brain damage. CP can occur as a result of risk factors and associated conditions in the prenatal, perinatal, and postnatal periods of the developing brain. Initially, CP was thought to be caused by hypoxia at birth or during the perinatal period. However, in most cases, the initial event of CP cannot be determined. Studies have indicated that the cause of CP is often difficult to determine. In approximately 30% of children with CP, no known etiology or risk factor can be identified. Approximately 75% of cases are associated with a prenatal cause, while perinatal and neonatal risk factors are responsible for 10–18% of cases. However, it is observed that most children with risk factors do not develop CP [10–12].

Risk factors associated with CP include maternal infection, difficult delivery, arterial defects, and asphyxia in the prenatal period, as well as trauma and cerebrovascular events in the postnatal period. Preterm birth is one of the greatest risk factors for the development of CP, with preterm children accounting for approximately 35% of CP cases. A neonate born prior to 28 weeks of gestational age is 50 times more likely to develop CP than a neonate born at term. Multiple births carry a fivefold increased risk of CP compared to single births. Other risk factors for CP include male gender and low socioeconomic status. Previously, genetic factors were thought to have a 1–2% effect on CP. However, recent studies have indicated that genetic factors are involved in approximately 30% of children diagnosed with CP [13–15].

5. Diagnosis

The diagnosis of CP is based on a combination of neurological examinations, neuroimaging findings, and clinical risk factors. Recent advances in technology have enabled earlier and more accurate diagnosis of CP, allowing early diagnosis and initiation of treatments that can improve long-term outcomes. It is noted that early diagnosis allows for the initiation of treatments and can improve long-term outcomes. Population studies indicate that parents generally prefer to find out earlier whether their child has CP or is at high risk for CP. A variety of screening tools and neurological assessments are employed to diagnose CP, with the objective of enabling earlier detection of high-risk children in the neonatal period and closer follow-up. Prior to 5 months of age, neonatal magnetic resonance imaging (MRI) is reported to be among the tools with the best predictive validity for the detection of CP [16, 17]. Consequently, it is imperative to implement more effective measures for early diagnosis and initiate treatments at an earlier stage. Neonatal MRI, Prechtl General Movement Assessment, and Hammersmith Infant Neurological Examination are important tools used for the diagnosis of CP in newborns. A standardized neurological examination and neuroimaging is recommended for CP in newborns. It is recommended to use the label 'high risk for CP' for babies with suspected CP. MRI findings indicating high risk for CP in newborns include white matter damage, damage to deep gray matter structures, cerebellar hemorrhage, and developmental brain malformations [18]. Some children with CP may have normal MRI or ultrasonography results in the neonatal period. In children with normal neuroimaging but persistent neurologic abnormalities, underlying genetic or metabolic causes should be investigated. In patients with CP, imaging is crucial for determining the types and extent of brain damage, as well as for assessing the risk of neurodevelopmental disability [19–21].

The assessment of spontaneous infant movements is a method employed in the diagnosis of motor dysfunctions. The General Movement Assessment (GMA), developed by Heinz Prechtl, is a predictive model used to describe infants' movements. A recent review of the GMA identified two movement patterns that are highly sensitive and specific for the diagnosis of spastic paresis: restricted synchronized general movements, which are characterized by rigid contraction and relaxation of muscles, and the lack of small amplitude fidgety movements that should be present in normal newborns. Other reviews have also reported that assessment with GMA in high-risk neonates provides high sensitivity and specificity in predicting spastic paresis. It is recommended that GMA be performed by providers who have completed standardized training in order to ensure accuracy and reliability [19, 22–24].

6. Early symptoms and classification

Early detection of cerebral palsy in infancy is paramount for initiating timely interventions and improving long-term outcomes. Several key indicators can aid in the recognition of CP during this critical period:

1. Neurobehavioral signs: Suspicious neurobehavioral signs may include excessive irritability, lethargy, poor sleep patterns, frequent vomiting, difficulty in being held or cuddled, and impaired visual attention.

2. Developmental reflexes: Monitoring the disappearance of developmental reflexes is crucial. Delayed or exaggerated disappearance of these reflexes, such as the tonic labyrinth reflex or abnormal response to vertical suspension, can serve as early indicators of motor disability.

3. Motor tone and posture: Evaluation of motor tone and posture provides valuable insights. Observing for poor head control, persistent or asymmetric hand fisting, and abnormal oromotor patterns (e.g., tongue thrusting or facial gestures) can help identify early motor signs. However, it's important to note that elevated neck extensor and axial tone may falsely indicate superior head control.

4. Motor milestones: Regular assessment of motor milestones is recommended by the American Academy of Pediatrics. Conducting developmental screenings at 9, 18, 30, and 48 months enables the early detection of any delays or abnormalities, facilitating prompt intervention and support.

By incorporating these systematic assessments into clinical practice, healthcare professionals can enhance their ability to detect CP in infancy, leading to earlier interventions and improved outcomes for affected children [25].

6.1 Cerebral palsy surveillance group of Europe (SCPE) classification system

The SCPE classification system is currently the most widely used classification system for the classification of CP. It classifies children with CP according to their clinical characteristics as follows:

a. Spastic type (unilateral or bilateral)

b. Dyskinetic type (dystonic, chorea-athetoid)

c. Ataxic

d. Unclassifiable (Mix)

A recent study by Himmelmann et al. reported that 40% of children with cerebral palsy exhibited unilateral spasticity (hemiparetic), 39% exhibited bilateral spasticity (diparetic and quadriparetic), 16% exhibited dyskinetic features, and 5% exhibited ataxic features [26–28]. It is not uncommon for one type of CP to exhibit features belonging to other types. In such cases, classification is based on the dominant feature. The "Classification Tree," created by the SCPE, facilitates the process of classification, making it more straightforward and accurate [26]. Although hypotonic CP has been previously defined, it is not included in contemporary classifications. The evolution of CP from hypotonia in early infancy to other subtypes such as spastic, dyskinetic, or ataxic CP is a common phenomenon. However, it's important to recognize that not all children follow this typical progression. In some cases, children may continue to exhibit hypotonia due to specific involvement of cerebro-cerebellar or extrapyramidal circuits. These circuits play crucial roles in motor control and coordination, and their impairment can result in persistent hypotonia.

6.1.1 Spastic cerebral palsy

Patients with spastic cerebral palsy present with upper motor neurone findings, including spasticity, hyperreflexia (with or without clonus), and an extensor plantar response [27–29]. Children with CP may exhibit various spastic syndromes, including spastic diplegia, characterized by gross motor problems primarily affecting the lower limbs but with preserved fine motor function in the upper limbs, often associated with periventricular leukomalacia and periventricular hemorrhagic infarction; spastic quadriplegia, presenting severe motor impairments affecting both upper and lower limbs equally, with minimal speech and language development, visual impairment, epilepsy, and feeding difficulties, often accompanied by multicystic encephalomalacia on magnetic resonance imaging; and spastic hemiplegia, featuring asymmetric motor impairment with the arm more affected than the leg, sometimes accompanied by athetotic posture, and commonly associated with sensory deficits reflected as poor muscle mass on the affected side without motor deficits [29].

In addition, mental impairment, hemianopia, and other visual problems may also be observed. Furthermore, behavioral problems including anxiety, defiance, and specific phobias are common among children with hemiplegic CP.

6.1.2 Dyskinetic syndromes

Dyskinetic CP can be further subclassified as choreo-athetoid and dystonic. Choreo-athetoid CP is characterized by rapid, irregular, unpredictable contractions of individual muscles/muscle groups, involving the face, bulbar muscles, proximal extremities, and fingers. In addition, there are slow writhing movements involving the distal muscles. Oropharyngeal difficulties may result from grimacing. Primitive reflexes usually persist into childhood. Dystonic CP is characterized by the simultaneous contraction of agonist and antagonist muscles. Pyramidal findings and dysarthria are frequently observed in conjunction with one another.

6.1.3 Ataxic CP

Ataxic CP represents a relatively infrequent manifestation necessitating careful differentiation from progressive neurodegenerative conditions. Delayed attainment of motor and language milestones commonly characterizes its clinical presentation. Notably, the ataxic symptoms tend to ameliorate with time, emphasizing the dynamic nature of this subtype within the spectrum of CP [29, 30].

7. Classification by functional ability

In addition to the SCPE classification method, functional classification systems are another classification method currently used for children with CP. These classification systems have been developed to provide information about the functional status of children with CP, to categorize the level of independence of children in different areas, to provide a holistic view, and to provide a common language within multidisciplinary and interdisciplinary study models. They make the classification using a simple ordinal scale. They classify Gross Motor Function Classification System (GMFCS), Manual Ability Classification System (MACS), Communication Function Classification System (CFCS), Eating and Drinking Function Classification System (EDACS), Visual Function Classification System (VFCS), and Speech Function System (VSS).

Of these classification systems, GMFCS, MACS, CFCS, EDACS, and VFCS consist of five levels, while VSS consists of four levels. However, all classification systems categorize functions with a similar logic. Level 1 refers to the level at which children are most functionally independent [31].

7.1 Gross motor function classification system

The GMFCS is a measure used to classify the gross motor function of people with cerebral palsy. This simple and sequential grading system provides a common language used in conjunction with the GMFCS. The GMFCS describes the mobility of the individual and the assistive devices used for mobility (walkers, crutches, canes, wheelchairs). This classification system is used to distinguish clinically significant differences in the assessment of motor function in children with CP. The GMFCS was originally designed for children aged 2–12 years but was later extended to the age range 12–18 years, making the levels more detailed. This revision allows age-appropriate classifications to be made, taking into account developmental milestones [32–34].

7.2 Manual ability classification system

In 2006, Eliasson et al. introduced the Manual Ability Classification System (MACS) as a counterpart to the Gross Motor Function Classification System (GMFCS), focusing specifically on upper extremity function. This simple ordinal classification system consists of five points and is tailored for children aged 4–18 years. The MACS serves as a validated tool for categorizing a child's habitual use of their hands and upper limbs in cases of cerebral palsy [28, 35].

7.3 Communication function classification system

The CFCS is a communication classification system developed by Hidecker et al. in 2011. This system is designed to assess the daily communication of people with cerebral palsy. It is estimated that 31–88% of people with CP have a comorbid communication disorder [36]. The CFCS is a five-point rating system and is designed to be compatible with other classification systems such as the GMFCS and MACS. The CFCS is a system that assesses both how information is expressed and how it is received. It covers all methods of communication and is suitable for people who cannot express themselves. The CFCS assesses a variety of communication methods including voice, manual signs, eye gaze, pictures, communication boards, and voice generating devices. The CFCS also considers both familiar and unfamiliar communication partners. In this way, the CFCS provides a comprehensive and descriptive assessment of communication [37].

7.4 Eating and drinking ability classification system

The Eating and Drinking Ability Classification System has been developed as a valid measure to assess the eating and drinking ability of children with cerebral palsy. People with CP are thought to have difficulties with eating and drinking. In 2014, Sellers et al. devised the EDACS, aimed at evaluating the nutritional skills of children diagnosed with cerebral palsy aged 3 years and older. The system assesses the safety and efficiency of eating and drinking. There is also an additional three-point ordinal scale to determine the level of assistance required: independent, requiring assistance, or dependent for eating. EDACS is similar and supplementary to the GMFCS, MACS, and CFCS. This classification system provides a comprehensive assessment of the eating and drinking needs of people with CP [38, 39].

8. Problems seen in cerebral palsy

The problems seen in cerebral palsy are quite complex, and different pictures can occur.

8.1 Range of motion problems

Although spasticity is a common finding in people with cerebral palsy, most people with CP have limb deformities and limited range of motion rather than spasticity. It is generally accepted that such movement limitations are caused by secondary changes in the muscles and soft tissues. In these patients, the limited range of motion, known as contracture, is treated by splinting, botulinum toxin type A injections, surgical lengthening of the spastic muscles, or tenotomy [40].

8.2 Muscle tone problems

Cerebral palsy is usually associated with developmental delay and muscle tone problems such as hypotonia, dystonia, and spasticity. The peripheral and central nervous systems produce muscle tone by reflex mechanisms. In hypotonia, the mechanism of muscle contraction is slower. It is characterized by a decrease in muscle tone, stretch reflexes, and primitive reflex patterns. Hypotonia can often be seen as a transitional stage to spasticity. The most prominent feature of these individuals is joint hypermobility. Motor problems in these individuals are usually characterized by inadequate head and trunk control, balance, and corrective and protective responses. In dystonia, involuntary muscle contractions are repeated continuously or intermittently, resulting in hypertonic movements and prolonged muscle contractions. This leads to abnormal posture in the proximal parts of the extremities, trunk and neck. Spasticity, another muscle problem, is known to be the main cause of CP in children. When a muscle is stretched, the neuromuscular system can respond automatically by changing muscle tone. This modulation of the stretch reflex is important for controlling movement and maintaining balance. Lance et al. defined spasticity as "a speed-dependent increase in the stretch reflex." Prolonged spasticity can lead to changes in anatomical structures, such as bone dislocation or transformation of muscle into fibrous tissue. Ineffective management of spasticity can lead to severe immobilization in addition to these detrimental effects [41–44].

Spasticity stands out as the predominant issue in cerebral palsy, demonstrating a tendency to affect the entirety of the body. Nonetheless, it typically exhibits heightened severity in the lower limbs among individuals with bilateral involvement, while in those with unilateral impairment, it is more prominently observed in the upper limbs. In children with CP, the gastrocsoleus, hamstrings, rectus femoris, adductors, and psoas muscles are usually affected in the lower limbs, while in the upper limbs, spasticity is seen in the shoulder external rotators, elbow, wrist and finger flexors, and elbow pronators. Spasticity impairs voluntary control, increases energy expenditure, and contributes to the development of secondary muscle and soft tissue contractures and skeletal deformities by preventing normal muscle stretching. Muscle contractures and skeletal deformities can lead to abnormal joint moments during gait [45–50].

8.3 Selectivity

People with cerebral palsy often experience problems such as reduced muscle strength, increased muscle tone/spasticity, and loss of motor control. Selectivity is a very important aspect of human movement and provides independent control of joint movement. Loss of selectivity can be described as "impaired isolated muscle activation during movement." Impaired selectivity is the inability to activate certain muscles without simultaneously activating other muscles. This can lead to a lack or excess of muscle activity and an inability to perform expected movements. Although impaired selectivity is associated with significant loss of function, the possible causes are not fully understood. However, it is thought that mirror movements occur due to bilateral cortical activation resulting from preserved ipsilateral corticospinal projections or insufficient interhemispheric inhibition. Impaired selectivity may interfere with isolated joint movements of flexor or extensor synergies, which may adversely affect functional movements such as walking and reaching. It is not clear which method is the most effective in treating selectivity [51–53].

8.4 Trunk stability and movement problems

One of the most important factors affecting the independence and quality of life of people with cerebral palsy is trunk control. Trunk control can be defined as the ability of the trunk muscles to maintain static and dynamic balance and to keep the body upright. In people with cerebral palsy, problems such as increased kyphosis, lumbar lordosis, and scoliosis can be seen with reduced head and trunk control. It has been reported that people with cerebral palsy increase their head and trunk movements during walking compared to their healthy peers, which may be due to reduced trunk stability. At the same time, trunk control is very important in situations that require upper and lower extremity activity, such as walking. Impaired trunk control may lead to increased trunk mobility during walking. In addition, trunk mobility may increase during upper extremity movements. Although there are studies reporting that poor upper extremity function limits postural control, it has been reported that there are many studies investigating upper extremity function in people with CP but a limited number of studies investigating the relationship between upper extremity function and trunk control. Therefore, the relationship between trunk control and upper extremity remains unclear [54–57].

8.5 Problems with functional independence

Causes such as spasticity, selectivity and sensory problems, muscle weakness, and secondary musculoskeletal problems negatively affect the level of functional independence of people with CP. Dressing, bathing, mobility, and bladder/bowel problems are reported to reduce the independence of people with cerebral palsy [58]. Therefore, it is also important to investigate the effect of a method used in people with CP on quality of life and functional independence.

8.6 Quality of life problems

Quality of life is a broad and multidimensional concept that encompasses the assessment of all positive and negative aspects of life. The World Health Organization defines quality of life as "an individual's expectations, goals, standards, concerns and perceptions of his or her position in life within the culture and value system in which he or she lives" [59, 60].

Given the diversity of problems associated with cerebral palsy, it is not surprising that these problems have a profound impact on the physical, social, and emotional health and well-being of people with CP and their parents. Children with cerebral palsy are four times more likely than their peers to experience physical problems such as muscle weakness and spasticity, as well as emotional and behavioral problems. Therefore, quality of life is very important as it is a subjective indicator of the well-being of children with CP in their life domains. The individual's well-being and functioning in daily life is becoming an important part of clinical assessment and can help determine the individual's quality of life and help health professionals decide how best to plan appropriate and individualized care interventions [61, 62].

9. Innovative therapeutic techniques and technologies

Technological advances have had a significant impact on the field of pediatric physiotherapy, providing new ways to improve outcomes for children with CP and other motor and movement disorders. Innovative techniques and technologies are being integrated into clinical practice to improve established techniques and provide more effective interventions. Innovative techniques in the context of physiotherapy refer to new and advanced methods used by practitioners to assess, treat, and rehabilitate patients with CP. These techniques frequently entail creative and tailored approaches that may encompass a spectrum of manual therapies, exercise regimens, and movement retraining strategies designed to address specific impairments and optimize functional outcomes for individuals with CP. Innovative technologies pertain to the utilization of cutting-edge tools, equipment, and digital resources to enhance the assessment, intervention, and monitoring of individuals with CP. These technologies encompass a vast array of wearable sensors, virtual reality systems, and assistive robots. The utilization of contemporary technology enables physiotherapists to provide more precise and personalized care, which in turn leads to enhanced outcomes for individuals with CP [63].

9.1 Virtual reality rehabilitation

Virtual reality (VR) is a technology that creates immersive, computer-generated environments that users can interact with. In the context of rehabilitation, VR provides a controlled and customizable environment for individuals to participate in therapeutic exercises. This technology allows the creation of virtual scenarios that mimic real-world situations or specific tasks related to the individual's rehabilitation goals [64]. The utilization of virtual reality in sensorimotor training entails the design of exercises and activities that necessitate the integration of sensory and motor skills within a virtual environment. For instance, a patient with cerebral palsy may utilize VR simulations to perform tasks involving reaching, grasping, balance, or gait training [65]. One of the principal advantages of VR-based training is the capacity to provide immediate and accurate feedback to the user. The virtual environment monitors the user's movements in real time, allowing for accurate assessment and adjustment of performance. This feedback loop helps people with CP to develop their motor skills and improve their coordination. Furthermore, VR can create a motivating and engaging therapy experience. The immersive nature of the technology can increase patient focus and engagement, which is particularly important for maintaining interest and adherence to rehabilitation programs over time. Furthermore, VR enables the creation of exercises that are tailored to the specific needs and abilities of the individual. Therapists can adjust parameters such as the level of difficulty, speed, and complexity of tasks to align with the patient's current skill level, with gradual progression as their abilities improve [66]. Research studies have demonstrated the efficacy of VR-based training for individuals with CP. Improvements have been observed in areas such as balance, coordination, muscle strength, and functional mobility [67].

9.2 Robot-assisted therapy

Robotic therapy is a form of rehabilitation that employs specialized robotic devices. These devices are designed to support and enhance the rehabilitation process. They are equipped with sensors and advanced control systems, which allow them to interact with patients in a controlled and precise manner. Robotic therapy for children with cerebral palsy can target different aspects of motor function, including mobility, muscle strength, coordination, and range of movement. Therapy sessions are typically supervised by trained healthcare professionals, such as physiotherapists, who work with the robot to guide and monitor the child's progress. One of the main advantages of robotic therapy is its ability to provide repetitive and consistent movements. The robot can repeat precise movements, which is essential to promote neuroplasticity, especially in individuals with neurological disorders such as CP. Furthermore, robotic therapy offers a level of customization that allows therapists to tailor treatment to the specific needs of each child. Therapy parameters such as the range of motion, resistance levels, and speed of movement can be adjusted to suit the child's current abilities and gradually increased as they develop [68]. The robotic devices used in therapy are equipped with sensors that provide real-time feedback on the child's performance. This immediate feedback enables therapists to monitor progress and implement necessary adjustments to optimize therapy sessions. Furthermore, it allows for objective measurement of improvements in motor skills over time. Additionally, robot-assisted therapy can be engaging and motivating for children. Interaction with the robot often resembles a game or play, which can enhance the child's willingness to participate in therapy and maintain interest and enthusiasm throughout the sessions [69]. A number of research studies have demonstrated the efficacy of robot-assisted therapy for children with cerebral palsy. These studies have indicated that robot-assisted therapy can improve muscle strength, motor control, functional mobility, and overall quality of life [70, 71].

9.3 Neuromuscular electrical stimulation

Another innovative technique employed in aediatric physical therapy is neuromuscular electrical stimulation (NMES). NMES involves the application of electrical impulses to specific muscles, which promotes muscle activation and strengthening. This technique may be particularly useful for children with cerebral palsy who may have difficulties with muscle recruitment and strength development. Yiğitoğlu and Kozanoğlu [72] conducted a prospective, randomized clinical trial to investigate the efficacy of electrical stimulation following botulinum toxin administration in children with spastic diplegic CP. The study randomly assigned participants to different treatment groups and evaluated the effect of combining electrical stimulation with botulinum toxin therapy on children with spastic diplegic CP. The findings of the study indicate that the addition of electrical stimulation when used in combination with botulinum toxin may have positive effects on motor function and general well-being of children with spastic diplegic CP. The authors therefore recommend further research in this area to confirm and extend these promising results [72].

9.4 Wearable sensors for movement analysis

A systematic review by Rozin Kleiner et al. [73] conducted a comprehensive evaluation of the feasibility and effectiveness of using wearable sensors to assess gait in people with CP in real-world, everyday settings. The researchers focused on the use of wearable sensors, which included a variety of devices that could collect data related to movement, posture, and other relevant parameters. These sensors were used to monitor gait patterns and assess motor functions in people with CP. The systematic review examines existing studies to assess the practicality and validity of the use of wearable sensors in everyday settings. This includes activities and environments encountered in everyday life rather than just controlled clinical or laboratory conditions. The review explores the potential benefits of wearable sensor technology, including its ability to provide continuous, objective, and ecologically valid data on gait performance. The authors discuss the relevance of such data for optimizing intervention strategies and monitoring progress in people with CP. However, the paper also addresses the challenges and limitations associated with the use of wearable sensors in real-world scenarios. Factors such as sensor placement, data processing, and participant compliance are considered [73].

9.5 Neurofeedback training

This is a training program that applies neurofeedback technology to children with CP. Neurofeedback provides real-time feedback on brain activity using the latest neuroimaging technology. This approach can be used to train specific brain functions related to motor control in children with CP. Previous research on brain-computer interface-based neurofeedback training demonstrated its effectiveness in improving motor outcomes and supported previous findings suggesting its potential to enhance neuroplasticity in adults recovering from stroke [74]. In recent times, associative learning paradigms have gained prominence and are recognized as particularly feasible and effective methods for neurorehabilitation. However, it is important to note that there is a notable lack of research focusing on children with CP. This highlights the urgent need for more studies in the field of pediatric neurorehabilitation, not only to improve methods and dosages but also to compare them with other evidence-based educational strategies.

9.6 Three-dimensional printing for customized orthotics

Previous research has investigated the use of three-dimensional (3D) printing technology to create customized orthodontic appliances to meet the specific needs of children with cerebral palsy [75]. These devices provide a more accurate fit and improved support. A study to develop and evaluate a customized 3D-printed dynamic upper limb orthosis for children with CP and severe hand impairment involved five participants with CP and unilateral upper limb involvement. The intervention involved the use of the customized orthosis in combination with occupational therapy sessions. The results demonstrated improvements in several assessments of upper limb function. The study concluded that the 3D-printed orthosis, when used in combination with occupational therapy, has the potential to improve upper limb function in children with severe hand impairment.

9.7 Telehealth and remote monitoring

Telehealth and remote monitoring can be employed in the physiotherapy of children with cerebral palsy using digital communication technologies and specialized equipment. This enables healthcare professionals to assess, monitor, and guide therapy sessions remotely. Video conferencing allows therapists to observe the child's movements, give instructions and provide real-time feedback on exercises. In addition, wearable sensors and smart devices can track the child's progress and provide valuable data for customized treatment plans. These technologies enhance accessibility, comfort, and continuity of care for children with CP, facilitating more effective and personalized rehabilitation interventions. A previous study examined the utilization of telemedicine in the management of children with CP, an application that demonstrated promise prior to 2020 but has received significant attention due to the COVID-19 pandemic [76]. A scoping review of the literature was conducted by systematically searching MEDLINE and PubMed in July 2021. The inclusion criteria were as follows: Primary research and systematic reviews focusing on telehealth interventions for children with CP, studies published between 2010 and 2021, and articles written in English. Some evidence suggested that the need for telehealth may vary depending on the child's developmental stage and functional level. Although there is mixed evidence on children's adherence to telehealth, telehealth has been reported to reduce carer burden. In general, telehealth interventions for the management of children with CP have demonstrated favorable outcomes, with comparable or improved outcomes compared to traditional face-to-face care.

9.8 Biofeedback systems

Biofeedback systems can be employed as an effective method of physical therapy for children with CP. These systems utilize electronic or computerized tools to provide real-time information about physiological processes such as muscle activity or body movements. In CP, biofeedback can be utilized to enhance motor control and coordination. One method of utilizing biofeedback is to incorporate electromyography sensors. These sensors measure muscle activity and allow therapists to provide the child with immediate feedback on muscle interaction patterns. This information assists the child in learning how to activate specific muscles more effectively, thereby enhancing their capacity to perform tasks [77].

9.9 Transcranial direct current stimulation

Transcranial direct current stimulation (tDCS) represents a non-invasive method of brain stimulation whereby a mild electrical current is applied to the scalp, seeking to regulate neuronal activity. This is done using a direct current stimulator, which produces a small electrical current. Two electrodes are used for stimulation: an anode (positive electrode) and a cathode (negative electrode). The anode is placed over the target area of the brain, while the cathode is placed elsewhere, usually on the opposite side of the head. The specific arrangement of the electrodes, known as the montage, depends on the desired outcome, as different montages can target different areas of the brain and have different effects on neuronal activity. The intensity of the current is typically between 1 and 2 mA, and the duration of stimulation can vary from a few minutes to an hour. Safety precautions are very important with tDCS, including avoiding contact with metal objects during stimulation and monitoring for any discomfort or skin irritation. Research studies often include a control group that receives a sham stimulation condition to account for placebo effects. After tDCS sessions, researchers assess effects on various outcome measures, such as changes in motor function or cognitive ability, depending on the aims of the study [78, 79].

10. Daily activities and participation in social life

The severity of motor impairment, sensory involvement, and cognitive and behavioral problems among children with CP is different for each child. Consequently, activity and participation levels of children with CP will also vary greatly. In the ICF-CY classification, activity and participation are included in the same domain, while in some studies, they are evaluated separately; in others, they are analyzed under a single heading [80–82].

Children with physical or neurological problems participate in activities and have similar demands as children with normal development. Children's participation in age-appropriate activities is an important indicator of quality of life and a fundamental right of every child. Children who actively participate in school life can gain educational and social benefits through this participation. Children with CP face more limitations in daily activities and social life compared to their typically developing peers. Consequently, participation in activities of daily living and appropriate education for children with CP represents a shared objective among parents, health professionals, service providers, and relevant organizations [82–84].

During the first 6 years of life, children discover themselves and the world by using their bodies and senses, moving and exploring their environment [85]. The period during which the child actively orientates toward their environment, attempts to explore the external world full of stimuli, and acquires the most basic skills of human life is referred to as the preschool period (24–60 months) [86]. This period represents a critical period during which the child develops at the highest level and learns with curiosity and thinking potential. The experiences acquired by the child through learning form the basis of their life in adulthood [87]. In this period, the rate of physical development is slower than in infancy. The acquisition of self-care skills, such as dressing, toileting, and using language, becomes a part of daily life in this period. The development of motor skills between the ages of 3 and 6 is closely related to physical development. In the preschool years, the child's primary means of expression is movement [88]. Therefore, movement is both meaningful and functional.

Preschool children with CP exhibit lower levels of body structure and function and activity and participation compared to their typically developing counterparts [89]. According to the ICF-CY, the number and impact of impairments in body structure and function are higher in children with CP compared to their typically developing peers. A multitude of factors, including socioeconomic level, gender, motor function, and CP type, influence activity and participation in these children [90]. They engage in a multitude of recreational and leisure activities, such as playing with toys, listening to stories, and drawing and coloring, which require minimal parental preparation and utilize few materials. These activities are sedentary and may not provide the same level of physical activity as swimming, gymnastics, and team sports. The level of participation in recreational activities of preschool children with CP is lower than that of children with normal development. The preschool children with CP who participate in the highest number of recreational activities are those who are able to walk independently and engage in activities that require physical exertion both at home and in their social environment. In contrast, the preschool children with CP who participate in the least number of activities are those with GMFCS IV and V levels, who are unable to move independently [91].

In order to fulfill activities of daily living, the child must possess physical and cognitive competence, as well as active skills. The term "activity" is a broad term that encompasses a multitude of concepts. "Ability" refers to the skills and abilities that the child can utilize in the daily environment. "Performance" refers to the child's optimal ability in a structured, standardized, and controlled environment in which the test is administered. Performance describes the skills and abilities that are a'tually used in daily life [92, 93]. Participation can be defined as being involved in life and being present in life. Participation can be modified by factors such as the child's preferences, motivation, and internal structure. Factors within the child, such as the child's ability to perform an activity and the physical and social environment affecting this activity, cause participation to be limited. For instance, participation can be analyzed in a multitude of domains, including participation in domestic activities, participation in educational and social settings, participation in everyday life, participation in social activities, and participation in leisure activities [92, 93].

It is of great importance to consider the participation of children with CP in social, daily life, and leisure time activities. Such participation is essential for the child to maintain their development in a healthy manner, to increase motivation, to interact with peers and other people in society, to develop functional abilities and social skills, to enjoy life, and to become more independent [94, 95]. It is of great importance to evaluate children with CP from a holistic perspective. The ICF-CY provides guidance on how to address this holistic perspective when evaluating and planning treatment approaches. It is of the utmost importance to ensure that children with CP are able to participate in social, daily, and leisure time activities, as this is a fundamental aspect of maintaining healthy development, increasing motivation, interacting with peers and other people in society, developing functional and social skills, enjoying life, and becoming more independent [94, 95]. In studies conducted with children with CP, it has been found that children have limitations in activity and participation due to difficulties in many activities, including mobility, personal care, play, and school activities [96–98]. Furthermore, studies have demonstrated that children with CP experience more limitations in social activities and participation in leisure time activities compared to their typically developing peers. The aforementioned limitations experienced by children may be dependent on a multitude of factors, including the level of impairment, motor and sensory problems, problems in body structure and function, age, environmental factors, functional abilities, and personal characteristics [88, 92, 97–99].

The ICF framework encompasses a plethora of parameters, including body structure and function, activity, participation, and environmental and personal factors. The body structure and function category encompasses a range of features, including selective motor control, muscle tone, pain, muscle strength, muscle structure, range of motion, posture, and trunk control. The activity category encompasses both fine and gross motor functional activities, such as self-care activities and activities of daily living. The participation category encompasses participation in social, community, and school life. In addition, the environmental factor category encompasses factors such as the physical condition of the home and the external environment, family, and friends. Personal factors encompass the child's fundamental characteristics, including age, personality traits, cognitive status, and motivation level. These five areas interact with each other, and it is evident that numerous factors converge to influence the health and functionality level of the child [88, 97–99].

Children with spastic CP exhibit a range of structural and functional impairments. These impairments result in activity limitations, hindering their ability to perform various activities. Furthermore, these children experience severe participation limitations, which prevent them from engaging in activities with their peers, writing in class, or going to the cinema. Participation limitations can be attributed to impairments in body structure and function, activity limitations, or personal and environmental factors. For instance, a child's ability to write in the classroom with the assistance of appropriate equipment represents a factor that facilitates participation. Conversely, for a child who is unable to attend the cinema due to a lack of suitable transportation, this constitutes a barrier to participation. Consequently, it is imperative to conduct a comprehensive assessment utilizing the ICF framework in order to make accurate determinations [88, 97–99].

11. Conclusions

- Neurological disorders such as cerebral palsy have varying effects on children's motor skills, sensory abilities, cognitive functions, and behavioral patterns. Therefore, the activity and participation levels of each child should be assessed individually.

- The participation of children with CP in daily life activities and education should be a shared goal among healthcare professionals, families, and relevant organizations.

- The preschool period is a critical phase where children undergo rapid development and acquire fundamental skills. Activities and participation during this period lay the foundation for the child's life.

- Children with CP in the preschool years tend to have lower body structure and function compared to typically developing peers, which can impact their activity and participation.

- The involvement of children with CP in social, daily, and leisure activities supports their development and enhances their enjoyment of life.

- Spastic CP children may experience activity and participation restrictions due to impairments in body structure and function. These limitations can be mitigated or eliminated with appropriate support and environmental factors.

These conclusions provide a foundational basis for evaluating and improving various aspects of the lives of children with CP.

Author details

Asiya Uzun
Wellness Centre, Gaziantep, Turkey

*Address all correspondence to: asiyeaaycicek@gmail.com

References

[1] Surveillance of Cerebral Palsy in Europe. Surveillance of cerebral palsy in Europe: A collaboration of cerebral palsy surveys and registers. Developmental Medicine and Child Neurology. 2000;**42**:816-824

[2] Smithers-Sheedy H, Badawi N, Blair E, et al. What constitutes cerebral palsy in the twenty-first century? Developmental Medicine and Child Neurology. 2014;**56**:323-328

[3] Rosenbaum P, Paneth N, Leviton A, Goldstein M, Bax M, Damiano D, et al. A report: The definition and classification of cerebral palsy April 2006. Developmental Medicine and Child Neurology. Supplement. 2007;**109**:8-14

[4] Morris C. Definition and classification of cerebral palsy: A historical perspective. Developmental Medicine and Child Neurology. Supplement. 2007;**109**:3-7

[5] Cans C. Surveillance of cerebral palsy in Europe: A collaboration of cerebral palsy surveys and registers. Developmental Medicine and Child Neurology. 2000;**42**(12):816-824

[6] McAdams RM, Juul SE. Cerebral palsy: Prevalence, predictability, andparental counseling. NeoReviews. 2011;**12**(10):e564-ee74

[7] Jonsson U, Eek MN, Sunnerhagen KS, Himmelmann K. Cerebral palsy prevalence, subtypes, and associated impairments: A population-based comparison study of adults and children. Developmental Medicine and Child Neurology. 2019;**61**(10):1162-1167

[8] Oskoui M, Coutinho F, Dykeman J, Jetté N, Pringsheim T. An update on the prevalence of cerebral palsy: A systematic review and meta-analysis. Developmental Medicine and Child Neurology. 2013;**55**(6):509-519

[9] McIntyre S, Goldsmith S, Webb A, Ehlinger V, Hollung SJ, McConnell K, et al. Global prevalence of cerebral palsy: A systematic analysis. Developmental Medicine and Child Neurology. 2022;**64**(12):1494-1506

[10] Sankar C, Mundkur N. Cerebral palsy-definition, classification, etiology and early diagnosis. Indian Journal of Pediatrics. 2005;**72**(10):865-868

[11] Vova J. Cerebral palsy: An overview of etiology, types and comorbidities. OBM Neurobiology. 2022;**6**(2):1-25

[12] MacLennan AH, Thompson SC, Gecz J. Cerebral palsy: Causes, pathways, and the role of genetic variants. American Journal of Obstetrics and Gynecology. 2015;**213**(6):779-788

[13] Kuban KC, Allred EN, O'Shea TM, Paneth N, Pagano M, Dammann O, et al. Cranial ultrasound lesions in the NICU predict cerebral palsy at age 2 years in children born at extremely low gestational age. Journal of Child Neurology. 2009;**24**(1):63-72

[14] Moreno-De-Luca A, Ledbetter DH, Martin CL. Genetic insights into the causes and classification of the cerebral palsies. Lancet Neurology. 2012;**11**(3):283-292

[15] Fahey MC, Maclennan AH, Kretzschmar D, Gecz J, Kruer MC. The genetic basis of cerebral palsy. Developmental Medicine and Child Neurology. 2017;**59**(5):462-469

[16] Baird G, McConachie H, Scrutton D. Parents' perceptions of

disclosure of the diagnosis of cerebral palsy. Archives of Disease in Childhood. 2000;**83**(6):475-480

[17] Spittle AJ, Morgan C, Olsen JE, et al. Early diagnosis and treatment of cerebral palsy in children with a history of preterm birth. Clinics in Perinatology. 2018;**45**(3):409-420

[18] Novak I, Morgan C, Adde L, et al. Early, accurate diagnosis and early intervention in cerebral palsy: Advances in diagnosis and treatment. JAMA Pediatrics. 2017;**171**(9):897-907

[19] Bosanquet M, Copeland L, Ware R, et al. A systematic review of tests to predict cerebral palsy in young children. Developmental Medicine and Child Neurology. 2013;**55**(5):418-426

[20] Ashwal S, Russman BS, Blasco PA, et al. Practice parameter: Diagnostic assessment of the child with cerebral palsy: Report of the quality standards subcommittee of the American Academy of Neurology and the Practice Committee of the Child Neurology Society. Neurology. 2004;**62**(6):851-863

[21] Korzeniewski SJ, Birbeck G, DeLano MC, et al. A systematic review of neuroimaging for cerebral palsy. Journal of Child Neurology. 2008;**23**(2):216-227

[22] Prechtl HF. Qualitative changes of spontaneous movements in fetus and preterm infant are a marker of neurological dysfunction. Early Human Development. 1990;**23**(3):151-158

[23] Kwong AKL, Fitzgerald TL, Doyle LW, et al. Predictive validity of spontaneous early infant movement for later cerebral palsy: A systematic review. Developmental Medicine and Child Neurology. 2018;**60**(5):480-489

[24] Einspieler C, Prechtl HF. Prechtl's assessment of general movements: A diagnostic tool for the functional assessment of the young nervous system. Mental Retardation and Developmental Disabilities Research Reviews. 2005;**11**(1):61-67

[25] Palmer FB. Strategies for the early diagnosis of cerebral palsy. The Journal of Pediatrics. 2004;**145**(Suppl. 2):S8-S11

[26] Cans C, Dolk H, Platt M, Colver A. Recommendations from the SCPE collaborative group for defining and classifying cerebral palsy. Developmental Medicine and Child Neurology. 2007;**49**:35-38

[27] Graham HK, Rosenbaum P, Paneth N, et al. Cerebral palsy. Nature Reviews Disease Primers. 2016;**2**:15082

[28] Himmelmann K, Horber V, De La Cruz J, Horridge K, Mejaski-Bosnjak V, Hollody K, et al. MRI classification system (MRICS) for children with cerebral palsy: Development, reliability, and recommendations. Developmental Medicine and Child Neurology. 2017;**59**(1):57-64

[29] Vossough A. Brain imaging: Magnetic resonance imaging. In: Pateliadis CP, editor. Cerebral Palsy: A Multidisciplinary Approach. 3rd ed. Cham, Switzerland: Springer International Publishing; 2018. pp. 113-131

[30] Jacobsson B, Hagberg G. Antenatal risk factors for cerebral palsy. Best Practice & Research Clinical Obstetrics & Gynaecology. 2004;**18**(3):425-436

[31] Paulson A, Vargus-Adams J. Overview of four functional classification systems commonly used in cerebral palsy. Children. 2017;**4**(4):30

[32] Palisano R, Rosenbaum P, Walter S, Russell D, Wood E, Galuppi B.

Development and reliability of a system to classify gross motor function in children with cerebral palsy. Developmental Medicine and Child Neurology. 1997;**39**:214-223

[33] Rosenbaum PL, Palisano RJ, Bartlett DJ, Galuppi BE, Russell DJ. Development of the gross motor function classification system for cerebral palsy. Developmental Medicine and Child Neurology. 2008;**50**:249-253

[34] Palisano R, Rosenbaum P, Bartlett D, Livingston M, Gmfcs-e&r. Gross motor function classification system expanded and revised. In: Canchild Centre for Childhood Disability Research. Hamilton, ON, Canada: Mcmaster University; Institute for Applied Health Sciences McMaster University; 2007. p. 15

[35] Eliasson AC, Krumlinde-Sundholm L, Rosblad B, Beckung E, Arner M, Ohrvall AM, et al. The manual ability classification system (macs) for children with cerebral palsy: Scale development and evidence of validity and reliability. Developmental Medicine and Child Neurology. 2006;**48**:549-554

[36] Andersen G, Mjøen TR, Vik T. Prevalence of speech problems and the use of augmentative and alternative communication in children with cerebral palsy: A registry-based study in Norway. SIG 12 Perspectives on Augmentative and Alternative Communication. 2010;**19**:12-20

[37] Hidecker MJ, Paneth N, Rosenbaum PL, Kent RD, Lillie J, E ulenberg JB, et al. Developing and validating the communication function classification system for individuals with cerebral palsy. Developmental Medicine and Child Neurology. 2011;**53**:704-710

[38] Reilly S, Skuse D, Poblete X. Prevalence of feeding problems and oral motor dysfunction in children with cerebral palsy: A community survey. The Journal of Pediatrics. 1996;**129**:877-882

[39] Sellers D, Mandy A, Pennington L, Hankins M, Morris C. Development and reliability of a system to classify the eating and drinking ability of people with cerebral palsy. Developmental Medicine and Child Neurology. 2014;**56**:245-251

[40] Papavasiliou AS. Management of motor problems in cerebral palsy: A critical update for the clinician. European Journal of Paediatric Neurology. 2009;**13**(5):387-396

[41] Nielsen JB, Petersen NT, Crone C, Sinkjaer T. Stretch reflex regulation in healthy subjects and patients with spasticity. Neuromodulation: Technology at the Neural Interface. 2005;**8**(1):49-57

[42] Bar-On L, Molenaers G, Aertbeliën E, Van Campenhout A, Feys H, Nuttin B, et al. Spasticity and its contribution to hypertonia in cerebral palsy. BioMed Research International. 2015;**7**(1):1-10

[43] Peck J, Urits I, Kassem H, Lee C, Robinson W, Cornett EM, et al. Interventional approaches to pain and spasticity related to cerebral palsy. Psychopharmacology Bulletin. 2020;**50**(41):108-120

[44] Lance JW. Symposium synopsis. In: Feldman RG, Young RR, Koella WP, editors. Spasticity: Disordered Motor Control. Chicago, IL: Year Book; 1980. pp. 485-494

[45] Flamand VH, Massé-Alarie H, Schneider C. Psychometric evidence of spasticity measurement tools in cerebral palsy children and adolescents: A systematic review. Journal of Rehabilitation Medicine. 2013;**45**(1):14-23

[46] Sakzewski L, Ziviani J, Boyd R. Systematic review and meta-analysis of therapeutic management of upper-limb dysfunction in children with congenital hemiplegia. Pediatrics. 2009;**123**(6):e1111-e1122

[47] Barnes MP. Upper Motor Neuone Syndrome and Spasticity: Clinical Management and Neurophysiology. Cambridge, UK: Cambridge University Press; 2008

[48] Klingels K, Demeyere I, Jaspers E, et al. Upper limb impairments and their impact on activity measures in children with unilateral cerebral palsy. European Journal of Paediatric Neurology. 2012;**16**(5):475-484

[49] Gage JR. The Identification and Treatment of Gait Problems in Cerebral Palsy. London: Mac Keith Press; 2009

[50] Morrell DS, Pearson JM, Sauser DD. Progressive bone and joint abnormalities of the spine and lower extremities in cerebral palsy. Radiographics. 2002;**22**(2):257-268

[51] Cahill-Rowley K, Rose J. Etiology of impaired selective motor control: Emerging evidence and its implications for research and treatment in cerebral palsy. Developmental Medicine and Child Neurology. 2014;**56**(6):522-528

[52] Kuo HC, Friel KM, Gordon AM. Neurophysiological mechanisms and functional impact of mirror movements in children with unilateral spastic cerebral palsy. Developmental Medicine and Child Neurology. 2018;**60**(2):155-161

[53] Fahr A, Keller JW, Van Hedel HJ. A systematic review of training methods that may improve selective voluntary motor control in children with spastic cerebral palsy. Frontiers in Neurology. 2020;**11**:572038

[54] Heyrman L, Desloovere K, Molenaers G, Verheyden G, Klingels K, Monbaliu E, et al. Clinical characteristics of impaired trunk control in children with spastic cerebral palsy. Research in Developmental Disabilities. 2013;**34**(1):327-334

[55] Winter DA. Human balance and posture control during standing and walking. Gait and Posture. 1995;**3**(4):193-214

[56] Romkes J, Peeters W, Oosterom AM, Molenaar S, Bakels I, Brunner R. Evaluating upper body movements during gait in healthy children and children with diplegic cerebral palsy. Journal of Pediatric Orthopaedics Part B. 2007;**16**(3):175-180

[57] Prosser LA, Lee SC, Barbe MF, VanSant AF, Lauer RT. Trunk and hip muscle activity in early walkers with and without cerebral palsy–A frequency analysis. Journal of Electromyography and Kinesiology. 2010;**20**(5):851-859

[58] Tseng M-H, Chen K-L, Shieh J-Y, Lu L, Huang C-Y. The determinants of daily function in children with cerebral palsy. Research in Developmental Disabilities. 2011;**32**(1):235-245

[59] Majnemer A, Shevell M, Rosenbaum P, Law M, Poulin C. Determinants of life quality in school-age children with cerebral palsy. The Journal of Pediatrics. 2007;**151**(5):470-475

[60] Group W. Study protocol for the World Health Organization project to develop a quality of life assessment instrument (WHOQOL). Quality of Life Research. 1993;**2**:153-159

[61] Sigurdardottir S, Indredavik MS, Eiriksdottir A, Einarsdottir K, Gudmundsson HS, Vik T. Behavioural and emotional symptoms of preschool

children with cerebral palsy: A population-based study. Developmental Medicine and Child Neurology. 2010;**52**(11):1056-1061

[62] Gilson KM, Davis E, Reddihough D, Graham K, Waters E. Quality of life in children with cerebral palsy: Implications for practice. Journal of Child Neurology. 2014;**29**(8):1134-1140

[63] Kim C. Comprehensive physiotherapy approaches for children with cerebral palsy: Overview and contemporary trends. Physical Therapy Korea. 2023;**30**(4):253-260

[64] Adamovich SV, Fluet GG, Tunik E, Merians AS. Sensorimotor training in virtual reality: A review. NeuroRehabilitation. 2009;**25**(1):29-44

[65] Liu C, Wang X, Chen R, Zhang J. The effects of virtual reality training on balance, gross motor function, and daily living ability in children with cerebral palsy: Systematic review and meta-analysis. JMIR Serious Games. 2022;**10**(4):e38972

[66] Nossa R, Gagliardi C, Panzeri D, Diella E, Maghini C, Genova C, et al. Could an immersive virtual reality training improve navigation skills in children with cerebral palsy? A pilot controlled study. Journal of Clinical Medicine. 2022;**11**(20):6146

[67] Arnoni JLB, Kleiner AFR, Lima CRG, de Campos AC, Rocha NACF. Nonimmersive virtual reality as complementary rehabilitation on functional mobility and gait in cerebral palsy: A randomized controlled clinical trial. Games for Health Journal. 2021;**10**(4):254-263

[68] Meneses Castaño C, Penagos P, Yamile JB. Effectiveness of robotic technology and virtual reality for the rehabilitation of motor function in cerebral palsy. Systematic review. Rehabilitacion (Madr). 2023;**57**(3):100752. Spanish

[69] Cortés-Pérez I, González-González N, Peinado-Rubia AB, Nieto- Escamez FA, Obrero-Gaitán E, García-López H. Efficacy of robot-assisted gait therapy compared to conventional therapy or treadmill training in children with cerebral palsy: A systematic review with meta-analysis. Sensors (Basel). 2022;**22**(24):9910

[70] Kawasaki S, Ohata K, Yoshida T, Yokoyama A, Yamada S. Gait improvements by assisting hip movements with the robot in children with cerebral palsy: A pilot randomized controlled trial. Journal of Neuroengineering and Rehabilitation. 2020;**17**(1):87

[71] Matsuda M, Iwasaki N, Mataki Y, Mutsuzaki H, Yoshikawa K, Takahashi K, et al. Robot-assisted training using hybrid assistive limb® for cerebral palsy. Brain and Development. 2018;**40**(8):642-648

[72] Yiğitoğlu P, Kozanoğlu E. Effectiveness of electrical stimulation after administration of botulinum toxin in children with spastic diplegic cerebral palsy: A prospective, randomized clinical study. Turkish Journal of Physical Medicine and Rehabilitation. 2019;**65**(1):16

[73] Rozin Kleiner AF, Bellomo A, Pagnussat AS, de Athayde CE, Silva A, Sforza C, et al. Wearable sensors, cerebral palsy and gait assessment in everyday environments: Is it a reality? - A systematic review. Functional Neurology. 2019;**34**(2):85-91

[74] Behboodi A, Lee WA, Hinchberger VS, Damiano DL. Determining optimal mobile neurofeedback methods for motor

neurorehabilitation in children and adults with non-progressive neurological disorders: A scoping review. Journal of Neuroengineering and Rehabilitation. 2022;**19**(1):104

[75] Ragni LB, Dlugacz SK, Sadowsky C, Cammarata G, Sala DA, Bill V, et al. Design and use of a 3D-printed dynamic upper extremity orthosis for children with cerebral palsy and severe upper extremity involvement: A pilot study. The American Journal of Occupational Therapy. 2023;**77**(4):7704205060

[76] Pagaki-Skaliora M, Morrow E, Theologis T. Telehealth and remote interventions for children with cerebral palsy: Scoping review. JMIR Rehabilitation and Assistive Technologies. 2022;**9**(4):e36842

[77] Conner BC, Lerner ZF. Improving ankle muscle recruitment via plantar pressure biofeedback during robot resisted gait training in cerebral palsy. IEEE International Conference on Rehabilitation Robotics. 2022:1-6

[78] Gillick BT, Feyma T, Menk J, Usset M, Vaith A, Wood TJ, et al. Safety and feasibility of transcranial direct current stimulation in pediatric hemiparesis: Randomized controlled preliminary study. Physical Therapy. 2015;**95**(3):337-349

[79] Organization WH. International Classification of Functioning, Disability, and Health: Children & Youth Version: ICF-CY. Switzerland: World Health Organization; 2007

[80] Voorman JM, Dallmeijer AJ, Schuengel C, Knol DL, Lankhorst GJ, Becher JG. Activities and participation of 9- to 13-year-old children with cerebral palsy. Clinical Rehabilitation. 2006;**20**(11):937-948

[81] Johnson A. Prevalence and characteristics of children with cerebral palsy in Europe. Developmental Medicine and Child Neurology. 2002;**44**(9):633-640

[82] Mc Manus V, Corcoran P, Perry IJ. Participation in everyday activities and quality of life in pre-teenage children living with cerebral palsy in south west Ireland. BMC Pediatrics. 2008;**8**:50

[83] Heah T, Case T, McGuire B, Law M. Successful participation: The lived experience among children with disabilities. Canadian Journal of Occupational Therapy. 2007;**74**(1):38-47

[84] Khetani MA, Graham JE, Davies PL, Law MC, Simeonsson RJ. Psychometric properties of the young children's participation and environment measure. Archives of Physical Medicine and Rehabilitation. 2015;**96**(2):307-316

[85] Aral N, Baran G. Çocuk gelişimi. İstanbul: Ya-Pa Yayınları; 2011

[86] Tuzcuoğlu N, Azkeskin KE, Küsmüs Gİ, Cengiz Ö. Okul öncesi dönem çocuklarının öz düzenleme becerileri ile benlik algıları arasındaki ilişkisinin incelenmesi. IBAD Sosyal Bilimler Dergisi. 2019:607-623

[87] Frankenburg WK, Dodds JB. The Denver developmental screening test. The Journal of Pediatrics. 1967;**71**(2):181-191

[88] Majnemer A, Shevell M, Law M, Birnbaum R, Chilingaryan G, Rosenbaum P, et al. Participation and enjoyment of leisure activities in school-aged childrenwith cerebral palsy. Developmental Medicine and Child Neurology. 2008;**50**(10):751-758

[89] Chiarello LA, Palisano RJ, Orlin MN, Chang HJ, Begnoche D, An M. Understanding participation of

preschool-age children with cerebral palsy. Journal of Early Intervention. 2012;**34**(1):3-19

[90] Wu KP, Chuang YF, Chen CL, Liu IS, Liu HT, Chen HC. Predictors of participation change in various areas for preschool children with cerebral palsy: A longitudinal study. Research in Developmental Disabilities. 2015;**37**:102-111

[91] Alsem MW, Ketelaar M, Verhoef M. The course of health-related quality of life of preschool children with cerebral palsy. Disability and Rehabilitation. 2013;**35**(8):686-693

[92] Imms C, Granlund M, Wilson PH, Steenbergen B, Rosenbaum PL, Gordon AM. Participation, both a means and an end: A conceptual analysis of processes and outcomes in childhood disability. Developmental Medicine and Child Neurology. 2017;**59**(1):16-25

[93] Holsbeeke L, Ketelaar M, Schoemaker MM, Gorter JW. Capacity, capability, and performance: Different constructs or three of a kind? Archives of Physical Medicine and Rehabilitation. 2009;**90**(5):849-855

[94] Majnemer A, Shikako-Thomas K, Chokron N, Law M, Shevell M, Chilingaryan G, et al. Leisure activity preferences for 6- to 12-year-old children with cerebral palsy. Developmental Medicine and Child Neurology. 2010;**52**(2):167-173

[95] Simpkins SD, Ripke M, Huston AC, Eccles JS. Predicting participation and outcomes in out-of-school activities: Similarities and differences across social ecologies. New Directions for Youth Development. 2005;**105**:51-69, 10-1

[96] Kim K, Kang JY, Jang DH. Relationship between mobility and self-care activity in children with cerebral palsy. Annals of Rehabilitation Medicine. 2017;**41**(2):266-272. 106

[97] Schenker R, Coster WJ, Parush S. Neuroimpairments, activity performance,and participation in children with cerebral palsy mainstreamed in elementaryschools. Developmental Medicine and Child Neurology. 2005;**47**(12):808-814

[98] Huang CY, Tseng MH, Chen KL, Shieh JY, Lu L. Determinants of schoolactivity performance in children with cerebral palsy: A multidimensionalapproach using the ICF-CY as a framework. Research in Developmental Disabilities. 2013;**34**(11):4025-4033

[99] Anaby D, Law M, Coster W, Bedell G, Khetani M, Avery L, et al. Themediating role of the environment in explaining participation of children andyouth with and without disabilities across home, school, and community. Archives of Physical Medicine and Rehabilitation. 2014;**95**(5):908-917

Section 3

Common Nephrological Disorders in Children

Chapter 4

Common Disorders in Paediatric Nephrology: Diagnosis, Prevention, and Management

Mirjam Močnik and Nataša Marčun Varda

Abstract

Paediatric nephrology is frequently seen as a challenging aspect of paediatric care and necessitating specialised expertise. Nevertheless, the typical issues encountered in paediatric nephrology, such as urinary tract infections and mild micturition disorders, often do not require the attention of a paediatric nephrologist and can be managed effectively by a general practitioner. Urinary tract infections frequently present to emergency centres. They commonly include acute pyelonephritis and uncomplicated cystitis, differentiated upon clinical presentation. Urinalysis, urine culture, acute phase reactants, and renal and bladder ultrasound are the mainstay for the diagnosis. Except for asymptomatic bacteriuria, antibiotic treatment is necessary in the management. Micturition disorders are more common in nephrological outpatient clinics and encompass a wide range of urinary issues, with primary nocturnal enuresis and various forms of daytime micturition problems being the most prevalent. These disorders can be classified as primary or secondary, as well as monosymptomatic or non-monosymptomatic. The diagnosis is based on history and voiding diary and supplemented with imaging and functional diagnostic procedures, as needed. The management primarily involves urotherapy, complemented with medications, if necessary.

Keywords: children, urinary tract infections, micturition disorders, management, prevention

1. Introduction

Paediatric nephrology encompasses a wide range of conditions necessitating specific treatment. From this perspective, the more prevalent conditions in this domain, such as urinary infections and micturition disorders, differ, as their basic treatment does not typically require the specialised expertise of a paediatric nephrologist but can be managed by a general paediatrician or primary care paediatrician. Therefore, this chapter aims to provide support and further education to all paediatric experts encountering these conditions due to their frequency, seeking additional validation or supplementation of the management without specialised knowledge in paediatric nephrology.

Urinary tract infections (UTI) and micturition disorders are prevalent childhood conditions frequently encountered in clinical settings. UTI are often observed in the emergency department, especially in febrile children with sudden onset symptoms, potentially indicating a severe infection. Prompt diagnosis and treatment are imperative to differentiate UTI from other bacterial infections and mitigate the risk of long-term complications, notably renal scarring.

Conversely, micturition disorders represent a common yet non-life-threatening nephrological conditions in paediatrics. These disorders typically manifest in outpatient settings and significantly affect a child's daily life and functionality, exerting a notable impact on their psychological well-being. Both UTI and micturition disorders are significant due to their frequency and their potential long-term implications for quality of life.

2. Urinary tract infections

UTI are among the most common bacterial infections in paediatrics [1] and are the most common serious bacterial illness in febrile children up to 2 years of age in the emergency setting [2]. The demographic characteristics appear to play a crucial role in epidemiological examinations of UTI. The greatest occurrence of febrile UTI is observed among boys under 3 months of age who are uncircumcised, followed by girls below 1 year of age [2]. However, due to the heterogeneous studies differing in age range, inclusion criteria, race, circumcision status, and location of enrolment, epidemiological data is inconclusive. Nevertheless, estimates suggest that by the age of seven, approximately 8% of girls and 2% of boys will experience at least one episode of UTI [3]. Up to 30% of patients experience recurrence of the infection during the first year after initial UTI [4]. Recurring UTI are suggestive for underlying kidney disorder, most commonly congenital anomalies of the kidney and urinary tract (CAKUT) [4].

The pathology is usually divided into febrile upper UTI (most commonly acute pyelonephritis) and lower UTI (most commonly cystitis) [1]. They differ in clinical presentation and management, as presented in **Table 1**. The infection may spread ascendingly, which is more common, and haematogenously, which is more frequently found in neonatal period. In this case, UTI may manifest as sepsis with nonspecific clinical features (mainly feeding problems, irritability, convulsions, pallor, hypothermia, and sometimes jaundice) [4]. Otherwise, acute pyelonephritis commonly manifests with a high temperature, abdominal or flank pain, sometimes accompanied by malaise, vomiting, or diarrhoea, and should be considered in every child with a fever of unknown aetiology [5]. Symptoms and signs indicative of lower urinary tract involvement comprise suprapubic or abdominal discomfort accompanied by tenderness, painful urination (dysuria), frequent urges to urinate, urgency, cloudy or foul-smelling urine, and recent onset of daytime wetting or bedwetting (nocturnal enuresis) [6].

Most commonly encountered bacteria, causing UTI, is *Escherichia coli*, responsible for 80–90% of cases, followed by *Proteus mirabilis, Klebsiella* spp., and *Staphylococcus saprophyticus* [4]. The presence of bacteria in the urine at specified quantitative counts (colony forming units, CFU) without having signs and symptoms is characteristic of asymptomatic bacteriuria, present in <1% of children [7]. Clinically, we differ it from UTI as presented in **Table 1**. Along with urine contamination, asymptomatic bacteriuria is a common confounding entity during the evaluation of a symptomatic child that was determined to not have a UTI. As a rule, it is not recommended to screen for or treat asymptomatic bacteriuria in children [8].

Characteristic	Acute pyelonephritis	Uncomplicated cystitis	Asymptomatic bacteriuria
Age distribution	More common in younger children	Typically in children aged >2 years	Across all age groups
Fever	>38°C	Afebrile or low-grade fever ≤38°C	Absent
Systemic symptoms	Common	Uncommon	Absent
Local symptoms	Flank pain and/or tenderness	Dysuria, urgency, frequency, urinary incontinence, suprapubic pain, or haematuria	Absent
Causative agent	Bacterial (*E. coli* is the commonest)	Bacterial (*E. coli* is the commonest), viral, fungal, and chemical	Bacterial
Gross haematuria	Uncommon	May have fresh blood and clots	Absent
Urine culture for bacteria	Positive	Positive (bacterial cause) or negative (non-bacterial cause)	Positive
Renal and bladder ultrasound	Normal or may reveal edema and hyperaemia of kidney	Normal or may reveal thickened urinary bladder wall, debris in the bladder	Unremarkable
Renal complications	Renal scarring	None	None
Antibiotic treatment	7–10 (14) days	3–5 days	None

Table 1.
Features distinguishing between acute pyelonephritis, uncomplicated cystitis, and asymptomatic bacteriuria.

2.1 Diagnosis

Accurate and reliable diagnosis of UTI in children is very important, due to immediate or long-term harm, namely renal scarring, with underdiagnosis and unnecessary treatment and potentially invasive diagnostic procedures with overdiagnosis. Basic diagnostics consists of urinalysis and urine culture [9].

Firstly, an appropriate urine sample must be obtained, usually clean midstream catch, if possible. The use of bag specimens is strongly discouraged due to their notably high rate of false positivity. If required in younger children, catheterisation or, rarely, suprapubic aspiration provides additional possibilities of urine sampling. With these two methods, the culture threshold (CFU/ml) might be lower [9].

Urinalysis has proven to be a crucial supplement to urine culture when identifying UTI. Evaluating inflammation through pyuria can assist in distinguishing between contamination/colonisation or asymptomatic bacteriuria, from infection [9]. While evidence indicates that pyuria can manifest without UTI, such as during fevers from other infections or conditions like Kawasaki disease or following intense physical activity, it is uncommon for it to be absent in genuine UTI cases [10]. Furthermore, urinalysis includes a urinary nitrite test, which, if positive, strongly suggests bacteriuria. However, the absence of nitrites does not rule out urinary tract infection [9, 10].

Along with pathologic urinalysis, urine culture should be positive with the presence of a single uropathogen in specified quantitative counts, demonstrated as CFU/ml [11].

The majority of paediatric laboratories adhere to thresholds ranging from 10^4 to 10^5 CFU/ml for clean catch/midstream urine samples and catheter urine samples [9]. Defining infections based on culture poses challenges due to asymptomatic bacteriuria or a contaminant, which can yield growth levels resembling infection. In a true UTI, the same pathogen might be detected also in blood cultures, especially in younger patients with haematogenous spread of infection [12].

Supplementary diagnostic tests of upper UTI, namely acute pyelonephritis, include acute phase reactants determination, such as C-reactive protein, white blood cell count, and erythrocyte sedimentation rate, which, when elevated, can help in the diagnosis of upper UTI, differentiating it from lower UTI and asymptomatic bacteriuria. It is important to mention that stand-alone are not neither completely sensitive nor specific for detecting UTI and its localisation and therefore should be used along with history and clinical examination [13].

Imaging diagnostic techniques, typically renal and bladder ultrasound, commonly aid in location determination, as well as potential abscess visualisation or renal/bladder malformation, suggestive for CAKUT, most commonly vesicoureteral reflux (VUR). In children with febrile UTI, renal and bladder ultrasonography should be performed as soon as possible [14]. If there are abnormalities, or UTI are recurring, voiding cystourethrogram is indicated, as well as some additional diagnostics if necessary [14, 15]. Also, in children with positive family history of CAKUT and an UTI, voiding cystourethrogram might be considered, since a large number of CAKUT are genetic in origin [16]. Otherwise, upper UTI is characterised with ultrasound as enlarged kidneys with hypoechoic parenchyma and loss of the normal corticomedullary junction [17]; meanwhile, in the later stages of cystitis, thick bladder wall with irregular surface is seen, and sometimes urine may contain fine suspended echoes [18].

2.2 Prevention

The mainstay of prevention, especially in children with increased risk for infection, such as VUR and other CAKUT, has historically been low-dose antibiotic prophylaxis [19]. Prolonged antibiotic therapy might decrease the likelihood of recurrent symptomatic UTI in children with a history of one or more prior UTI. However, the potential advantage needs to be weighed against the heightened risk of microbial resistance, which must be carefully considered [19]. Even more, recent systematic review showed that low-dose continuous antibiotic prophylaxis plays some limited role in preventing recurrences, mainly in children with significant obstructive uropathies until surgical correction, and was not recommended in children with a previous UTI, recurrent UTI, VUR of any grade, isolated hydronephrosis, and neurogenic bladder [20].

Consequently, other interventions for prevention of UTI in children are being researched, most commonly probiotics, D-mannose, vitamin A, cranberry, nasturtium, horseradish, and others, but yielded insufficient evidence on their effect versus antibiotics [21–23]. Other preventive measures include satisfactory liquid consumption, intermittent catheterisation in patients with incomplete bladder emptying, and bladder bowel dysfunction management [14].

In children with UTI and some potential functional voiding problems, non-pharmacological preventive approaches of voiding and defecation have to be implemented.

2.3 Management

The management of UTI depends on its presentation and localisation.

Asymptomatic bacteriuria is characterised by the absence of an inflammatory reaction, occurring at all ages and usually resolves spontaneously in a few months to a couple of years [24]. In otherwise healthy children, treatment is not recommended because it promotes antimicrobial resistance and other adverse effects [24].

Acute pyelonephritis and cystitis require antimicrobial treatment. The decision between oral and parenteral treatment should hinge upon factors including patient age, clinical suspicion of urosepsis, aversion to fluids, food, and oral medication, as well as the presence of vomiting, diarrhoea, and complicated pyelonephritis. In neonates and infants under 2 months old, it is advisable to opt for parenteral antibiotic therapy due to the heightened risk of urosepsis and severe pyelonephritis. These cases may also involve electrolyte imbalances leading to potentially life-threatening hyponatraemia and hyperkalaemia associated with pseudohypoaldosteronism. Clinicians should remain vigilant for anatomical abnormalities, such as obstructive conditions, which may contribute to these complications [25, 26].

Prompt and efficient treatment of UTI can reduce the likelihood of infection spreading and resulting in renal scarring. Research indicates that shorter antibiotic regimens (lasting 1–3 days) yield less favourable outcomes when compared to longer courses lasting 7–14 days [10, 27]. Nevertheless, uncomplicated cystitis may be managed effectively with antibiotic regimens lasting 3–5 days [28]. For young infants, it might be worthwhile to contemplate a brief period of parenteral treatment followed by an early transition to oral antibiotics. In cases where outpatient treatment is preferred, it is imperative to ensure active monitoring, medical oversight, and readiness to modify therapy if needed [25].

The selection of an antimicrobial for empirical therapy should be performed by the local prevalence of resistant uropathogens. However, particularly in young febrile children at high risk of renal involvement, it is prudent to opt for an antimicrobial with a low resistance profile among organisms. Presently, the majority of uropathogens demonstrate susceptibility to third-generation cephalosporins. For afebrile children, it would be more appropriate to consider first-generation cephalosporins, trimethoprim-sulfamethoxazole, or nitrofurantoin. Notably, the use of amoxicillin is discouraged due to widespread resistance among uropathogens [24].

Management also involves addressing complications associated with UTI, which parallel those seen in any febrile illness in young children. These complications may include dehydration, electrolyte imbalances, and febrile seizures. Although renal complications stemming from acute pyelonephritis are uncommon in otherwise healthy children, they may involve the development of a renal abscess or the complete blockage of a pre-existing partial ureteropelvic junction. Acute kidney injury might arise due to dehydration or the administration of nonsteroidal anti-inflammatory drugs like ibuprofen, which can also lead to diminished renal function by inducing papillary necrosis or interstitial nephritis. Additionally, interstitial nephritis may be caused by the antibiotic used to treat UTI. Urosepsis is a potential complication, particularly in cases of Gram-negative infections [24]. As UTI can be associated with a CAKUT or micturition problems, additional diagnostics has to be performed as appropriate [1].

The most significant long-term complication of acute pyelonephritis is renal scarring, with reported prevalence approximately around 15% [29]. This prevalence ranges from 3% after the first UTI to 29% after more than three febrile UTI [24].

Although renal scarring may not show clinical symptoms in the majority of children, it can result in hypertension, proteinuria, and a gradual deterioration in renal function, particularly in instances of significant bilateral scarring [30]. Delayed onset of antibiotic therapy is linked to a heightened risk of scarring, with children whose treatment begins within 24 hours of fever onset having a 74% lower likelihood of developing new renal scarring compared to those whose treatment is initiated after 72 hours of fever onset [31].

3. Micturition disorders

Urinary issues in children, known as micturition disorders, encompass a range of problems including nocturnal enuresis, incontinence, urgency, nocturia, pollakisuria, hesitancy, straining, weak or intermittent stream, dysuria, and retention. These disorders can be classified as primary or secondary, as well as monosymptomatic or non-monosymptomatic [32, 33].

The cause of micturition disorders in children is complex and not fully understood. Several studies have attempted to identify early risk factors in children experiencing nighttime or daytime incontinence, but their findings have often been unclear or even contradictory. Research indicates that children with micturition disorders and low birthweight tend to have a lower estimated bladder capacity compared to children of the same age. Low birthweight is also linked to other perinatal factors like low gestational age (which is directly linked to low birthweight) and APGAR score, both of which may impact further development, including micturition [34]. Additionally, age, gender, and the mother's level of education are significant risk factors for enuresis, with the prevalence of primary nocturnal enuresis being notably higher in children with a positive family history of enuresis, particularly when present in the fathers' history [35].

The most prevalent urinary issue seen in children is primary nocturnal enuresis, characterised by bedwetting in a child over the age of 5, with at least one incident per month persisting for a minimum of three consecutive months. In its primary form, this condition denotes a child who has not consistently stayed dry at night since infancy. Secondary primary nocturnal enuresis occurs when bedwetting resumes after a period of at least 6 months of dryness. Additionally, monosymptomatic nocturnal enuresis is characterised by bedwetting without accompanying symptoms of daytime urinary issues, whereas the presence of such symptoms leads to the classification of non-monosymptomatic nocturnal enuresis [33].

The high occurrence rate of primary nocturnal enuresis indicates its common presence, with approximately 16% of five-year-olds estimated to experience bedwetting. Even at the age of 7, close to 10% continue to exhibit frequent bedwetting (more than three nights per week) [36, 37]. Additionally, another study demonstrated the prevalence of bedwetting less than two nights per week in 30% of 4.5-year-olds and 8% of 9.5-year-olds, and the prevalence of bedwetting more than two nights per week in 8% of 4.5-year-olds and 1.5% of 9.5-year-old children [38]. However, the prevalence of bedwetting diminishes, as children grow older. Additionally, bedwetting is more prevalent among boys [36, 37]. Conversely, daytime urinary incontinence during childhood is frequently underestimated and receives less effective treatment. According to one study, it was identified in 15.5% of children aged 4.5 and in 4.9% of those aged 9.5 [39]. In another population-based study, daily urinary incontinence occurrences within the last 6 months were reported in 16.9% of children [40].

Incontinence can manifest in two main ways: less frequently as continuous incontinence, suggesting an underlying anatomical or neurological condition, or intermittent incontinence, which is more common. These forms can be further categorised as primary or secondary, as well as monosymptomatic or non-monosymptomatic [33]. Daytime incontinence can be accompanied by several other micturition disorders, which can also be present as stand-alone. *Urgency* refers to the sudden and unexpected experience of an immediate and compelling need to void. *Nocturia* is the complaint that the child has to wake at night to void. *Hesitancy* refers to the challenge in starting urination when the child feels the urge to urinate. *Straining* involves the child reporting the need to exert significant effort to raise intra-abdominal pressure in order to start and sustain urination. *Dysuria* is the complaint of burning or discomfort during micturition. *Voiding stream* can also be *weak* or *intermittent*. Intermittency implies micturition that is not continuous but rather has several discrete stop-and-start spurts. *Urinary retention* describes the feeling of being unable to urinate despite continuous attempts, even with a fully distended bladder. *Pollakisuria* is defined by increased frequency of urination with small urine volume [33]. Normal voiding frequency ranges between 3 to 8 times per day with voiding ≥8 times per day defining increased daytime urinary frequency and voiding ≤3 times per day decreased daytime urinary frequency.

A number of micturition disorders, summarised in **Table 2**, manifest with daily urinary incontinence and other symptoms [33].

3.1 Diagnosis

The identification of micturition disorders relies on reviewing medical history and conducting clinical assessments. Through the patient's medical background, we can differentiate between monosymptomatic and non-monosymptomatic disorders and pinpoint the primary micturition issue. It is crucial to consider potential systemic conditions like renal or neurological diseases, as well as diabetes mellitus, which may influence the onset of micturition disorders [36].

During assessment of a child with a micturition disorder, a completed questionnaire and voiding diary are required, where the patient records their fluid intake, micturition frequency, timing and quantity of urination episodes, micturition patterns, and defecation frequency. By analysing this recorded data, we can assess the child's bladder capacity and compare it with the anticipated capacity for his/her age. For ages 4–12, this expected capacity is calculated using the equation: 30 × (age in years + 1), up to a maximum of 390 ml. A reduced bladder capacity is indicated if the estimated maximum urine per micturition is less than 65% of the expected bladder capacity for the child's age. Nocturnal polyuria is identified if the volume of urine produced at night exceeds 130% of the expected bladder capacity for the child's age [33, 36].

During the clinical assessment, specific findings are typically absent, yet we remain vigilant for potential indicators such as an abdominal mass (indicating an enlarged bladder or constipation), anatomical variations in the genital region, and external manifestations associated with neurogenic bladder dysfunction [36].

For each child, a basic urine analysis is conducted. Glycosuria may suggest diabetes, while proteinuria could indicate chronic kidney disease. Attention is also given to the possible presence of pyuria and the urine's specific gravity. Furthermore, a routine ultrasound examination of the urinary tract is often conducted to evaluate post-void residual urine volume. An elevated residual volume is noted when urinary retention surpasses 30 ml or 21% of bladder capacity in children aged 4–6 years or exceeds

Micturition disorder	Definition	Clinical manifestations
Overactive bladder	Overactivity of detrusor, seen in cystometry	Urgency, frequent voiding, nocturia, incontinence, and absence of UTI
Underactive bladder	Underactivity of detrusor, seen in cystometry (not always present with the same clinical manifestations)	Straining is needed to start, continue, and end voiding, increased bladder volume, and urine residual volume
Holding manoeuvres	Habitual retention of urine	Decreased frequency of voiding, urgency, and overflow incontinence
Dysfunctional micturition (the term is used for neurologically healthy children)	Habitual contractions of the urethral sphincter and pelvic floor muscles	Intermittent stream
Bladder outlet obstruction	Urinary flow obstruction during urination (mechanical/functional)	Weak stream
Stress incontinence	Urinary incontinence with small amounts of urine during physical exertion or other activity which increases intra-abdominal pressure	Urinary incontinence with coughing, sneezing, etc.
Vaginal reflux	It is caused by urinating with adducted legs, in which the urine is trapped in the vaginal introitus; it can result from labia adhesions due to local inflammation	Daily incontinence in moderate amounts immediately after urination
Laughter incontinence	Urinary incontinence during or immediately after laughing	
Extreme daytime frequency	Frequent need to urinate during the day	Pollakisuria, urinating at least once per hour and small urine volumes
Bladder neck dysfunction	Difficult or too slow opening of the bladder neck, despite normal or increased detrusor contractions	Weak stream
Bladder and bowel dysfunction	The simultaneous presence of bladder and bowel disorder (constipation, encopresis)	

Table 2.
Frequent daytime micturition disorders.

20 ml or 15% of bladder capacity in children aged 7–12 years. Ultrasound is also employed to evaluate constipation. Further invasive tests are determined based on the patient's symptoms, although they should not be conducted in cases of monosymptomatic nocturnal enuresis [37, 41].

In cases of micturition disorders, urine flow recording or uroflowmetry alongside urodynamic tests are commonly employed. Uroflowmetry is utilised to measure micturition duration, urine volume, and to delineate the shape of the urine curve [33]. It is imperative that the volume of urine is adequate, as indicated by the curve at a volume exceeding 50% of the calculated urinary bladder capacity. To enhance reliability, multiple measurements are consistently conducted. A typical curve exhibits a bell shape. However, a columnar or sudden, high-amplitude curve of brief duration suggests an overactive bladder. Conversely, a staccato curve, irregular yet continuous, implies a dissonance between the bladder and the sphincter. An intermittent curve manifests as flow with numerous peaks and complete halts, indicative of an underactive bladder or dysfunctional micturition. Additionally, a plateau-shaped curve, characterised by a flattened, low-amplitude, and prolonged pattern, signals a blockage in the outflow tract from the urinary bladder [33].

The urodynamic assessment involves evaluating both the filling and emptying phases of the urinary bladder. Using cystometry during the filling phase, we assess the sensory function of the bladder, detrusor function, bladder compliance, and bladder capacity. In the emptying phase, cystometry examines the relationship between pressure and volume during urination, detrusor function during urination, and urethral function during urination. This examination is conducted when there is suspicion of a neuropathic bladder, as well as in cases of obstruction, dilated ureters, bladder neck dysfunction, lack of response to treatment, history of neurological conditions, and anatomical abnormalities [33].

3.2 Prevention

Preventive measures for micturition disorders are often limited due to the various factors that influence a child's development. Primary enuresis is primarily attributed to pathophysiological factors such as an altered diuretic hormone profile, arousal failure, and delayed bladder maturation, with significant influence from genetic factors. Nevertheless, somatic and psychosocial environmental factors play a significant modulatory role. Addressing potential coexisting conditions like constipation and obesity may prove beneficial in preventing the onset of enuresis [42, 43]. Good bladder control necessitates appropriate toilet training at a suitable age [44]. Particular attention should be directed towards children with preexisting conditions, predisposing them to an elevated risk of micturition disorders, such as anatomical abnormalities and nervous system diseases. Regular assessment of voiding patterns and prompt intervention if necessary are crucial in their care.

3.3 Management

The primary treatment approach is urotherapy, characterised as non-surgical and non-pharmacological interventions aimed at addressing lower urinary tract disorders in children and adolescents. Urotherapy, a specialised practice, has emerged as the cornerstone therapy, not only for daytime urinary incontinence but also for addressing issues such as nocturnal enuresis, functional constipation, and faecal incontinence [45].

Urotherapy encompasses both standard and specific approaches. Standard urotherapy involves educating children and parents about micturition disorders, dispelling myths surrounding them, and providing guidance on behavioural modifications. These modifications may include ensuring adequate fluid intake during the day while restricting it in the evening for those experiencing nocturnal enuresis, encouraging regular urination intervals and pre-bedtime voiding, discouraging restraining manoeuvers, promoting optimal urination posture, advocating for a balanced diet and regular bowel movements, maintaining a diary, and attending regular check-ups. Support and encouragement have to be offered throughout this process [45, 46].

Tailored measures are implemented to address the individual's specific incontinence disorder. For instance, if there are associated issues with defecation, the primary focus will be on treating those problems before addressing urinary concerns [45, 46].

Specific urotherapy encompasses a range of treatment modalities tailored to the individual's needs. These may include:

1. Biofeedback: utilising a feedback loop method to help individuals gain control over their urinary function by providing real-time information about physiological processes. This form of treatment is primarily indicated for dysfunctional micturition. The method not only focuses on training relaxation of the pelvic floor muscles but also educates individuals about the activity of the abdominal muscles. Additionally, it involves visualising the electromyographic activity of the pelvic floor muscles. This visualisation can be combined with real-time urine flow measurement display or interactive computer games, enhancing engagement and effectiveness of the treatment process [47].

2. Neuromodulation: employing techniques to modulate nerve activity and alter bladder function, often through electrical stimulation. This treatment can be administered through various methods, including transcutaneous, intravesical, endoanal, and anogenital ones. Techniques may involve stimulating the posterior tibial nerve or implanting a sacral nerve pulse generator. The electric current is believed to directly affect the central nervous system, facilitating the reactivation of pelvic floor muscles, modulating bladder function, and improving control of the external urethral sphincter and pelvic floor. It also aims to establish balance and coordination of sacral reflexes. However, research findings do not consistently demonstrate immediate effectiveness of this treatment [48, 49].

3. Intermittent catheterisation: a procedure involving periodic insertion of a catheter into the bladder to empty urine, particularly useful in cases of urinary retention or incomplete bladder emptying.

4. Cognitive-behavioural therapy: addressing psychological factors influencing urinary function through therapeutic techniques aimed at modifying behaviour and thought patterns, including increasing motivation for treatment and adherence to urotherapy, alleviating stress and feelings of guilt associated with incontinence through counselling [46].

5. Psychotherapy: in-depth therapy sessions aimed at exploring and addressing psychological issues contributing to urinary problems. Urinary incontinence is frequently associated with attention deficit hyperactivity disorder and personality disorders [50].

6. Specific group programs: offering specialised group interventions tailored to children with unresponsive urinary disorders, providing support, education, and targeted interventions within a group setting.

7. Bedwetting alarm: the night waking alarm system activates when a sensor positioned in the underwear detects urine leakage. Upon activation, a loud sound signal prompts the child to wake up. The child is then expected to turn off the alarm, fully empty the bladder in the toilet, change clothes, and reinstall the sensor. This mechanism operates on the principle of a conditioned reflex. The ultimate objective is to develop an awareness of bladder fullness, suppress its immediate emptying, and consequently enhance the ability to retain urine during the night.

Effective treatment is greatly influenced by the motivation and cooperation of the child and the entire family [37].

These specific urotherapy approaches aim to address the unique needs of individuals with urinary disorders, employing a multidisciplinary approach to optimise treatment outcomes.

Urotherapy can be complemented and combined with pharmacological and surgical interventions, if needed.

Desmopressin is commonly prescribed in cases of persistent primary nocturnal enuresis that are unresponsive to urotherapy. It is an analog of antidiuretic hormone with extended action, functioning by promoting increased water reabsorption, resulting in urine with higher concentration and reduced volume. It is typically administered to the child in the evening, approximately 1 hour before bedtime. It is important for the child to refrain from drinking fluids for 1 hour before taking the medication and for 8 hours afterward. Desmopressin exclusively operates during the night it is administered, necessitating daily intake. Concurrently, adherence to standard urotherapy guidelines regarding fluid intake and urination is essential for optimal outcomes [37].

Pharmacological therapy is also indicated for daily micturition disorders with overactive bladder and bladder outlet obstruction. In the first case, muscarinic receptor blockers (oxybutynin, tolterodine, solifenacin, and propiverine) can be considered, and in the second case, alpha-adrenergic receptor blockers. In the treatment of overactive bladder, oxybutynin is most often used, but the others listed are also effective, however, are not yet approved for use in all countries. Adverse effects of treatment with muscarinic receptor blockers include dry mouth, facial flushing, tachycardia, difficulty concentrating, constipation, and visual disturbances [46]. Alpha-adrenergic receptor blockers also have limited approval, although their effectiveness has been proven. By blocking the alpha-adrenergic receptors in the area of the urinary bladder, they lower the outflow resistance from the bladder and improve its emptying. Adverse effects (hypotension, fatigue, and muscle weakness) are less pronounced when taking the drug in the morning [51, 52].

Surgical interventions for micturition disorders are infrequent in paediatric cases but may be considered for patients with genitourinary tract anomalies [53]. One potential option is the use of botulinum toxin, which can be applied in children with neurogenic bladder and in cases of non-neurogenic micturition disorders that do not respond to standard treatments [54].

4. Conclusions

UTI and micturition disorders are frequently encountered in paediatric nephrology. Both conditions can have long-term implications for a child's health. Achieving an accurate diagnosis can be challenging due to various factors that must be taken into consideration. Therefore, comprehensive management including prevention is essential, although preventive measures may be limited. A comprehensive approach is crucial for achieving optimal outcomes.

Conflict of interest

The authors declare no conflict of interest.

Author details

Mirjam Močnik[1]* and Nataša Marčun Varda[2]

1 Department of Paediatrics, University Medical Centre Maribor, Maribor, Slovenia

2 Department of Paediatrics, University Medical Centre Maribor and Medical Faculty, University of Maribor, Maribor, Slovenia

*Address all correspondence to: mirjammocnik91@gmail.com

References

[1] Tullus K, Shaikh N. Urinary tract infections in children. Lancet. 2020;**395**:1659-1668. DOI: 10.1016/S0140-6736(20)30676-0

[2] Bhat RG, Katy TA, Place FC. Pediatric urinary tract infections. Emergency Medicine Clinics of North America. 2011;**29**:637-653. DOI: 10.1016/j.emc.2011.04.004

[3] White B. Diagnosis and treatment of urinary tract infections in children. American Family Physician. 2011;**83**:409-415

[4] Simoes e Silva AC, Oliveira EA, Mak RH. Urinary tract infection in pediatrics: An overview. Journal de Pediatria. 2020;**96**:65-79. DOI: 10.1016/j.jped.2019.10.006

[5] Miyahara M, Osaki K, Aoki K. Unusual acute pediatric pyelonephritis presenting with cluster convulsions by possible central nervous system lesion: A case report. Cureus. 2022;**14**:e27654. DOI: 10.7759/cureus.27654

[6] Leung AKC, Wong AHC, Leung AAM, Hon KL. Urinary tract infection in children. Recent Patents on Inflammation & Allergy Drug Discovery. 2019;**13**:2-18. DOI: 10.2174/1872213X13666181228154940

[7] Shaikh N, Osio VA, Wessel CB, Jeong JH. Prevalence of asymptomatic bacteriuria in children: A meta-analysis. The Journal of Pediatrics. 2020;**217**:110-117.e4. DOI: 10.1016/j.jpeds.2019.10.019

[8] Nicolle LE, Gupta K, Bradley SF, Colgan R, DeMuri GP, Drekonja D, et al. Clinical practice guideline for the management of asymptomatic bacteriuria: 2019 update by the Infectious Diseases Society of America. Clinical Infectious Diseases. 2019;**68**:e83-e110. DOI: 10.1093/cid/ciy1121

[9] Doern CD, Richardson SE. Diagnosis of urinary tract infections in children. Journal of Clinical Microbiology. 2016;**54**:2233-2242. DOI: 10.1128/JCM.00189-16

[10] Roberts KB. Subcommittee on urinary tract infection, steering committee on quality improvement and management. Urinary tract infection: Clinical practice guideline for the diagnosis and management of the initial UTI in febrile infants and children 2 to 24 months. Pediatrics. 2011;**128**:595-610. DOI: 10.1542/peds.2011-1330

[11] Hoberman A, Wald ER, Reynolds EA, Penchansky L, Charron M. Pyuria and bacteriuria in urine specimens obtained by catheter from young children with fever. The Journal of Pediatrics. 1994;**124**:513-519. DOI: 10.1016/s0022-3476(05)83127-0

[12] Pitetti RD, Choi S. Utility of blood cultures in febrile children with UTI. The American Journal of Emergency Medicine. 2002;**20**:271-274. DOI: 10.1053/ajem.2002.33786

[13] Ayazi P, Mahyar A, Daneshi MM, Jahani Hashemi H, Pirouzi M, Esmailzadehha N. Diagnostic accuracy of the quantitative c-reactive protein, erythrocyte sedimentation rate and white blood cell count in urinary tract infections among infants and children. Malaysian Journal of Medical Sciences. 2013;**20**:40-46

[14] Yang SS, Tsai JD, Kanematsu A, Han CH. Asian guidelines for urinary tract infection in children. Journal of Infection and Chemotherapy.

2021;**27**:1543-1554. DOI: 10.1016/j.jiac.2021.07.014

[15] Nelson CP, Johnson EK, Logvinenko T, Chow JS. Ultrasound as a screening test for genitourinary anomalies in children with UTI. Pediatrics. 2014;**133**:e394-e403. DOI: 10.1542/peds.2013-2109

[16] Kolvenbach CM, Shril S, Hildebrandt F. The genetics and pathogenesis of CAKUT. Nature Reviews. Nephrology. 2023;**19**:709-720. DOI: 10.1038/s41581-023-00742-9

[17] Sim KC. Ultrasonography of acute flank pain: A focus on renal stones and acute pyelonephritis. Ultrasonography. 2018;**37**:345-354. DOI: 10.14366/usg.17051

[18] Bala KG, Chou YH. Ultrasonography of the urinary bladder. Journal of Medical Ultrasound. 2010;**18**:105-114. DOI: 10.1016/S0929-6441(10)60015-X

[19] Williams G, Craig JC. Long-term antibiotics for preventing recurrent urinary tract infection in children. Cochrane Database of Systematic Reviews. 2019;**4**:CD001534. DOI: 10.1002/14651858.CD001534.pub4

[20] Autore G, Bernardi L, Ghidini F, La Scola C, Berardi A, Biasucci G, et al. Antibiotic prophylaxis for the prevention of urinary tract infections in children: Guideline and recommendations from the Emilia-Romagna Pediatric Urinary Tract Infections (UTI-Ped-ER) Study Group. Antibiotics (Basel). 2023;**12**:1040. DOI: 10.3390/antibiotics12061040

[21] Meen J, Thomas CC, Kumar J, Raut S, Hari P. Non-antibiotic interventions for prevention of urinary tract infections in children: A systematic review and meta-analysis of randomized controlled trials. European Journal of Pediatrics. 2021;**180**:3535-3545. DOI: 10.1007/s00431-021-04091-2

[22] Williams G, Craig JC. Prevention of recurrent urinary tract infection in children. Current Opinion in Infectious Diseases. 2009;**22**:72-76. DOI: 10.1097/QCO.0b013e328320a885

[23] Cooper TE, Teng C, Howell M, Teixeira-Pinto A, Jaure A, Wong G. D-mannose for preventing and treating urinary tract infections. Cochrane Database of Systematic Reviews. 2022;**8**:CD013608. DOI: 10.1002/14651858.CD013608.pub2

[24] Mattoo TK, Shaikh N, Nelson CP. Contemporary management of urinary tract infection in children. Pediatrics. 2021;**147**:e2020012138. DOI: 10.1542/peds.2020-012138

[25] t Hoen LA, Bogaert G, Radmayr C, Dogan HS, RJM N, Quaedackers J, et al. Update of the EAU/ESPU guidelines on urinary tract infections in children. Journal of Pediatric Urology. 2021;**17**:200-207. DOI: 10.1016/j.jpurol.2021.01.037

[26] Nandagopal R, Vaidyanathan P, Kaplowitz P. Transient pseudohypoaldosteronism due to urinary tract infection in infancy: A report of 4 cases. International Journal of Pediatric Endocrinology. 2009;**2009**:195728. DOI: 10.1155/2009/195728

[27] Moreira MVB, de Freitas LR, Fonseca LM, Moreira MJB, Balieiro CCA, Marques IR, et al. Shorter versus longer-course of antibiotic therapy for urinary tract infections in pediatric population: An updated meta-analysis. European Journal of Pediatrics. 2024;**183**:2037-2047. DOI: 10.1007/s00431-024-05512-8

[28] Robinson JL, Le Saux N. Management of urinary tract infections in children

in an era of increasing antimicrobial resistance. Expert Review of Anti-Infective Therapy. 2016;**14**:809-816. DOI: 10.1080/14787210.2016.1206816

[29] Snodgrass WT, Shah A, Yang M, Kwon J, Villanueva C, Traylor J, et al. Prevalence and risk factors for renal scars in children with febrile UTI and/or VUR: A cross-sectional observational study of 565 consecutive patients. Journal of Pediatric Urology. 2013;**9**:856-863. DOI: 10.1016/j.jpurol.2012.11.019

[30] Mattoo TK. Vesicoureteral reflux and reflux nephropathy. Advances in Chronic Kidney Disease. 2011;**18**:348-354. DOI: 10.1053/j.ackd.2011.07.006

[31] Shaikh N, Mattoo TK, Keren R, Ivanova A, Cui G, Moxey-Mims M, et al. Early antibiotic treatment for pediatric febrile urinary tract infection and renal scarring. JAMA Pediatrics. 2016;**170**:848-854. DOI: 10.1001/jamapediatrics.2016.1181

[32] Baird DC, Seehusen DA, Bode DV. Enuresis in children: A case based approach. American Family Physician. 2014;**90**:560-568

[33] Austin PF, Bauer SB, Bower W, Chase J, Franco I, Hoebeke P, et al. The standardization of terminology of lower urinary tract function in children and adolescents: Update report from the Standardization Committee of the International Children's Continence Society. The Journal of Urology. 2014;**191**:1863-1865.e13. DOI: 10.1016/j.juro.2014.01.110

[34] Berk K, Powirtowska M, Blahuszewska A, Korzeniecka-Kozerska A. Retrospective evaluation of early risk factors in children with different types of micturition disorders. Acta Paediatrica. 2019;**108**:1151-1155. DOI: 10.1111/apa.14659

[35] Azhir A, Frajzadegan Z, Adibi A, Hedayatpoor B, Fazel A, Divband A. An epidemiological study of enuresis among primary school children in Isfahan, Iran. Saudi Medical Journal. 2006;**27**:1572-1577

[36] Vande Walle J, Rittig S, Bauer S, Eggert P, Marschall-Kehrel D, Tekgul S, et al. Practical consensus guidelines for the management of enuresis. European Journal of Pediatrics. 2012;**171**:971-983. DOI: 10.1007/s00431-012-1687-7

[37] Tu ND, Baskin LS, Arnhym AM. Nocturnal enuresis in children: Etiology and evaluation. 2024. Available from: https://www.uptodate.com/contents/nocturnal-enuresis-in-children-etiology-and-evaluation

[38] Butler RJ, Golding J, Northstone K, ALSPAC Study Team. Nocturnal enuresis at 7.5 years old: Prevalence and analysis of clinical signs. BJU International. 2005;**96**:404-410. DOI: 10.1111/j.1464-410X.2005.05640.x

[39] Swithinbank LV, Heron J, von Gontard A, Abrams P. The natural history of daytime urinary incontinence in children: A large British cohort. Acta Paediatrica. 2010;**99**:1031-1036. DOI: 10.1111/j.1651-2227.2010.01739.x

[40] Sureshkumar P, Jones M, Cumming R, Craig J. A population based study of 2,856 school-age children with urinary incontinence. The Journal of Urology. 2009;**181**:808-815. DOI: 10.1016/j.juro.2008.10.044

[41] Neveus T, Eggert P, Evans J, Macedo A, Rittig S, Tekgül S, et al. Evaluation of and treatment for monosymptomatic enuresis: A standardization document from the International Children's Continence Society. The Journal of Urology. 2010;**183**:441-447. DOI: 10.1016/j.juro.2009.10.043

[42] Haid B, Tekgül S. Primary and secondary enuresis: Pathophysiology, diagnosis, and treatment. European Urology Focus. 2017;**3**:198-206. DOI: 10.1016/j.euf.2017.08.010

[43] Breinbjerg A, Jørgensen CS, Borg B, Rittig S, Kamperis K, Christensen JH. The genetics of incontinence: A scoping review. Clinical Genetics. 2023;**104**:22-62. DOI: 10.1111/cge.14331

[44] Rogers J. Daytime wetting in children and acquisition of bladder control. Nursing Children and Young People. 2013;**25**:26-33. DOI: 10.7748/ncyp2013.07.25.6.26.e195

[45] Nieuwhof-Leppink AJ, Hussong J, Chase J, Larsson J, Renson C, Hoebeke P, et al. Definitions, indications and practice of urotherapy in children and adolescents: A standardization document of the International Children's Continence Society (ICCS). Journal of Pediatric Urology. 2021;**17**:172-181. DOI: 10.1016/j.jpurol.2020.11.006

[46] Chang SJ, Van Laecke E, Bauer SB, von Gontard A, Bagli D, Bower WF, et al. Treatment of daytime urinary incontinence: A standardization document from the International Children's Continence Society. Neurourology and Urodynamics. 2017;**36**:43-50. DOI: 10.1002/nau.22911

[47] Koenig JF, McKenna PH. Biofeedback therapy for dysfunctional voiding in children. Current Urology Reports. 2011;**12**:144-152. DOI: 10.1007/s11934-010-0166-9

[48] O'Sullivan H, Kelly G, Toale J, Cascio S. Comparing the outcomes of parasacral transcutaneous electrical nerve stimulation for the treatment of lower urinary tract dysfunction in children: A systematic review and meta-analysis of randomized controlled trials. Neurourology and Urodynamics. 2021;**40**:570-581. DOI: 10.1002/nau.24601

[49] Borch L, Rittig S, Kamperis K, Mahler B, Djurhuus JC, Hagstroem S. No immediate effect on urodynamic parameters during transcutaneous electrical nerve stimulation (TENS) in children with overactive bladder and daytime incontinence—A randomized, double-blind, placebo-controlled study. Neurourology and Urodynamics. 2017;**36**:1788-1795. DOI: 10.1002/nau.23179

[50] von Gontard A, Baeyens D, Van Hoecke E, Warzak WJ, Bachmann C. Psychological and psychiatric issues in urinary and fecal incontinence. The Journal of Urology. 2011;**185**:1432-1436. DOI: 10.1016/j.juro.2010.11.051

[51] Kramer SA, Rathbun SR, Elkins D, Karnes RJ, Husmann DA. Double-blind placebo controlled study of alpha-adrenergic receptor antagonists (doxazosin) for treatment of voiding dysfunction in the pediatric population. The Journal of Urology. 2005;**173**:2121-2124. DOI: 10.1097/01.ju.0000157689.98314.69

[52] Austin P. The role of alpha blockers in children with dysfunctional voiding. Scientific World Journal. 2009;**9**:880-883. DOI: 10.1100/tsw.2009.98

[53] Nakamura S, Kawai S, Kubo T, Kihara T, Mori K, Nakai H. Transurethral incision of congenital obstructive lesions in the posterior urethra in boys and its effect on urinary incontinence and urodynamic study. BJU International. 2011;**107**:1304-1311. DOI: 10.1111/j.1464-410X.2010.09578.x

[54] Hassouna T, Gleason JM, Lorenzo AJ. Botulinum toxin A's expanding role in the management of pediatric lower urinary tract dysfunction. Current Urology Reports. 2014;**15**:426. DOI: 10.1007/s11934-014-0426-1

Section 4

Common Disorders of Upper Respiratory Disorders in Children

Chapter 5

Common Ear, Nose, and Throat Disorders in Childhood

Dharanya Srinivasan and Kalaiarasi Raja

Abstract

This chapter provides a comprehensive overview of the most prevalent Ear, Nose, and Throat (ENT) disorders encountered in pediatric populations. Drawing insights from medical literature, the chapter delves into the multifaceted landscape of ENT disorders affecting children, exploring their etiology, clinical manifestations, diagnostic approaches, and contemporary management strategies. The discussion encompasses a wide spectrum of conditions, including otitis media, adenotonsillitis, and pediatric stridor. Emphasis is placed on the unique challenges posed by these disorders in the pediatric population, considering factors that affect physical and psychosocial development and age-specific treatment considerations. This chapter also highlights the importance of interdisciplinary collaboration between pediatricians, otolaryngologists, and other healthcare professionals in delivering optimal care for children with ENT disorders. Through a synthesis of evidence-based recommendations and practical clinical insights, this chapter aims to serve as a valuable resource for healthcare practitioners and medical students involved in the care of pediatric patients with ENT conditions.

Keywords: adenotonsillitis, acute otitis media, pediatric stridor, hearing loss, otitis media with effusion

1. Introduction

Children, with their unique physiology and evolving immune systems, are predisposed to a spectrum of Ear, Nose, and Throat (ENT) disorders that demand a specialized approach. Within the realm of pediatric healthcare, the intricate dynamics of ENT disorders play a significant role in shaping their overall health and quality of life. This chapter aims to illuminate the landscape of common ENT disorders in childhood, providing a nuanced understanding of the intricate interplay between pediatric anatomy and physiology and the myriad challenges that can arise in this vulnerable population. Etiopathogenesis, clinical manifestations, and contemporary management strategies of common ENT disorders affecting the pediatric population have also been discussed.

This chapter encompasses a diverse array of conditions, including acute otitis media, evaluation and management of pediatric stridor, and adenotonsillitis. A holistic and interdisciplinary approach between pediatricians, otolaryngologists, audiologists, and other healthcare professionals is essential in navigating the intricate web of symptoms, diagnostic considerations, and treatment modalities.

2. Acute otitis media

2.1 Definition

Acute otitis media (AOM) is defined as the rapid onset of signs and symptoms, such as otalgia and fever, due to acute inflammation of the middle ear cleft. Symptoms include pain in the ear, ear discharge, irritability, insomnia, and anorexia. Signs include fever, otorrhea, erythema of the tympanic membrane (TM), full or bulging opaque TM, and impaired TM mobility [1].

It emerges as a widely prevalent condition in early childhood, often leading to referral to otolaryngologists. While the majority of primary healthcare providers effectively manage most AOM cases, children experiencing recurring episodes, severe symptoms, or AOM-related complications which may need swift evaluation by otolaryngologists, potentially leading to surgical interventions. Despite the widespread occurrence of AOM and the use of tympanostomy tubes, achieving a consensus on the optimal surgical approach for children with AOM remains an ongoing challenge.

As we delve into the key concepts in the management of AOM in children, we particularly focus on the evolving microbiological trend observed over the past 2 decades. Emphasis is placed on the crucial aspect of accurate diagnosis, employing stringent criteria and refining the selection of children deemed suitable for observation without immediate antibiotic intervention upon initial AOM diagnosis.

2.2 Epidemiology

AOM stands as a major health concern among children, with substantial implications for both public health and healthcare expenditure in many countries. Peak incidence is between 6 and 24 months of age [2, 3]. AOM incidence rates vary across different age groups, reflecting the susceptibility and prevalence within each demographic. Incidence rates range from 20 to 30% or higher in children less than 2 years of age, depending on geographical and socioeconomic factors [4]. AOM remains common in preschool-aged children, although the incidence tends to decrease slightly compared to infants. Incidence rates in this age group typically range from 15 to 25%, with variations influenced by factors such as exposure to environmental pathogens and daycare attendance [5]. The incidence of AOM tends to decline further in school-going children between 6 and 12 years of age, with incidence rates ranging from 5 to 15% [6]. AOM is less common in adolescents and adults compared to younger age groups. Incidence rates in adolescents and adults are generally lower, often falling below 5% [7]. Another postulated reason for the decline is that as children become older, maturation of their immune system occurs. It is important to understand that these incidence rates may vary based on geographical location, socioeconomic factors, access to healthcare, vaccination rates, and other variables. Additionally, modifications in antibiotic prescribing practices and the prevalence of bacterial strains resistant to antibiotics can influence AOM incidence rates over time.

Antibiotics, prescribed more frequently for AOM than any other childhood illness, play a central role in its management [8]. The epidemiology of AOM has witnessed

DOI: http://dx.doi.org/10.5772/intechopen.1006071

noteworthy changes in trends over the past decade. Despite the prevalence of the condition, there has been a decrease in physician visits for suspected AOM globally and in the United States [5, 9]. The reasons for this decline are multifaceted, potentially influenced by public awareness campaigns regarding the viral etiology and mode of spread of Upper Respiratory Tract Infections (URTI) and the launch of vaccines such as the 7-valent pneumococcal vaccine (PCV7) and influenza vaccines [10]. The dissemination and adoption of best clinical practices and guidelines may also have contributed to the observed decrease in clinician visits.

2.3 Pathophysiology

AOM frequently, though not always, arises following a viral URTI [11]. Inflammatory processes cause edema in the nasal cavities and nasopharynx, leading to blockage of the eustachian tube. This obstruction leads to the development of negative pressure in the middle ear, followed by middle ear effusion. Microbe-laden secretions from the nasal and nasopharyngeal mucosa migrate into the middle ear due to the pressure differential, becoming entrapped and potentially fostering bacterial replication and infection. Young children face an elevated risk for AOM due to heightened viral exposure, immunological naivety, and inherent eustachian tube dysfunction [12]. Recurrent attacks of sore throat, URTIs, and exanthematous fevers like measles, diphtheria or whooping cough, adenotonsillitis, chronic rhinosinusitis, allergic rhinitis, cleft palate can act as predisposing factors.

The 2013 American Academy of Pediatrics (AAP) guidelines advocate for various preventive health interventions to decrease the incidence of AOM. Over the past 2 decades, the microbiology of AOM has transformed and been influenced by the widespread adoption of pneumococcal vaccination programs. Despite *Streptococcus pneumoniae*, nontypeable *Haemophilus influenza*, and *Moraxella catarrhalis* persisting as the major bacterial culprits, the introduction of the heptavalent PCV7 in 2000 led to a decline in the recovery of *Streptococcus pneumoniae* in AOM cases. However, nonvaccine pneumococcal serotypes have emerged in tympanocentesis and nasopharyngeal colonization studies, equating the incidence of *Streptococcus pneumoniae* with that of *Hemophilus influenza*, while *Moraxella catarrhalis* becomes less frequent. The subsequent licensing of the 13-valent *Streptococcus pneumoniae* vaccine (PCV13) in 2010 is expected to further modify the microbiological landscape of AOM. PCV7 vaccination led to a decline in physician visits for AOM, though subsequent serotype replacement emerged, necessitating consideration for PCV13 vaccination [13–16]. Furthermore, the influenza vaccine is advised for children above 6 months of age. Given the association between influenza and AOM, particularly due to upper respiratory mucosa inflammation, the influenza vaccine can significantly decrease the frequency of AOM with approximately 55% efficacy.

2.4 Pathological stages of AOM and clinical features

2.4.1 Stage of tubal occlusion

The initial phase involves tubal occlusion, marked by nasopharyngeal edema obstructing the eustachian tube, resulting in negative intratympanic pressure. TM retraction and subtle effusion characterize this stage, accompanied by minor symptoms of deafness and earache without notable fever.

2.4.2 Stage of presuppuration

Advancing to the presuppuration stage, prolonged tubal occlusion invites pyogenic organisms, instigating inflammation in the middle ear. Intense earache, deafness, and tinnitus become prominent, with a feverish and restless child. Signs include a congested TM and a cart-wheel appearance due to blood vessel prominence. Tuning fork tests confirm conductive deafness (**Figure 1**).

2.4.3 Stage of suppuration

The subsequent suppuration stage is characterized by the formation of pus in the mastoid air cell system and middle ear, causing excruciating otalgia, increased hard of hearing, and potential fever. TM bulging indicates imminent rupture with a visible yellow spot.

2.4.4 Stage of resolution

Resolution follows TM rupture, leading to symptom relief as pus is evacuated. Patients may present with blood-stained discharge, progressing to mucopurulent, with a small perforation visible. The hyperemia diminishes, returning the membrane to a normal appearance.

2.4.5 Stage of complications

Complications may arise if the infection persists, extending beyond the confines of the middle ear and mastoid air cell system. Intratemporal complications such as acute mastoiditis, subperiosteal abscess, facial paralysis, labyrinthitis, petrositis, and

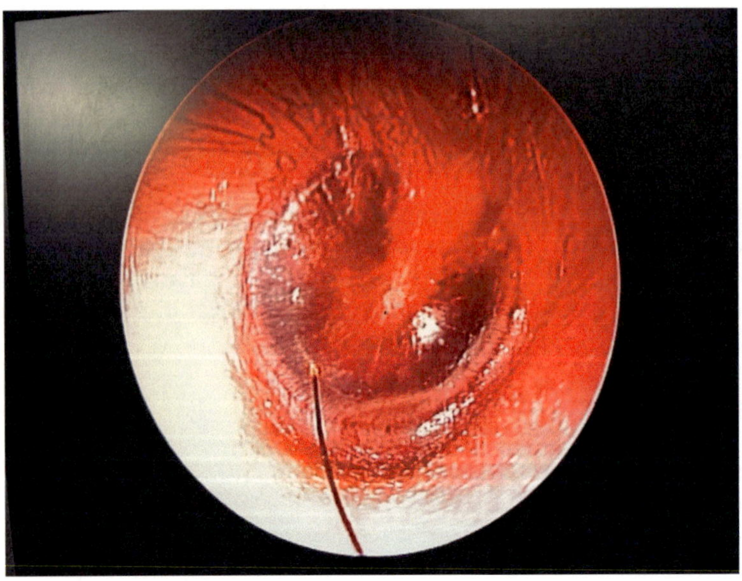

Figure 1.
Stage of presuppuration of AOM—signs of congested tympanic membrane with prominent blood vessels are shown.

intracranial complications such as extradural abscess, meningitis, brain abscess, or lateral sinus thrombophlebitis can manifest in cases of high virulence or poor patient resistance. Vigilant management is crucial to prevent such complications.

2.5 Diagnosis

The diagnosis of AOM poses significant challenges owing to the absence of a definitive gold standard diagnostic method apart from tympanocentesis and culture of middle ear fluid. The lack of a diagnostic benchmark fuels ongoing debate regarding the most accurate clinical means of identifying acute middle ear infections. The complexity arises from the diverse array of clinical presentations that evolve throughout the disease course, compounded by practical difficulties in examining the ears of young children, potentially uncooperative children, particularly when cerumen occlusion is present. Furthermore, the symptomatology of AOM, including fever, otalgia, irritability, and insomnia, often overlap with manifestations of other conditions, such as viral illnesses, further complicating diagnosis. In light of these diagnostic challenges, it becomes imperative to adopt a nuanced approach that integrates clinical judgment with available diagnostic tools and considers individual patient characteristics.

The initial step in diagnosing otitis media involves a thorough physical examination, including the use of an otoscope, preferably a pneumatic otoscopy. Laboratory studies are typically unnecessary. Imaging studies are generally not recommended unless there are concerns about intratemporal or intracranial complications. However, if complications are suspected, high-resolution computed tomography (HRCT) of the temporal bones can identify various conditions, such as mastoiditis, meningitis, or sigmoid sinus thrombophlebitis. Additionally, contrast-enhanced CT of the brain can be combined to rule out intracranial complications. Tympanocentesis, though reserved for extreme or refractory cases, may be employed to confirm the presence of middle ear fluid and to culture pathogens. Additionally, tests like tympanometry and acoustic reflectometry can aid in evaluating middle-ear effusion.

Employing otoscopy, preferably pneumatic otoscopy, and tympanometry, in conjunction with a thorough assessment of symptoms and medical history can improve diagnostic precision. The 2013 AAP guidelines on managing an AOM underscored diagnostic criteria centered on otoscopic examination. This marked a more stringent approach compared to the 2004 guidelines, with a focus on achieving greater diagnostic accuracy. According to the 2013 guidelines, diagnosing AOM is crucial and justified in children presenting with *moderate to severe bulging of the TM, new onset of otorrhea, or mild TM bulging accompanied by recent ear pain or notable TM erythema*. Importantly, the guidelines specify that AOM should not be diagnosed unless middle-ear effusion is present [17–21]. The guidelines also suggested various terminologies of AOM based on severity:

- *Uncomplicated AOM*—AOM without otorrhea
- *Severe AOM*—AOM with the presence of moderate to severe otalgia *or* fever equal to or higher than 39°C
- *Nonsevere AOM*—AOM with the presence of mild otalgia and a temperature below 39°C [17]

2.6 Treatment

2.6.1 Antibiotics of choice and duration

Every infant under 2 years old showing clinical features of AOM should be administered an antibiotic effective against the three primary bacterial pathogens that are implicated in AOM, *S. pneumoniae*, *H. influenzae*, and *M. catarrhalis*. Children above the age of 2 years who have "severe" AOM (i.e., moderate to severe otalgia or fever ≥39°C) should also receive antimicrobial therapy. The option of observation may be considered for a child older than 2 years who has "nonsevere" AOM (i.e., mild otalgia and fever <39°C in the past 24 hours) (**Table 1**).

High-dose amoxicillin, administered at a dosage of 80–90 mg/kg per day, stands as the recommended first-line treatment in the 2013 guidelines for AOM.

For individuals sensitive to penicillin, second- or third-generation cephalosporins, including intramuscular ceftriaxone, represent viable alternatives. Additional agents, particularly relevant for penicillin-sensitive patients or instances of amoxicillin failure, include second and third-generation cephalosporins and clindamycin. Patients exhibiting no improvement within 48–72 hours of their initial treatment regimen should undergo reassessment, with consideration given to alternative therapy. In these situations, the primary treatment choices typically include amoxicillin-clavulanate and intramuscular or intravenous ceftriaxone. Second-line options may involve clindamycin alone or combination therapy using clindamycin along with a third-generation cephalosporin. In challenging cases, tympanocentesis may be contemplated for drainage and culture-directed therapy [17, 22].

2.6.2 Supportive therapy

Analgesics: Once the diagnosis of acute otitis media is established, the goal of treatment is pain management and antibiotics to curb the infectious process. Nonsteroidal anti-inflammatory drugs (NSAIDs) such as acetaminophen and ibuprofen can be used to achieve pain control.

Decongestant nasal drops and antipyretics with antihistaminics are added to reduce edema and congestion of the Eustachian tube and tackle pain.

Tympanostomy tubes or ventilation tubes, also known as grommets, are tubes inserted in the TM following myringotomy (radial incision made in the anteroinferior

Age (months)	Certain diagnosis*	Uncertain diagnosis
<6	• Antibiotics	• Antibiotics
6–24	• Antibiotics	• Antibiotics if severe • Observe if not severe
>24	• Antibiotics if severe • Observe if not severe**	• Observe

**Certain diagnoses: middle-ear effusion, rapid onset, and middle-ear inflammation.*
***Nonsevere: mild otalgia; temperature <39°C orally or <39.5°C rectally in past 24 hours.*
Adapted from Refs. [17, 18].

Table 1.
Guidelines for management of acute otitis media—American Academy of Pediatrics and American Academy of Family Physicians.

quadrant of TM) and are meant to improve middle-ear ventilation. These are specifically recommended for children "at risk" of developing acute otitis media such as children with craniofacial syndromes, cleft palate, and Down's syndrome [23].

3. Pediatric stridor

3.1 Definition

Stridor, a high-pitched sound during breathing, is a clinical sign rather than a diagnosis, often signaling partial airway obstruction in children [24].

Stridor warrants careful evaluation to determine its cause and severity. In this section, we review the evolving landscape of various causes of pediatric stridor coupled with its evaluation and management.

3.2 Epidemiology

Pediatric stridor has a varied epidemiology influenced by age, geographic location, and underlying etiologies. In infancy, the overall incidence of stridor is estimated to be around 1–2% in the general population. Laryngomalacia, a congenital anomaly characterized by supraglottic collapse during inspiration, is the most common cause of stridor in infants, accounting for approximately 60–75% of cases. Other congenital anomalies such as vocal cord paralysis, subglottic stenosis, laryngeal webs, atresia, and subglottic hemangiomas contribute to a smaller proportion of cases. In older children, infectious or inflammatory conditions like croup and epiglottitis are more prevalent causes of stridor. Croup peaks in its incidence between 6 and 36 months of age, contributing to approximately 3,50,000–4,00,000 annual casualty visits related to the condition. Annually, croup affects approximately 2–6% of infants and children, with a slightly higher prevalence observed among males, at a ratio of 1.4:1, compared to females. Additionally, foreign body aspiration accounts for over 17,000 emergency department visits yearly in the United States, predominantly affecting children under the age of 3 [25–28].

3.3 Pathophysiology and etiology

The physics of stridor involves Poiseuille's law and the Bernoulli principle. Changes in airway radius, as seen in conditions like laryngomalacia, result in turbulent airflow and negative pressure, leading to airway collapse and the characteristic stridor sound [28]. Stridor can originate at various levels of the airway, such as the supraglottis, glottis, subglottis, and trachea, each presenting unique characteristics. Inspiratory stridor suggests a supraglottic or glottic etiology, expiratory stridor is typically due to a tracheal or bronchial obstruction, and biphasic stridor generally indicates subglottic pathology (**Figure 2**) [29].

Causes can range from a transient and benign condition to a critical manifestation of impending respiratory failure (**Table 2**). Laryngomalacia, a common cause of neonatal stridor, may require supraglottoplasty for severe cases. Vocal cord paralysis, whether unilateral or bilateral, presents with varying degrees of airway obstruction and may necessitate surgical interventions. Croup, recurrent croup, subglottic stenosis, and subglottic hemangioma are among the infectious, inflammatory, or structural causes that clinicians consider in the differential diagnosis.

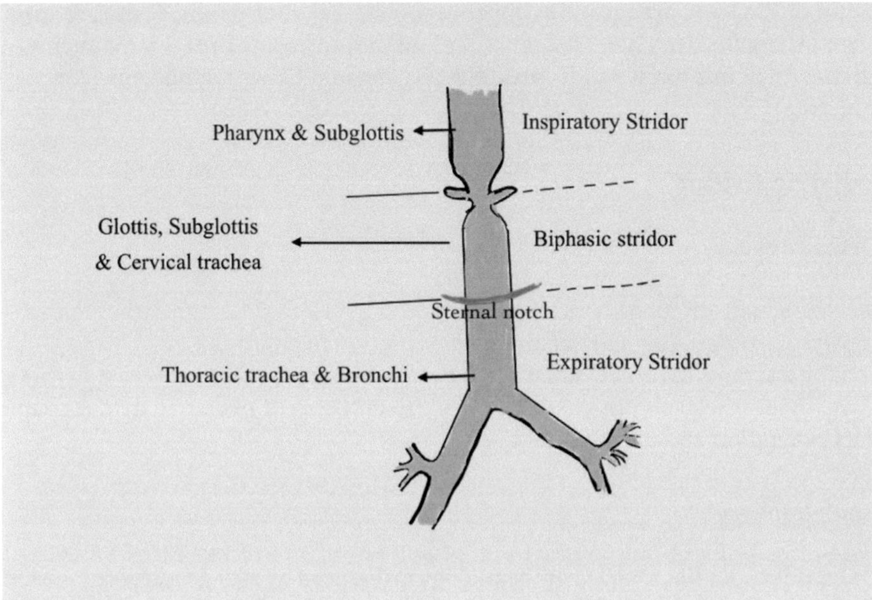

Figure 2.
Types of stridor.

3.4 Laryngomalacia

Laryngomalacia is a common congenital condition characterized by the collapse of the supraglottic structures during inspiration, leading to airway obstruction. It is the most common cause of stridor in infants and typically manifests within the first few weeks of life. It affects approximately 1 in 2000 live births. While the exact etiology remains unclear, it is believed to result from immaturity or softness of the laryngeal cartilages, leading to dynamic collapse during breathing.

Clinical features of laryngomalacia include high-pitched inspiratory stridor, which worsens with agitation, crying, feeding, or supine positioning noticed before 2 weeks of age. Typically, the noisy breathing subsides when the child is placed in the prone position. Infants may also exhibit retractions, feeding difficulties, failure to thrive, and occasionally, cyanosis or apnea episodes. Diagnosis is primarily clinical, based on history and physical examination, although flexible laryngoscopy may be performed to confirm the diagnosis and evaluate the severity of airway collapse.

Management of laryngomalacia is typically conservative, with reassurance and supportive care for mild cases. However, severe cases may require intervention to alleviate airway obstruction and improve symptoms. This can include positioning techniques, such as prone or lateral positioning during sleep, to optimize airway patency. Surgical intervention, such as supraglottoplasty, may be considered for severe and refractory cases or those associated with significant feeding difficulties, failure to thrive, and obstructive sleep apnea [27, 30–34].

3.5 Acute epiglottitis

This acute condition is caused by *Hemophilus influenzae b*. Though there is a rapid decline in the incidence due to widespread vaccination with *Hemophilus influenzae b*,

Pharynx/hypopharynx
• Vallecular cyst • Vascular malformation • Laryngopharyngeal reflux
Supraglottis
• Laryngomalacia • Laryngoscope • Acute epiglottitis • Vascular malformation • Stenosis
Glottis
• Vocal cord paralysis (Bilateral > unilateral) • Intubation injury • Laryngeal cleft • Glottic web • Stenosis • Laryngeal trauma
Subglottis
• Subglottic hemangioma • Croup • Intubation granuloma • Acquired stenosis • Cyst • Congenital cricoid malformation • Foreign body
Tracheobronchus
• Tracheomalacia • Foreign body • Complete tracheal rings • Stenosis • Vascular compression • Bacterial tracheitis • Neck/chest mass

Table 2.
Causes of stridor based on anatomical subsites.

a high level of suspicion to diagnose this condition should be present as it is an acute airway emergency. After widespread *Hemophilus influenzae* vaccination, group A β-hemolytic Streptococci infections have surpassed *Hemophilus influenzae type B* (Hib) as the predominant cause of acute epiglottitis, with variations in occurrence and management between children and adults.

Clinical presentation is classic with a 2–7-year-old with sudden occurrence of high-grade fever, difficulty in swallowing, and severe sore throat. The child appears to be toxic and stridulous with drooling of saliva, assuming a *Tripod position* (sitting up with neck in extension and leaning forward position using arms to support shoulder girdle aid in breathing). Lateral radiograph of soft tissue neck reveals *"thumb sign,"* which is severe inflammation of epiglottis with potential for imminent airway compromise. When acute epiglottitis is suspected, pharyngeal examination with tongue depressor is contraindicated as it may precipitate airway obstruction, although fibreoptic airway endoscopy done in a controlled pediatric Intensive care setting can aid in diagnosis.

Management is to secure the airway by endotracheal intubation by experienced personnel in the intensive care unit set up. Definitive treatment includes intravenous antibiotics (third-generation cephalosporins) until the swelling of the epiglottis reduces, usually within 36 hours [35–38].

3.6 Croup

Acute laryngotracheal bronchitis (croup) stands out as the primary culprit behind acute stridor in young children and toddlers, often stemming from a viral infection caused by parainfluenza viruses I (most common), II, and III accounting for 80% of cases affecting the larynx and upper trachea. The virus infects the epithelial cells of laryngotracheal mucosa, causing edema and glandular over-secretion. Pathognomonic signs include stridor accompanied by a distinctive barking cough and upper respiratory infection. Diagnosis is further confirmed by the characteristic radiographic "steeple sign," obviating the need for laryngoscopy in most cases. Westley Croup scoring system is used for indicating disease severity in which higher scores are given for the presence of cyanosis and altered mental status (**Table 3**). Treatment strategies encompass supportive measures like oxygenation, humidification with nebulized epinephrine, and intravenous corticosteroids. Intravenous corticosteroids are the mainstay of treatment as exert a systemic anti-inflammatory effect and reduction in mucosal edema. Nebulized epinephrine not only reduces mucosal edema by its alpha agonistic effect causing vasoconstriction but also aids in bronchodilatation [39, 40].

However, recurrent croup can signal an underlying anatomical airway issue, heightening the risk of persistent stridor due to a narrowed airway. Conditions such as subglottic cysts, hemangiomas, or congenital stenosis may contribute to persistent stridor characterized by a narrow airway diameter. Chronic inflammation of the upper airway from gastrointestinal sources, particularly eosinophilic esophagitis (EoE), has also been linked to recurrent croup. When recurrent croup intensifies in severity and frequency, especially with age, further investigation through airway endoscopy is recommended. This may unveil subtle structural abnormalities, like grade 1 subglottic stenosis, and identify inflammatory triggers that exacerbate symptoms [41–43].

Pinpointing these inflammatory triggers can be challenging, and while most children naturally outgrow croup symptoms as their airways mature, recurrent cases should prompt a closer look. Parents are crucial partners in this process, requiring reassurance and guidance. In cases where no serious structural abnormality is identified, parents can be encouraged to seek symptomatic relief. Some children may benefit from steroid prescriptions to control symptoms and prevent hospitalization, but careful monitoring and limitation of steroid usage frequency are essential.

Distinguishing features between croup and epiglottitis is included in **Table 4**.

S. no	Indicator of disease severity	Level of severity	Score
1.	Stridor	None	0
		Only with agitation/excitement	1
		At rest with stethoscope	2
		At rest without stethoscope	3
2.	Retraction	None	0
		Mild	1
		Moderate	2
		Severe	3
3.	Air entry	Normal	0
		Decreased	1
		Severely decreased	2
4.	Cyanosis	None	0
		With agitation	4
		At rest	5
5.	Level of consciousness	Normal	0
		Altered mental status	5

Mild respiratory distress = score <3; moderate respiratory distress = score 3–6; severe respiratory distress = score >6.

Table 3.
Westley croup scoring system.

S. no	Clinical features	Croup	Epiglottitis
1.	Age	1–2 years	2–7 years
2.	Cause	Parainfluenza viruses	*Hemophilus influenzae b*
3.	Prodrome	1–2 days Coryza	Rapid onset within hours with sore throat, dysphagia, drooling
4.	Fever	<38°C	>38°C
5.	Appearance	Lethargic	Pale and toxic, drooling and dysphagia, sitting with neck extended (*Tripod position*)
6.	Stridor	Barking cough, loud stridor	Muffled stridor
7.	Hypoxia	Unusual	Frequent
8.	Severity	<5% of hospitalized cases require intubation	All patients require intubation

Table 4.
Distinguishing features between croup and epiglottitis.

3.7 Observation and initial evaluation

The assessment of a stridulous patient begins with a thorough history, focusing on the onset, duration, and accompanying symptoms. Assessment should be done as quickly as possible. The pediatric assessment triangle encompasses appearance,

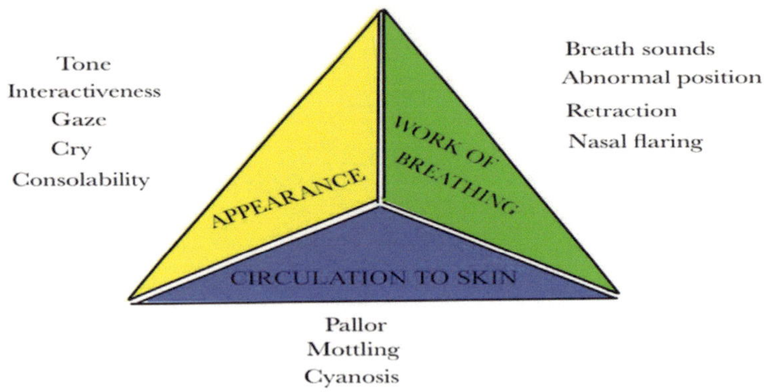

Figure 3.
Pediatric assessment triangle.

work of breathing, and circulation to skin (**Figure 3**). Acute-onset stridor is often associated with infectious, inflammatory, or foreign body causes, while chronic or gradual onset may be indicative of stable but restricted airways. In the emergency department, clinicians prioritize assessing vital signs, most importantly oxygenation, pulse rate, respiratory rate and effort. Airway and chest radiographs are performed to identify the level of obstruction, and a rapid evaluation helps determine the need for urgent intervention [44].

3.8 Physical examination

Observation of the phase of stridor in concurrence with the respiratory cycle, combined with struggling respiratory effort, aids in identifying patients at risk for impending respiratory failure. Retractions in the suprasternal and intercostal regions along with the use of accessory muscles of respiration indicate increased respiratory effort. Mental status changes suggest advancing hypoxia or hypercarbia. A comprehensive head and neck examination helps pinpoint the source of stridor, considering conditions like micrognathia, hemangiomas, or facial masses [27].

3.9 Diagnostic modalities

Diagnostic radiography, including airway radiographs and advanced imaging like CT or MRI, plays a crucial role in identifying airway lesions and evaluating anatomical abnormalities. Multidisciplinary assessments involving otolaryngologists, pulmonologists, and gastroenterologists contribute to a comprehensive understanding of the patient's condition. Awake fiberoptic nasopharyngoscopy and laryngoscopy provide real-time visualization, aiding in the diagnosis of conditions such as laryngomalacia, vocal cord paralysis, and laryngopharyngeal reflux.

3.10 Prevention

Preventive measures, such as widespread influenza vaccination, have significantly reduced the occurrence of acute epiglottitis. Despite a decline in neonatal-acquired subglottic stenosis due to improved intubation practices, surviving infants may have complex medical comorbidities affecting their management.

3.11 Treatment approaches

Fiberoptic airway endoscopy is a significant advancement in addressing obstructive airway diseases and emphasizes the need for collaborative efforts among pediatricians, anesthetists, and otorhinolaryngologists as it has to be performed in a controlled setting. Thus, integrating airway endoscopy into existing management protocols for childhood stridor is essential.

Treatment modalities are tailored according to the specific etiologies and the severity of the disease condition. Initial management often includes assessment of airway patency and oxygenation, followed by interventions to alleviate airway obstruction. Securing the airway is the most crucial step in managing various causes of pediatric stridor. Laryngomalacia management ranges from conservative management for mild cases of laryngomalacia to surgical interventions like supraglottoplasty for severe laryngomalacia. Following airway control, Acute epiglottitis is treated with IV antibiotics and croup is managed with intravenous corticosteroids and nebulized racemic epinephrine. Procedures such as adenotonsillectomy, supraglottoplasty, or airway reconstruction may be performed depending on the specific diagnosis and anatomical considerations.

Overall, the management of pediatric stridor requires a multidisciplinary approach involving pediatricians, otolaryngologists, anesthesiologists, and respiratory therapists to ensure appropriate assessment and treatment tailored to the individual child's needs [38–40, 44].

3.12 Conclusion

Pediatric stridor demands a comprehensive and multidisciplinary approach for accurate diagnosis and optimal management. Timely recognition of potential airway compromise is crucial to prevent respiratory failure and associated complications. Advances in diagnostic techniques and treatment modalities, coupled with a collaborative effort among various medical specialties, contribute to improved outcomes for children with stridor. Early intervention and a tailored treatment plan can significantly impact the quality of life for affected individuals and alleviate the potential risks associated with upper airway obstruction [45].

4. Adenotonsillitis

4.1 Applied anatomy

Palatine tonsils are paired lymphoid structures that are located in the lateral wall of the oropharynx between the anterior and posterior pillars. The anterior pillar is constituted by the palatoglossus muscle and the palatopharyngeus muscle constitutes the posterior pillar. Each tonsil has a medial and a lateral surface, with the medial surface covered by nonkeratinizing stratified squamous epithelium. This epithelium intends into the tonsillar substance forming crypts. Crypta magna is the most prominent crypt which represents the embryological origin, ventral part of the second pharyngeal pouch. The lateral surface of the tonsil is covered by a well-defined fibrous capsule with an intervening loose areolar tissue between the capsule and the bed of the tonsil. These whitish fibrous strands represent the plane of dissection during tonsillectomy [46, 47].

4.2 Blood supply of tonsil

The arterial supply of tonsil is depicted in **Figure 4**. Tonsillar branch of facial artery is the main arterial supply of tonsil. Venous drainage from the tonsils enters the paratonsillar vein which then joins the common facial vein and pharyngeal venous plexus.

4.3 Developmental anatomy

It encompasses the immunological activation timeline, structural modifications, enlargements, and involution processes. Understanding the fetal development and alterations within the first 10 years of age can assist in making informed surgical decisions (**Table 1**).

During intrauterine development, the tonsil's epithelium covering the medial surface and crypts originates from the second branchial pouch. Solid epithelial cores form in the lateral walls of these pouches, branching into primary and secondary tonsillar crypts. Mature crypt epithelium, revealed by transmission electron microscopy, is porous, allowing lymphocytes to *mediate immune responses.*

Pharyngeal tonsils which are a part of the mucosa-associated lymphoid tissue, develop monocellular populations similar to Peyer's patches in the gut. Lymphocytes invade the lamina propria around the 16th week postconception. The tonsil lacks afferent lymphatics, with dendritic cells in crypt epithelium transporting antigens.

Immune stimulation begins postnatally, leading to terminal differentiation of effector B-cells and the formation of secondary follicles with active germinal centers. This rapid germinal center proliferation dominates the 1st decade, resulting in tonsillar enlargement without invasion of surrounding tissues.

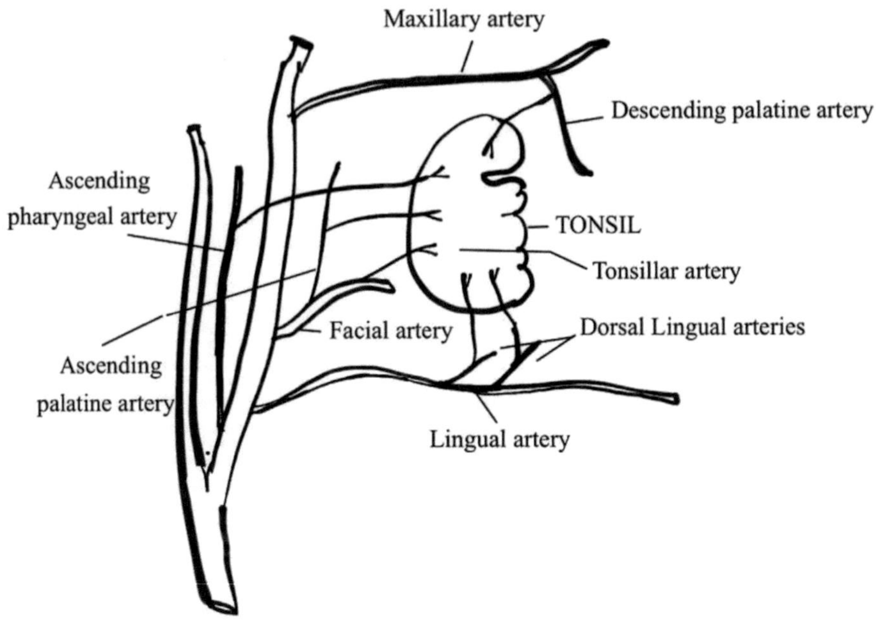

Figure 4.
Arterial supply of tonsil.

The tonsillar capsule arises from deep layers of the lamina propria, forming a continuous membrane except on the medial, cryptic surface. Unlike lymph nodes, the tonsil's parenchyma consists of densely packed fronds with a fibrovascular core, lymphoid tissue, and crypt epithelium.

In the 2nd decade, the B-cell component undergoes involution, with smaller germinal centers and increased fibrous tissue in trabeculae and capsules. The tonsil regresses, disappearing behind the anterior tonsillar pillar by the 7th decade, surrounded by fibrous connective tissue, making its outline less distinct. Fatty degeneration begins around 25 years and progresses with age [48–52].

4.4 Acute tonsillitis

4.4.1 Definition

Acute tonsillitis is a common inflammatory condition that involves acute inflammation of the tonsils. It is characterized by sore throat, difficulty in swallowing, fever, and enlarged tonsils. Timely and appropriate management, including antimicrobial therapy, is crucial to prevent complications and ensure a favorable outcome. It can be classified as:

1. Acute catarrhal or superficial tonsillitis: associated with generalized pharyngitis, often seen in viral infections.

2. Acute follicular tonsillitis: infection extends into the crypts, filling them with purulent material, resulting in yellowish spots at the crypt openings.

3. Acute parenchymatous tonsillitis: affects the tonsillar parenchyma, leading to uniform enlargement and redness.

4. Acute membranous tonsillitis: a stage beyond follicular tonsillitis, where exudation from crypts coalesce to form a membrane over the tonsillar surface.

4.4.2 Epidemiology

Acute tonsillitis commonly affects school-going children and adults, being rare in infants and those above 50 years. It primarily affects children and adolescents, with an incidence that peaks between the ages of 5 and 15 years. However, it can also occur in adults, especially those who are immunocompromised. The epidemiology of acute tonsillitis is influenced by various factors, including viral and bacterial pathogens, socioeconomic status, and environmental factors such as overcrowding. *Hemolytic streptococcus* is the most common infecting organism, contributing to approximately 15–30% of cases in children and 5–15% in adults. Other potential causes include *staphylococci*, *pneumococci*, or *Hemophilus influenzae*. Viral causes, including adenovirus, influenza virus, parainfluenza virus, and Epstein-Barr virus, are responsible for the majority of cases, especially in the adult population. The spread of acute tonsillitis is facilitated by close contact with infected individuals and can lead to outbreaks in settings such as schools and daycare centers. Early recognition and appropriate management, including antibiotic therapy when indicated, are essential for preventing complications and reducing the transmission of the disease [53–55].

4.4.3 Clinical features

Symptoms vary in severity and include sore throat, difficulty swallowing, fever, earache (possibly due to acute otitis media), and marked constitutional symptoms such as headache, body aches, malaise, and constipation.

Signs of acute tonsillitis include halitosis, coated tongue, hyperemia of pillars, soft palate, and uvula. Tonsils appear enlarged and congested, with yellow spots exuding out of crypts (follicular tonsillitis) or a wipeable whitish membrane (membranous tonsillitis). Enlarged and tender jugulodigastric lymph nodes may be present.

4.4.4 Treatment

Treatment involves bed rest, adequate hydration, antipyretics, and analgesics (aspirin or paracetamol) to alleviate pain and reduce fever. Antimicrobial therapy, typically with penicillin or erythromycin for penicillin-allergic individuals, is recommended and should be continued for a week to 10 days.

4.4.5 Complications

- Chronic tonsillitis: incomplete resolution leading to recurrent acute attacks.
- Peritonsillar abscess: collection of pus around the tonsils.
- Parapharyngeal abscess: abscess formation near the throat.
- Cervical abscess: suppuration of jugulodigastric nodes.
- Acute otitis media: recurrent attacks may coincide with tonsillitis.
- rheumatic fever: associated with Group A beta-hemolytic Streptococci.
- Acute glomerulonephritis: rare complication.
- Subacute bacterial endocarditis: possible in patients with valvular heart disease.

4.4.6 Chronic tonsillitis

It is characterized by persistent and chronic inflammation of the tonsils, most commonly occurring as a complication of acute tonsillitis. The condition may also emerge subclinically, affecting predominantly children and young adults.

Clinical symptoms of chronic tonsillitis encompass recurrent attacks of sore throats causing frequent school absenteeism and poor scholastic performance, chronic throat irritation with cough, halitosis, and, in severe cases, thick speech, swallowing difficulty, and nocturnal apneic spells.

4.4.7 Cardinal features of chronic adenotonsillitis

1. Crescentic residual anterior tonsillar pillar congestion

2. Bilateral, nontender, enlarged, and jugulodigastic nodes (Wood's node)

3. *Septic Squeeze test positive (Irwin Moore sign)*—performed with two tongue depressors with one depressing the anterior two-third of tongue and another one applying pressure over the anterior tonsillar pillar. A positive test is a cheesy material extruding out of the tonsillar crypt when the test is performed.

Most of these children have associated adenoid hypertrophy which can be clinically evident as adenoid facies. *Classical features of adenoid facies* include an elongated dull-looking face with a pinched upper lip, pinched nostrils, a high-arched palate, and overcrowding of upper teeth.

Treatment strategies involve conservative measures, focusing on overall health, diet, and addressing concurrent infections in the nose, paranasal sinuses, and teeth. Tonsillectomy is indicated when the tonsils significantly hinder normal functions or trigger recurrent attacks. Complications may arise, including peritonsillar abscess, parapharyngeal abscess, intratonsillar abscess, tonsilloliths, tonsillar cysts, and systemic infections.

4.5 Pediatric tonsillectomy

In recent years, pediatric tonsillectomy has changed its approach and considerations. The shift is notable, with more children undergoing the procedure for obstructive sleep apnea rather than recurrent pharyngitis. Advanced instrumentation that is available now enables less invasive surgical techniques. Systematic reviews by organizations like the Cochrane Collaboration have played a pivotal role in establishing best clinical practices for preoperative assessment and postoperative care. With approximately 100 million tonsillectomies performed worldwide over the past century, this procedure remains a vital intervention, particularly for obstructive sleep apnea and sleep-disordered breathing in children.

4.5.1 Indications for pediatric tonsillectomy

As per the Paradise criteria, tonsillectomy may be indicated for patients experiencing recurrent episodes of sore throat—history of at least seven documented episodes of sore throat in the preceding year, at least five documented episodes in each of the past 2 years, or at least three documented episodes in each of the past 3 years. Additionally, the presence of certain clinical features during these episodes, such as a temperature exceeding 100.9°F (38.3°C), cervical adenopathy, exudate over tonsil, or a culture that is positive for group A β-hemolytic Streptococcus, qualifies as counting toward an episode [56, 57].

4.5.2 Relative indications

Adenotonsillectomy in children proves effective for various other conditions such as recurrent sore throat attacks due to chronic tonsillitis, peritonsillar cellulitis or abscess, PANDAS (Pediatric Autoimmune Neuropsychiatric Disorders Associated with Streptococcal Infections), Periodic fever, aphthous stomatitis, pharyngitis and cervical adenitis syndrome (PFAPA), febrile seizures associated with high-grade fever (during an attack of acute tonsillitis), halitosis due to chronic adenotonsillitis, dental malocclusion due to adenoid facies, cryptic tonsils, prevention of rheumatic fever recurrences, and control of pharyngeal streptococcal carriage. Despite its efficacy, tonsillectomy remains a challenging entity for children and their caregivers, involving risks such as immediate or delayed hemorrhage and a low but existing mortality rate.

Complications and discomfort associated with pediatric tonsillectomy primarily stem from the injury due to surgery and the subsequent inflammatory healing process. Research into cutaneous wound healing mechanisms offers insights, indicating that the cold steel technique produces minimal collateral tissue damage and promotes rapid healing.

Optimal hydration and addressing dehydration have been linked to a reduction in postoperative tonsillectomy pain. According to reports, comforting the child by placing them on the lap of their parents emerges as a highly effective nonpharmacological approach for alleviating postoperative pain at home for daycare adenotonsillectomy [58, 59].

Thus, clinical decision-making should thoroughly analyze the potential benefits against the discomforts and risks associated with tonsillectomy.

In conclusion, pediatric tonsillectomy, while a well-established and effective intervention, necessitates a careful balance between potential benefits and associated challenges. Ongoing research and advancements in surgical techniques and postoperative care present opportunities for further improving outcomes and reducing the traumatic impact on children and their families.

5. Conclusion

In conclusion, this chapter underscores the multifaceted challenges these conditions present in both physical and psychosocial realms, as well as the critical importance of tailored treatment approaches that address age-specific needs. Throughout childhood, these disorders can significantly impact a child's development, from impairing sensory perception to hindering speech and language development and even affecting social interactions and self-esteem.

In managing these complex conditions, interdisciplinary collaborations between pediatricians, otolaryngologists, and various healthcare professionals are paramount. Pediatricians provide comprehensive care, understanding the child's medical history, developmental milestones, and family dynamics. Otolaryngologists offer specialized expertise in diagnosing and treating ENT disorders, ensuring that treatment plans are tailored to the child's unique physiological and developmental needs.

By working together in an interdisciplinary framework, healthcare professionals can provide holistic care that addresses not only the physical symptoms but also the psychosocial impact of ENT disorders on children and their families. Thus, the pursuit of excellence in the care of children with ENT disorders requires a commitment to ongoing research, collaboration, and a patient-centered approach, ensuring the best possible outcomes for the youngest members of our community. Early recognition and appropriate management of common ENT diseases are essential to prevent complications and improve patient outcomes. Regular ENT check-ups and prompt medical attention for symptoms can help in the early detection and effective treatment of these conditions.

Acknowledgements

The author acknowledges the assistance of AI tool (ChatGPT, an AI language model based on the GPT-4 architecture developed by OpenAI) for language polishing of the manuscript.

Conflict of interest

The authors declare no conflict of interest.

Author details

Dharanya Srinivasan and Kalaiarasi Raja*
Department of ENT, JIPMER, Puducherry, India

*Address all correspondence to: kalaiarasi004@gmail.com

References

[1] Bluestone CD. Definitions, terminology, and classification. In: Rosenfeld RM, Bluestone CD, editors. Evidence-Based Otitis Media. 2nd ed. Hamilton, ON: BC Decker; 2003. pp. 120-135

[2] Danishyar A, Ashurst JV. Acute otitis media. In: StatPearls. Treasure Island (FL): StatPearls Publishing; 2022. p. 2022

[3] Meherali S, Campbell A, Hartling L, Scott S. Understanding parents' experiences and information needs on pediatric acute otitis media: A qualitative study. Journal of Patient Experience. 2019;**6**(1):53-61

[4] Rosenfeld RM. Clinical practice guideline: Acute otitis media in children. Otolaryngology-Head and Neck Surgery. 2016;**154**(suppl. 1):S1-S41

[5] Monasta L, Ronfani L, Marchetti F, Montico M, Vecchi Brumatti L, Bavcar A, et al. Burden of disease caused by otitis media: Systematic review and global estimates. PLoS One. 2012;**7**(4):e36226

[6] Rovers MM, Schilder AG, Zielhuis GA, Rosenfeld RM. Otitis media. The Lancet. 2004;**363**(9407):465-473

[7] Teele DW, Klein JO, Rosner B. Epidemiology of otitis media during the first seven years of life in children in greater Boston: A prospective, cohort study. The Journal of Infectious Diseases. 1989;**160**(1):83-94

[8] Soni A. Ear Infections (Otitis Media) in Children (0-17): Use and Expenditures, 2006. Rockville (MD): Agency for Healthcare Research and Quality; 2008. Statistical Brief No. 228

[9] Grijalva CG, Nuorti JP, Griffin MR. Antibiotic prescription rates for acute respiratory tract infections in US ambulatory settings. JAMA. 2009;**302**(7):758-766

[10] Fireman B, Black SH, Shinefield HR, Lee J, Lewis E, Ray P. Impact of the pneumococcal conjugate vaccine on otitis media. The Pediatric Infectious Disease Journal. 2003;**22**:10-16

[11] Winther B, Alper CM, Mandel EM, et al. Temporal relationships between colds, upper respiratory viruses detected by polymerase chain reaction, and otitis media in young children followed through a typical cold season. Pediatrics. 2007;**119**(6):1069-1075

[12] Bluestone CD, Swarts JD. Human evolutionary history: Consequences for the pathogenesis of otitis media. Otolaryngology and Head and Neck Surgery. 2010;**143**(6):739-744

[13] Casey JR, Adlowitz DG, Pichichero ME. New patterns in the pathogens causing acute otitis media six to eight years after the introduction of the pneumococcal conjugate vaccine. The Pediatric Infectious Disease Journal. 2010;**29**(4):304-309

[14] Grubb MS, Spaugh DC. Microbiology of acute otitis media, Puget Sound region, 2005-2009. La Clinica Pediatrica. 2010;**49**(8):727-730

[15] Centers for Disease Control and Prevention. Licensure of a 13-valent pneumo-conjugate vaccine (PCV13) and recommendations for use among children—Advisory Committee on Immunization Practices (ACIP), 2010. MMWR Morbidity and Mortality Weekly Report. 2010;**59**(9):258-261

[16] Homme JH. Acute otitis media and group a streptococcal pharyngitis:

A review for the general pediatric practitioner. Pediatric Annals. 2019;**48**(9):e343-e348

[17] Lieberthal AS, Carroll AE, Chonmaitree T, Ganiats TG, Hoberman A, Jackson MA, et al. The diagnosis and management of acute otitis media. Pediatrics. 2013;**131**(3):e964-e999

[18] American Academy of Pediatrics Subcommittee on Management of Acute Otitis Media. Diagnosis and management of acute otitis media. Pediatrics. 2004;**113**(5):1451-1465

[19] Chiappini E, Ciarcià M, Bortone B, Doria M, Becherucci P, Marseglia GL, et al. Italian panel for the management of acute otitis media in children. Updated guidelines for the management of acute otitis media in children by the Italian society of pediatrics: Diagnosis. The Pediatric Infectious Disease Journal. 2019;**38**(12S Suppl.):S3-S9

[20] Penido Nde O, Borin A, Iha LC, Suguri VM, Onishi E, Fukuda Y, et al. Intracranial complications of otitis media: 15 years of experience in 33 patients. Otolaryngology and Head and Neck Surgery. 2005;**132**(1):37-42

[21] Mattos JL, Colman KL, Casselbrant ML, Chi DH. Intratemporal and intracranial complications of acute otitis media in a pediatric population. International Journal of Pediatric Otorhinolaryngology. 2014;**78**(12):2161-2164

[22] Paradise JL. Short-course antimicrobial treatment for acute otitis media: Not best for infants and young children. Journal of the American Medical Association. 1997;**278**:1640-1642

[23] Rosenfeld RM, Culpepper L, Doyle KJ, et al. Clinical practice guideline: Otitis media with effusion. Otolaryngology and Head and Neck Surgery. 2004;**130**(Suppl. 5):S95-S118

[24] Sicari V, Zabbo CP. Stridor in children. In: StatPearls. Treasure Island (FL): StatPearls Publishing; 2023. p. 2024

[25] Holinger LD, Eibling DE. Stridor in infants and children: Etiology, evaluation, and management. The Laryngoscope. 1989;**99**(1):1-10. DOI: 10.1288/00005537-198901000-00001

[26] Leung R, Berkowitz RG. Stridor in children: A diagnostic approach. Australian Family Physician. 2017;**46**(1-2):45-49

[27] Thompson DM. Laryngomalacia: Factors that influence disease severity and outcomes of management. Current Opinion in Otolaryngology and Head and Neck Surgery. 2010;**18**(6):564-570. DOI: 10.1097/MOO.0b013e32833f16a9

[28] Ida JB, Thompson DM. Pediatric stridor. Otolaryngologic Clinics of North America. 2014;**47**(5):795-819. DOI: 10.1016/j.otc.2014.06.005. Epub 2014 Aug 7

[29] Hirschberg J, Szende T. Pathological Cry, Stridor and Cough in Infants. A Clinical-Acoustic Study with Gramophone Record Attached. Budapest: Academy Publishers; 1982

[30] Lane RW, Weider DJ, Steinem C, Marin-Padilla M. Laryngomalacia. A review and case report of surgical treatment with resolution of pectus excavatum. Archives of Otolaryngology. 1984;**110**(8):546-551. DOI: 10.1001/archotol.1984.00800340058017

[31] Cohen SR, Thompson JW. Surgical treatment of severe laryngomalacia. The Laryngoscope. 2004;**114**(11):

2060-2067. DOI: 10.1097/01.mlg.0000149445.08098.21

[32] Richter GT, Thompson DM. The surgical management of laryngomalacia. Otolaryngologic Clinics of North America. 2008;**41**(5):837-864, vii. DOI: 10.1016/j.otc.2008.04.013

[33] Jain D, Jain S. Management of stridor in severe laryngomalacia: A review article. Cureus. 2022;**14**(9):e29585. DOI: 10.7759/cureus.29585

[34] Damm M, Eckel HE, Jungehülsing M, Roth B. Management of acute inflammatory childhood stridor. Otolaryngology and Head and Neck Surgery. 1999;**121**(5):633-638. DOI: 10.1016/S0194-5998(99)70071-9

[35] Charles R, Fadden M, Brook J. Acute epiglottitis. BMJ. 2013;**347**:f5235. DOI: 10.1136/bmj.f5235

[36] Abdallah C. Acute epiglottitis: Trends, diagnosis, and management. Saudi Journal of Anaesthesia. 2012;**6**(3):279-281. DOI: 10.4103/1658-354X.101222

[37] McEwan J, Giridharan W, Clarke RW, Shears P. Paediatric acute epiglottitis: Not a disappearing entity. International Journal of Pediatric Otorhinolaryngology. 2003;**67**(4):317-321. DOI: 10.1016/s0165-5876(02)00393-2

[38] Damm M, Eckel HE, Jungehülsing M, Roth B. Airway endoscopy in the interdisciplinary management of acute epiglottitis. International Journal of Pediatric Otorhinolaryngology. 1996;**38**(1):41-51. DOI: 10.1016/s0165-5876(96)01417-6

[39] Russel KF, Liang Y, O'Gorman K, et al. Glucocorticoids for croup. Cochrane Database of Systematic Reviews. 2011;**1**:CD001955

[40] Bjornson C, Russell KF, Vandermeer B, et al. Nebulized epinephrine for croup in children. Cochrane Database of Systematic Reviews. 2013;**12**:CD006822

[41] Zoorob R, Sidani M, Murray J. Croup: An overview. American Family Physician. 2011;**83**:1067-1073

[42] Cooper T, Kuruvilla G, Persad R, et al. Atypical croup: Association with airway lesions, atopy, and esophagitis. Otolaryngology and Head and Neck Surgery. 2012;**147**:209-214

[43] Jabbour N, Parker NP, Finkelstein M, et al. Incidence of operative endoscopy findings in recurrent croup. Otolaryngology and Head and Neck Surgery. 2011;**144**:596-601

[44] Amin MR, Friedmann DR. Simulation-based training in advanced airway skills in an otolaryngology residency program. Laryngoscope. 2013;**123**:629-634

[45] Rutter MJ, Cotton RT. Pediatric stridor. Otolaryngologic Clinics of North America. 2008;**41**(2):321-337. DOI: 10.1016/j.otc.2007.11.007

[46] Isaacson G. Pediatric tonsillectomy: An evidence-based approach. Otolaryngologic Clinics of North America. 2014;**47**(5):673-690. DOI: 10.1016/j.otc.2014.06.011. Epub 2014 Aug 7

[47] Dhingra PL, Dhingra S. Diseases of Ear, Nose, and Throat-EBook. Amsterdam, The Netherlands: Elsevier Health Sciences; 2017

[48] Isaacson G, Parikh T. Developmental anatomy of the tonsil and its implications for intracapsular tonsillectomy. International Journal of Pediatric Otorhinolaryngology. 2008;**72**(1):89-96

[49] Choi G, Suh YL, Lee HM, et al. Prenatal and postnatal changes of the human tonsillar crypt epithelium. Acta Oto-Laryngologica. Supplementum. 1996;**523**:28-33

[50] Boyaka PN, Wright PF, Marinaro M, et al. Human nasopharyngeal-associated lymphoreticular tissues. Functional analysis of subepithelial and intraepithelial B and T cells from adenoids and tonsils. The American Journal of Pathology. 2000;**157**:2023-2035

[51] von Gaudecker B. Development and functional anatomy of the human tonsilla palatina. Acta Oto-Laryngologica. Supplementum. 1988;**454**:28-32

[52] Brandtzaeg P. Immunology of tonsils and adenoids: Everything the ENT surgeon needs to know. International Journal of Pediatric Otorhinolaryngology. 2003;**67** (Suppl. 1):S69-S76

[53] Brook I. Acute bacterial adenotonsillitis: Microbiology and diagnosis. The Journal of Laryngology and Otology. 2010;**124**(1):3-9. DOI: 10.1017/S0022215109991555

[54] Van Staaij BK, van den Akker EH, Rovers MM, Hordijk GJ, Hoes AW, Schilder AG. Effectiveness of adenotonsillectomy in children with mild symptoms of throat infections or adenotonsillar hypertrophy: Open, randomized controlled trial. BMJ. 2004;**329**(7467):651. DOI: 10.1136/bmj.38210.827917.7C

[55] Windfuhr JP, Toepfner N, Steffen G, Waldfahrer F, Berner R. Clinical practice guideline: Tonsillitis II. Surgical management. European Archives of Oto-Rhino-Laryngology. 2016;**273**(4):989-1009. DOI: 10.1007/s00405-015-3808-8

[56] Paradise JL, Bluestone CD, Bachman RZ, et al. Efficacy of tonsillectomy for recurrent throat infection in severely affected children. Results of parallel randomized and nonrandomized clinical trials. The New England Journal of Medicine. 1984;**310**(11):674-683

[57] Paradise JL, Bluestone CD, Colborn DK, et al. Tonsillectomy and adenotonsillectomy for recurrent throat infection in moderately affected children. Pediatrics. 2002;**110**(1 Pt 1):7-15

[58] Klemetti S, Kinnunen I, Suominen T, et al. The effect of preoperative fasting on postoperative pain, nausea, and vomiting in pediatric ambulatory tonsillectomy. International Journal of Pediatric Otorhinolaryngology. 2009;**73**:263-273

[59] Kankkunen P, Vehvilainen-Julkunen K, Pietila AM, et al. Is the sufficiency of discharge instructions related to children's postoperative pain at home after day surgery? Scandinavian Journal of Caring Sciences. 2003;**17**:365-372

Section 5

Common Benign Vascular Tumors in Children

Chapter 6

Periocular Hemangioma: Clinicopathological Aspects

Hind M. Alkatan, Dalal R. Fatani, Hala A. Helmi, Rakan Alsaad, Rahaf Altwijri and Munirah Aldofyan

Abstract

Hemangiomas are pathologically considered to be developmental hamartomatous lesions. In the periocular region, capillary hemangioma is commonly encountered in infants and children, and it is of particular importance because of its critical location if involving the eyelid with obstruction of the visual axis. In this chapter, we aim to briefly discuss the pathogenesis and etiology of such lesions, describe the histopathological features, and the diagnostic immunohistochemical stains used, with differentiating features between infantile hemangioma and capillary hemangioma in adults. In the periocular region, the clinical appearance and manifestations depend on three primary locations of the hemangioma: the superficial, subcutaneous, and deep orbital hemangiomas. Treatment options are similar to hemangioma elsewhere, however, as mentioned above, early treatment may be advocated to avoid developing amblyopia (lazy eye) because of visual deprivation or obstruction. The most used therapy in the periocular region is beta-blockers, either orally or locally. Intralesional steroids and sclerosing agents may also be used. Surgical intervention is reserved for deep orbital-selected lesions.

Keywords: periocular, hemangioma, vascular, capillary, blood vessels, hamartoma, angiogenesis, pathogenesis, histopathology, amblyopia, beta-blocker, corticosteroid

1. Introduction

Periocular hemangioma is a known benign hamartoma characterized by capillary proliferation and endothelial hyperplasia [1]. Although the exact incidence of periocular hemangioma is unknown, it is one of the most common benign orbital tumors of infants and young children, affecting up to 5% of infants under the age of 1 year [1–5].

The majority of the time, periocular hemangioma is identified by clinical observation. It can be presented at birth with a precursor sign as telangiectatic patches with a pale halo, erythematous patches, pale patches, and bruise-like macules that rapidly proliferate with the highest growth in the first 3 months of life that slowly involute afterward [6]. Almost all periocular hemangiomas are discovered before the age of 6 months. It manifests as soft, blue lumps under the skin or as strawberry-colored masses that enlarge when the patient cries [1, 7]. Based on the extent of skin involvement, periorbital hemangiomas can be categorized as superficial, deep, or mixed [6].

Although periocular hemangiomas have a regression pattern with age, they can cause serious ocular problems most importantly, amblyopia which is known as "lazy eye." Infantile hemangioma can cause amblyopia by different mechanisms and one of the main causes is an abnormal visual axis development in the early years of child life. Partial or complete visual axis occlusion also causes imperfection in the curvature of the eye resulting in blurred distance and near vision (astigmatism), asymmetric refractive error between the two eyes (anisometropia), and eye misalignment commonly called strabismus [3, 6–9].

In this chapter, we aim to briefly discuss the pathogenesis and etiology of such lesions, describe the histopathological findings, and the diagnostic immunohistochemical stains (IHC) used, with a demonstration of the correlating clinical features. Treatment options will be also discussed briefly.

2. Periocular hemangioma etiology and pathogenesis

2.1 Risk factors and etiological theories

Understanding the pathogenesis and risk factors associated with this condition is essential for its early diagnosis and appropriate management.

Certain risk factors such as female gender, prematurity, and history of chorionic-villus sampling or pre-eclampsia during pregnancy have been shown to increase the risk of developing infantile hemangiomas [10]. Infantile hemangioma pathogenesis remains unclear; however, multiple theories have been suggested.

Etiological theories:

1. Embryonic origin: According to this theory, periocular hemangiomas are believed to originate during embryonic development. It suggests that abnormal blood vessels develop due to an error or abnormality in the formation of blood vessels during the early stages of fetal development [11]. This is further supported by the location of facial hemangiomas at areas of mesenchymal and ectodermal fusion [12, 13]. Additionally, the proliferation in hemangiomas exhibits an increased rate of mitosis. This can be induced by certain vasculogenic stem cells like hemangioma-derived stem cells (hemeSCs) [14, 15].

2. Genetic factors: Genetic factors are also thought to play a role in the pathogenesis of periocular hemangiomas. Certain genetic mutations or alterations may contribute to the development of abnormal blood vessels in the eye region. Studies have identified specific gene mutations, such as in the Glucose transporter -1 gene (GLUT-1) that may be associated with the formation of hemangiomas [14, 16]. Other theories suggest a mutation in the genes encoding growth and hormonal factors [13, 17, 18].

3. Hormonal factors: Hormonal factors, particularly estrogen, have been proposed as potential contributors to the development of periocular hemangiomas. It has been observed that these tumors occur more frequently in females than males, and they often exhibit rapid growth during periods of hormonal changes such as infancy and pregnancy. Estrogen is believed to promote the proliferation of endothelial cells, which may contribute to hemangioma formation [19–21].

4. Placental factors: Some studies suggest that periocular hemangiomas may be influenced by placental factors. It is hypothesized that certain placental trophoblasts or hormones produced by the placenta can stimulate the growth of blood vessels in the eye region, leading to the development of periocular hemangiomas [13, 19]. The placenta produces 2-methoxyestradiol which is an angiogenesis inhibitor and it is believed to be downregulated in cases of infantile hemangioma (IH) [22, 23].

5. Growth factors: Capillary proliferation is enhanced by vascular proliferative angiogenesis markers such as vascular endothelial growth factor (VEGF). VEGF-A is classically elevated in the proliferative phase of the disease and decreased in the involutional phase; thus, suggesting it has a pivotal role in the disease process. Similarly, insulin-like growth factor-2 (IGF-2) also regulates the growth and proliferation of the hemangioma. It is further hypothesized that IGF-2 production is derived by cell hypoxia from low oxygen levels [14, 24] Basic Fibroblast growth factor (bFGF) is also elevated in hemangioma cases [25].

2.2 Pathogenesis

As mentioned, the exact pathogenesis of periocular hemangioma remains unclear to date. As the disease is characterized by a proliferative phase followed by an involutional phase, studies often compare the biomarkers between these phases to better understand the disease process.

The proliferative phase shows active inflammation as it exhibits an increase in the number of T lymphocytes and pro-inflammatory cytokines [26]. Matrix metalloproteinase-9 (MMP-9) regulates the extracellular matrix components and can indirectly regulate the angiogenesis process through the release of VEGF [27].

Interferon beta levels were noted to be decreased in cases of IH in its proliferative phase, suggesting its therapeutic role in the resolution of disease [25].

In the involutional phase, mast cells exhibit an increase in number suggesting a role in the regression of the hemangiomas [28].

Hypoxia a recognized trigger for new blood vessel formation, plays a significant part in the development of hemangiomas. It stimulates the production of hypoxia-inducible factor-1 alpha (HIF-1a), which in turn triggers the activation of VEGF and Stromal-Derived Factor-1 alpha (SDF-1a), thereby encouraging the growth of endothelial cells [19, 29]. VEGF can also be influenced by certain inflammatory cytokines such as Interleukin-6 (IL-6) and Interleukin-8 (IL-8). While both IL-6 and IL-8 were significantly increased in hemangioma cells, only anti-IL-6 resulted in suppression of proliferation [30].

Therefore, comprehending the intricate relationship between the vasculogenic process, angiogenesis, and inflammatory markers sheds light on the underlying mechanisms driving the infantile hemangioma pathogenesis. This is crucial for directing future treatment options for infantile hemangioma and targeting research efforts.

3. Histopathological features and diagnosis

In the periocular region, most ophthalmologists use the term capillary hemangioma for infantile vascular lesions that develop in early infancy while lobular capillary hemangioma is known to occur as acquired lesions in adults [31]. Lobular capillary hemangioma has been described since 1897 followed in 1904 by the evolution of the so called "pyogenic granuloma," which represents exuberant granulation tissue [32].

In that context, pyogenic granuloma has been added to the category of lobular capillary hemangioma despite the characteristic clinical and morphological features that differentiate the two entities. Histopathologically, all hemangiomas exhibit microscopic features characterized by varying-sized lobules of proliferating capillary-like blood vessels lined by plump endothelial cells with intervening variable amounts of fibrous stroma [31, 32].

Congenital hemangiomas manifest in two types: the non-involuting type and the rapidly involuting type, each displaying distinct characteristics [31, 33]. Non-involuting congenital hemangiomas present large vascular channels with features of arteriovenous malformations, whereas rapidly involuting congenital hemangiomas showcase prominent fibrosis accompanied by calcification, intralesional hemorrhage, hemosiderin deposition, and atrophic dermis or epidermis [31, 33].

Infantile hemangiomas are different in terms of natural history, presentation, histopathological characteristics, and treatment. Infantile hemangiomas exhibit microscopic variations depending on their phase [31]. The growth phase manifests large, mitotically active endothelial cells with discrete capillary lumina, while the maturation phase displays flattened endothelial cells with widened capillary lumina [31]. Involuted infantile hemangiomas demonstrate progressive fibrosis and fatty replacement. Lobular capillary hemangiomas reveal characteristic hyperplastic clusters of capillaries separated by fibrosis [31].

Immunohistochemical (IHC) staining reveals that endothelial cells in all tumors uniformly test positive for CD-34 [31]. However, when stained with GLUT-1, different types of hemangiomas exhibit varied results. Congenital hemangiomas and

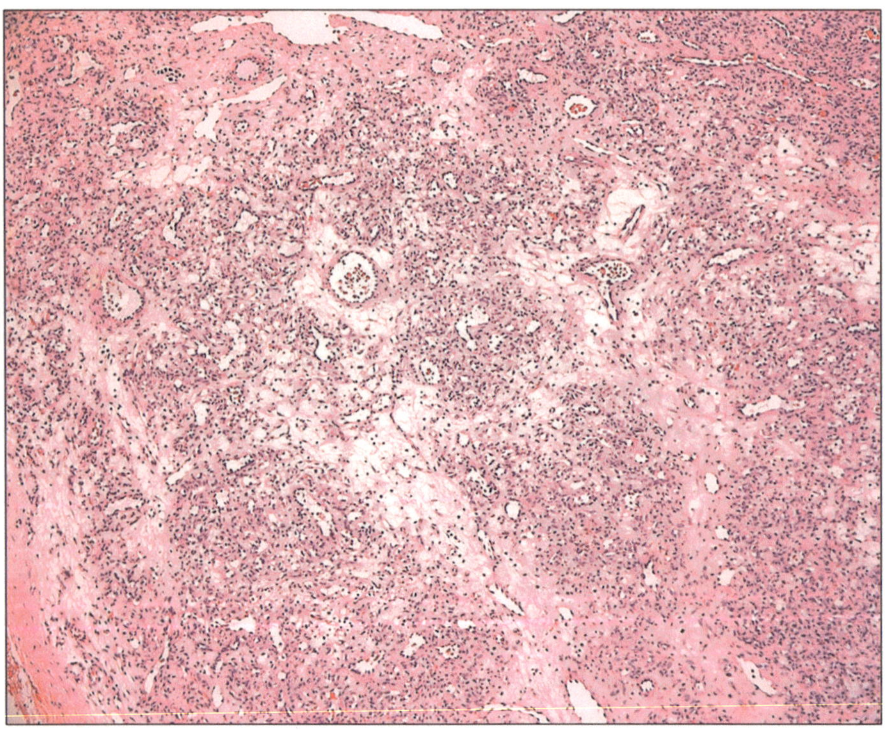

Figure 1.
Lower power histopathological appearance of an infantile lobular capillary hemangioma of the upper eyelid (Original magnification X50 Hematoxylin & Eosin).

Lobular Adult hemangiomas test negative for GLUT-1, whereas infantile hemangiomas yield a positive staining for GLUT-1 [16, 31].

The histopathological features and the IHC staining of the capillary-like proliferation are shown below (**Figures 1–3**).

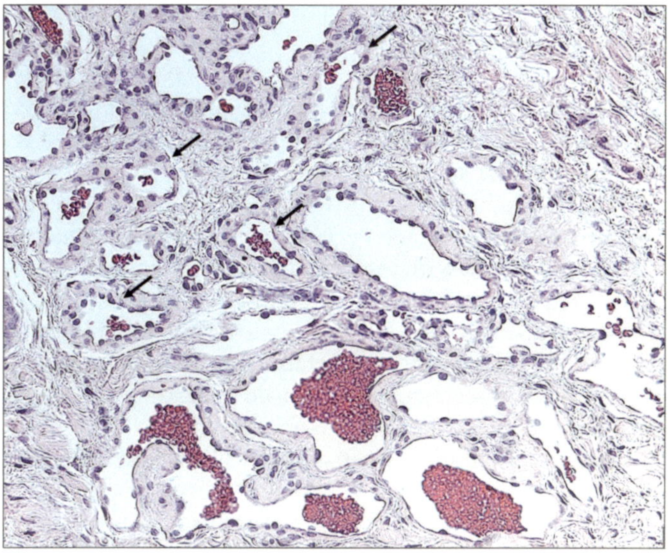

Figure 2.
Higher power histopathological appearance of the proliferating capillary blood vessels (black arrows) within fibro-collagenous stroma in an infantile hemangioma (Original magnification X400 Hematoxylin & Eosin).

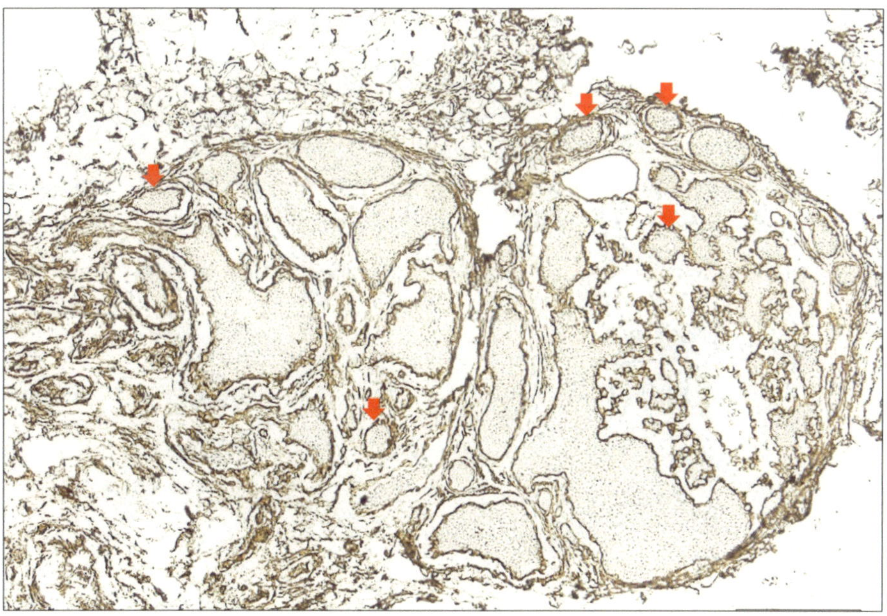

Figure 3.
The proliferating capillary blood vessels in an infantile hemangioma outlined using endothelial cells immunohistochemical marker, some of which are marked with red arrowheads (Original magnification X200 CD34).

4. Clinicopathological correlation

Periocular capillary hemangiomas typically manifest within the initial months of an infant's life, with nearly half of cases apparent at birth [7]. They commonly undergo a phase of rapid proliferation within 3–6 months of onset, followed by a stabilization period and subsequent regression. This involution phase typically occurs between the ages of 2–5 years [7, 34].

Haik et al. classified periocular capillary hemangiomas into three distinct clinical presentations: the superficial strawberry nevus, the subcutaneous hemangioma, and the deep orbital tumor [4]. This classification is based on the depth of the lesion and the subsequent resultant color variations. The more superficial lesions are bright red (strawberry-like) in appearance while the deeper lesions give a more purple/blue appearance. In some cases, the lesion is very deep resulting in normal skin color making the diagnosis more difficult with the need for orbital imaging [35]. Superficial hemangiomas tend to appear and regress sooner than deeper hemangiomas [36]. Superficial lesions typically emerge a few months after birth as reddish papules or nodules that may exhibit a flat or uneven surface (**Figure 4**). Therefore, applying pressure to these lesions to assess blanching can aid in distinguishing them from a port-wine stain in individuals with Sturge–Weber syndrome [37].

Another classification of infantile hemangioma is based on their anatomic distribution ranging from focal localized lesion, segmental involving a larger embryonic territory, or multifocal extending to different anatomical areas. Focal hemangiomas are most common, with unilateral upper eyelid involvement being the most frequent location [34, 36, 37]. Segmented hemangiomas were reported in 13% of cases and they usually follow a distinct pattern on the face similar to the dermatomal distribution like frontal, maxillary, or mandibular configuration. Multifocal involvement can be seen in 3.6% and is often associated with hemangioma syndromes [36].

In cases with deep orbital hemangiomas, anterior displacement of the eye may induce proptosis and expose the cornea to potential damage, and in severe cases, optic nerve impairment may occur from external mass compression [7, 34]. Approximately 60% of patients with eyelid involvement in superficial hemangiomas develop amblyopia [34]. This occurs via two mechanisms: (1) the mass-induced deformation of the highly flexible infantile sclera and cornea leads to anisometropia from resultant astigmatism, and (2) the enlarging eyelid mass obstructs the visual axis, depriving the infant of clear vision [4].

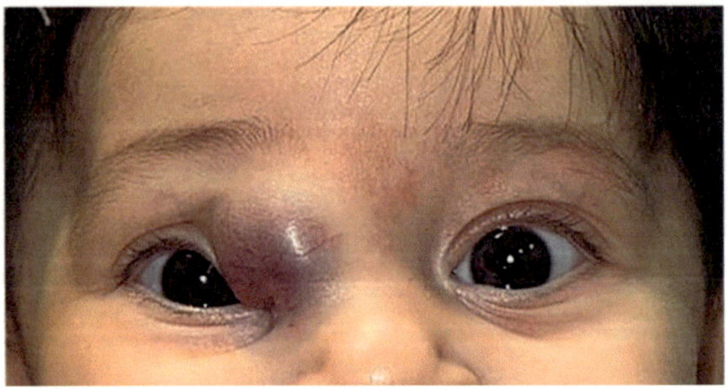

Figure 4.
External photo of a 9-month-old girl with mixed deep and superficial periocular hemangioma inducing mechanical right medial upper eyelid ptosis. Kindly note the clear visual axis, which is not obstructed by the lesion.

It is important to note that periocular hemangiomas can also be a component of systemic diseases. One of the prominent hematological abnormalities associated with extensive capillary hemangiomas is Kasabach–Merrit syndrome (KMS). This syndrome is characterized by the entrapment and consumption of platelets and/or fibrinogen, resulting in coagulopathy that can lead to sudden and substantial hemorrhages [4, 7]. KMS may even be fatal when significant hemorrhage results in heart failure and secondary multiorgan failure with a mortality rate ranging from 12 to 30%. These patients may require blood transfusions in the form of fresh frozen plasma with the addition of high-dose steroids, antifibrinolytics, and antithrombotic [38]. Another significant systemic condition is PHACE syndrome. PHACE is an abbreviation that stands for:

P = posterior fossa anomalies of the brain and cerebellum.
H = Hemangioma both cutaneous and visceral.
A = Arterial anomalies affecting the arteries of brain neck or chest.
C = Cardiac anomalies from major heart defects or large vessel abnormalities.
E = Eyes including anatomical irregularities and visual disturbances.

In infants with substantial segmental facial hemangiomas, the estimated incidence of PHACE syndrome is around 20% [37, 39]. PHACES should be considered in infants with large segmental hemangiomas over the head, neck, and chest areas. A distinct feature of PHACE syndrome is the ulceration of the hemangiomas from the rapid proliferation. Certain life-threatening complications are associated with PHACE syndrome such as arterial ischemic stroke (AIS), cerebral infarction, and aortic changes like aortic coarctation and aneurysms. Infants with PHACE syndrome may suffer from significant hypothyroidism in the early years of life which may threaten their neurological development.

Extensive hemangiomas may form in the respiratory tract such as subglottic hemangiomas where special care needs to be taken to maintain the airway and prevent respiratory failure in such cases [40].

It is therefore important to diagnose any underlying systemic conditions associated with infantile hemangiomas to ensure early and adequate intervention and management.

5. Periocular hemangioma management considerations

5.1 Treatment options and indications

Periocular hemangiomas are self-limiting disorders that undergo natural spontaneous resolution with age. This phenomenon supports the general practice of observation without treatment, especially when the hemangioma is of small size and does not result in disfiguration [40].

There are certain indications that warrant the initiating of treatment in periocular hemangioma. Indications to treat include life-threatening or vision-threatening sequalae in addition to psychological distress from cosmetic disfigurement or dissatisfaction. Periocular hemangiomas may be associated with serious life-threatening complications like high cardiac output failure or bleeding disorder from consumptive coagulopathies. In such cases, treatment is considered mandatory and lifesaving. Furthermore, vision-threatening complications can lead to occlusive or refractive amblyopia, either through direct mechanical ptosis obstructing the visual axis or mechanical distortion of the cornea resulting in unilateral refractive changes. In such scenarios, treatment is also imperative. Although there is controversy on whether treatment of periocular hemangioma reverses the astigmatism or refractive error; it is often done to limit the progression of these corneal changes. Studies did document successful refractive error reduction and improvement in visual acuity after treatment of hemangiomas as well as amblyopia treatment with spectacles and occlusion [41]. Other nonfunctional causes such as major facial disfigurement is another indication for treatment as it may psychologically impact the child and family.

5.2 Medical management and expected outcomes

There are different treatment options available including local and systemic medical management as well as surgical options [16]. Observation remains the most common management plan for patients with periocular hemangioma [40].

The most recent and widely accepted medical approach to managing periocular hemangioma is the administration of systemic beta-blockers. This was first introduced in the management of hemangiomas in 2008 as an incidental finding in children receiving oral propranolol for cardiac disease. Due to its rapid efficacy in promoting hemangioma regression and the favorable safety profile associated with beta-blockers, this treatment approach has gained significant traction and is now regarded as the primary treatment of choice.

The chemical structure of propranolol has a similarity to catecholamines and, thus, competes with B-adrenergic receptors. While the precise mechanisms underlying the action of propranolol in hemangioma regression remain unclear, it is proposed that propranolol's blockade of catecholamines leads to suppression of angiogenesis via the downregulation of key factors such as HIF-I alpha, VEGF-A, MMPs, and IL-6, potentially contributing to hemangioma regression [37, 42]. Propranolol has a membrane-stabilizing action with blockage of sodium and calcium channels in high dosages. The main effect on infantile hemangioma is believed to be through the regulation of the renin-angiotensin system (RAS) via a biological effect since angiotensin is known to promote the proliferation of capillaries [36]. Additionally, beta-blockers are known to decrease nitric oxide levels, resulting in vasoconstriction, particularly during the early stages of treatment.

Propranolol is administered 1–3 mg/kg/day in a titration regimen starting from 0.5 mg/kg/day in three doses. This requires a multidisciplinary approach as it is strongly recommended that patients undergo regular follow-ups with their general pediatrician and cardiologist to monitor for possible side effects such as bradycardia, hypotension, hypoglycemia, hyperkalemia, and other sleep disturbances. Admission and close observation during the initiation of treatment have also been strongly recommended [43, 44]. However, infants who develop adverse effects that necessitate cessation of propranolol treatment may reach only 4%, therefore, it is still considered to be safe and effective [42].

Another method for beta-blocker administration is topical application, typically reserved for superficial hemangiomas, although successful outcomes in deeper lesions have been reported [45]. Timolol maleate usually in a 0.5% solution or gel form is administered twice daily on the lesion and is continued until complete regression is achieved. Results are often visible after 4–8 weeks of treatment [37, 46]. Topical Timolol can be started in the first few months of life and can prevent hemangioma growth and prevent the future need for oral therapy from disease sequalae [47].

Propranolol cream 5% twice daily for 24 weeks showed an efficacy of up to 68.8%. Potential side effects reported include mild elevation in liver enzymes, eczema, urticaria, and infectious dermatitis [48].

Furthermore, the local form of beta-blocker treatment is Intralesional Propranolol injection. With this modality, regression is noted within the first 24 hours and continues for 3 weeks post-administration. The recommended dose is 0.2 ml up to 1 ml (1 mg/ml) depending on the lesion size [49].

Prior to the emergence of beta-blockers as a primary therapeutic approach in the management of periocular hemangioma, corticosteroids were considered the cornerstone of therapy. Corticosteroids also work by inhibiting VEGF-A production as well as suppression of MMP-1 and IL-6 thereby mitigating the vasculogenic process [50]. The recommended effective dose for systemic corticosteroid therapy is 2–3 mg/kg/day for 2 weeks. However, the use of corticosteroids in the treatment of periocular hemangiomas declined in popularity due to the undesirable side effects associated with their administration, including growth retardation, adrenal insufficiency, hypertension, hyperglycemia, weight gain, gastritis, and immune suppression [37, 51].

Intralesional steroids continue to be a viable option in managing periocular hemangiomas. The recommended dosage typically involves a 1–5 ml injection of Triamcinolone (40 mg/ml), with or without Betamethasone (4 mg/ml). It is essential to exercise caution and administer the injection slowly as this may adversely result in central retinal artery or vein occlusion. Other less serious side effects include localized fat atrophy and skin necrosis [51].

For cases where hemangiomas are unresponsive to treatment or when there are contraindications to the aforementioned modalities, Interferon alpha-2a and -2b can be considered. INFa-2a or -2b has antiangiogenic properties decreasing the proliferation of the endothelial cells within the hemangioma vasculature with a success rate of 80–100% in hemangioma reduction [52, 53]. The recommended dose is 1–3 million units/m2 of body surface. This also requires regular follow-ups with a pediatrician. The reported adverse side effects include flu-like symptoms, transient neutropenia, liver toxicity, and neurotoxicity [54]. In cases of severe vision-threatening lesions that are unresponsive, treatment with chemotherapy such as vincristine and alkylating agents like cyclophosphamide under the care of oncologists may be promising. The exact mechanism of these agents in the treatment of infantile hemangiomas is yet to be established [53].

Local injection of the sclerosing agent, bleomycin has been reported to be successful in the treatment of cutaneous hemangiomas. This agent works by creating fibrosis which is believed to induce regression of the lesion. Although there are limited studies on the efficacy and safety of bleomycin in periocular hemangioma, some reported up to 60–100% regression of these lesions [55].

Surgical options can be implored for deep localized lesions. Hemangiomas are vascular in nature and not encapsulated; making them difficult to be excised completely with a high risk of bleeding. When the choice of surgery is made, the procedure must be done under the care of specialized surgeons and should be done with care to avoid significant blood loss and maintain the anatomical integrity of adjacent structures. Such options are usually reserved for sight-threatening lesions that failed to respond to the aforementioned medical management options [40, 56].

Superficial lesions may be treated with a pulse dye laser. This modality has limited penetration when lesions are deeper than 1.2 mm but has a high safety profile and can reduce overall redness as well regression of vascular components when given every 2–4 weeks intervals. Resultant scarring and skin atrophy with hypopigmentation may be encountered [57].

Brauer et al. conducted a study comparing various laser therapies for hemangiomas. According to their findings, pulse dye laser (PDL) is preferred in their practice due to its excellent tolerance and high safety profile, even among individuals with higher Fitzpatrick skin types. Nd: YAG laser can be used for thicker and deeper hemangiomas because of its ability to penetrate deeper tissue layers, although it often leads to more scarring and pigmentation issues [58, 59]. Additionally, a combination of Nd: YAG therapy and systemic corticosteroids has been reported to achieve a high success rate with minimal risk of complications [41].

6. Conclusion

Periocular hemangioma is a prevalent benign hamartoma among infants and young children, characterized by distinct clinical features and natural course. Its pathogenesis is multifactorial, with embryonic, genetic, hormonal, and placental factors contributing to its development. Despite being generally self-limiting with a pattern of regression, periocular hemangiomas necessitate careful clinical attention due to potential complications such as amblyopia and systemic associations like Kasabach–Merritt and PHACES syndrome.

Clinically, periocular hemangiomas are categorized based on their depth and presentation, each with unique diagnostic and management challenges. The management of periocular hemangioma has evolved significantly, with systemic beta-blockers, particularly propranolol, emerging as a first-line treatment. This shift is due to their efficacy, safety profile, and ability to address both functional and cosmetic outcomes effectively.

Additionally, other treatment modalities like topical beta-blockers, corticosteroids, intralesional injections, and surgical interventions remain relevant in specific contexts. The management of these lesions necessitates a multidisciplinary approach involving pediatricians, ophthalmologists, dermatologists, and other specialists to ensure comprehensive care.

Ongoing research into their pathogenesis and treatment will continue to refine strategies, improving outcomes for affected infants and children.

Acknowledgements

This work was supported by the College of Medicine Research Center, Deanship of Scientific Research, King Saud University, Riyadh, Saudi Arabia.

Conflict of interest

Authors do not have conflict of interest or any financial disclosures related to the above work or any of the listed items in this chapter.

Author details

Hind M. Alkatan[1,2,3*], Dalal R. Fatani[4], Hala A. Helmi[5,6], Rakan Alsaad[1], Rahaf Altwijri[1] and Munirah Aldofyan[1]

1 Ophthalmology Department, College of Medicine, King Saud University, Riyadh, Saudi Arabia

2 Pathology and Laboratory Medicine Department, College of Medicine, King Saud University, Riyadh, Saudi Arabia

3 King Saud University Medical City, King Saud University, Riyadh, Saudi Arabia

4 Oculoplastic and Orbit Surgery, King Khaled Eye Specialist Hospital, Riyadh, Saudi Arabia

5 Department of Ophthalmology, McGill University, Montreal, Canada

6 Ophthalmology Department, King Faisal Specialist Hospital and Research Center, Riyadh, Saudi Arabia

*Address all correspondence to: hindkatan@yahoo.com

References

[1] Wasserman BN, Medow NB, Homa-Palladino M, Hoehn ME. Treatment of periocular capillary hemangiomas. Journal of AAPOS. 2004;**8**(2):175-181. DOI: 10.1016/j.jaapos.2003.12.002

[2] Capillary Hemangioma. Available from: https://eyewiki.aao.org/Capillary_Hemangioma [Accessed: January 2, 2024]

[3] Bruckner AL, Frieden IJ. Infantile hemangiomas. Journal of the American Academy of Dermatology. 2006;**55**(4):671-682. DOI: 10.1016/j.jaad.2006.05.017

[4] Haik BG, Karcioglu ZA, Gordon RA, Pechous BP. Capillary hemangioma (infantile periocular hemangioma). Survey of Ophthalmology. 1994;**38**(5):399-426. DOI: 10.1016/0039-6257(94)90172-4

[5] Tambe K, Munshi V, Dewsbery C, Ainsworth JR, Willshaw H, Parulekar MV. Relationship of infantile periocular hemangioma depth to growth and regression pattern. Journal of AAPOS. 2009;**13**(6):567-570. DOI: 10.1016/j.jaapos.2009.09.014

[6] Spence-Shishido AA, Good WV, Baselga E, Frieden IJ. Hemangiomas and the eye. Clinics in Dermatology. 2015;**33**(2):170-182. DOI: 10.1016/j.clindermatol.2014.10.009

[7] Bang GM, Setabutr P. Periocular capillary hemangiomas: Indications and options for treatment. Middle East African Journal of Ophthalmology. 2010;**17**(2):121-128. DOI: 10.4103/0974-9233.63071

[8] Callahan AB, Yoon MK. Infantile hemangiomas: A review. Saudi Journal of Ophthalmology. 2012;**26**(3):283-291. DOI: 10.1016/j.sjopt.2012.05.004. Epub 2012 May 23

[9] Schwartz SR, Blei F, Ceisler E, Steele M, Furlan L, Kodsi S. Risk factors for amblyopia in children with capillary hemangiomas of the eyelids and orbit. Journal of AAPOS. 2006;**10**(3):262-268. DOI: 10.1016/j.jaapos.2006.01.210

[10] Itinteang T, Withers AH, Davis PF, Tan ST. Biology of infantile hemangioma. Frontiers in Surgery. 2014;**1**:38. DOI: 10.3389/fsurg.2014.00038

[11] Sarangi S, Mukherjee D. Current concepts in the pathogenesis and management of vascular lesions - A brief review. International Journal of Approximate Reasoning. 2017;**5**:1469-1475

[12] Waner M, North PE, Scherer KA, Frieden IJ, Waner A, Mihm MC Jr. The nonrandom distribution of facial hemangiomas. Archives of Dermatology. 2003;**139**(7):869-875. DOI: 10.1001/archderm.139.7.869

[13] Barnés CM, Christison-Lagay EA, Folkman J. The placenta theory and the origin of infantile hemangioma. Lymphatic Research and Biology. 2007;**5**(4):245-255. DOI: 10.1089/lrb.2007.1018

[14] Phung TL, Hochman M. Pathogenesis of infantile hemangioma. Facial Plastic Surgery. 2012;**28**(6):554-562. DOI: 10.1055/s-0032-1329930. Epub 2012 November 27

[15] Sun Y, Qiu F, Hu C, Guo Y, Lei S. Hemangioma endothelial cells and hemangioma stem cells in infantile hemangioma. Annals of Plastic Surgery.

2022;**88**(2):244-249. DOI: 10.1097/SAP.0000000000002835

[16] North PE, Waner M, Mizeracki A, Mihm MC Jr. GLUT1: A newly discovered immunohistochemical marker for juvenile hemangiomas. Human Pathology. 2000;**31**(1):11-22. DOI: 10.1016/s0046-8177(00)80192-6

[17] Walter JW, North PE, Waner M, Mizeracki A, Blei F, Walker JW, et al. Somatic mutation of vascular endothelial growth factor receptors in juvenile hemangioma. Genes, Chromosomes & Cancer. 2002;**33**(3):295-303. DOI: 10.1002/gcc.10028

[18] Boye E, Yu Y, Paranya G, Mulliken JB, Olsen BR, Bischoff J. Clonality and altered behavior of endothelial cells from hemangiomas. The Journal of Clinical Investigation. 2001;**107**(6):745-752. DOI: 10.1172/JCI11432

[19] Chang EI et al. Hypoxia, hormones, and endothelial progenitor cells in hemangioma. Lymphatic Research and Biology. 2007;**5**(4):237-243

[20] Sun Z et al. Possibilities and potential roles of estrogen in the pathogenesis of proliferation hemangiomas formation. Medical Hypotheses. 2008;**71**(2):286-292

[21] Lui W, Zhang S, Hu T, Wei F, Gao Y, Cheng N. Sex hormone receptors of hemangiomas in children. Chinese Medical Journal. 1997;**110**(5):349-351

[22] Mooberry SL. New insights into 2-methoxyestradiol, a promising antiangiogenic and antitumor agent. Current Opinion in Oncology. 2003;**15**(6):425-430. DOI: 10.1097/00001622-200311000-00004

[23] Friedlander SF, Ritter MR, Friedlander M. Recent progress in our understanding of the pathogenesis of infantile hemangiomas. Lymphatic Research and Biology. 2005;**3**(4):219-225. DOI: 10.1089/lrb.2005.3.219

[24] Ritter MR, Reinisch J, Friedlander SF, Friedlander M. Myeloid cells in infantile hemangioma. The American Journal of Pathology. 2006;**168**(2):621-628. DOI: 10.2353/ajpath.2006.050618

[25] Bielenberg DR, Bucana CD, Sanchez R, Mulliken JB, Folkman J, Fidler IJ. Progressive growth of infantile cutaneous hemangiomas is directly correlated with hyperplasia and angiogenesis of adjacent epidermis and inversely correlated with expression of the endogenous angiogenesis inhibitor, IFN-beta. International Journal of Oncology. 1999;**14**(3):401-408

[26] Ritter MR, Moreno SK, Dorrell MI, Rubens J, Ney J, Friedlander DF, et al. Identifying potential regulators of infantile hemangioma progression through large-scale expression analysis: A possible role for the immune system and indoleamine 2,3 dioxygenase (IDO) during involution. Lymphatic Research and Biology. 2003;**1**(4):291-299. DOI: 10.1089/153968503322758094

[27] Yin RR, Hao D, Chen P. Expression and correlation of MMP-9, VEGF, and p16 in infantile hemangioma. European Review for Medical and Pharmacological Sciences. 2018;**22**(15):4806-4811. DOI: 10.26355/eurrev_201808_15615

[28] Tan ST, Wallis RA, He Y, Davis PF. Mast cells and hemangioma. Plastic and Reconstructive Surgery. 2004;**113**(3):999-1011. DOI: 10.1097/01.prs.0000105683.10752.a6

[29] Pugh CW, Ratcliffe PJ. Regulation of angiogenesis by hypoxia: Role of the HIF system. Nature Medicine. 2003;**9**(6):677-684. DOI: 10.1038/nm0603-677

[30] Fu X, Zhai S, Yuan J. Interleukin-6 (IL-6) triggers the malignancy of hemangioma cells via activation of HIF-1α/VEGFA signals. European Journal of Pharmacology. 2018;**841**:82-89. DOI: 10.1016/j.ejphar.2018.10.022. Epub 2018 October 19

[31] Bejjanki KM, Mishra DK, Kaliki S. Periocular lobular capillary hemangioma in adults: A clinicopathological study. Middle East African Journal of Ophthalmology. 2019;**26**(3):138-140. DOI: 10.4103/meajo.MEAJO_42_19

[32] Stagner AM, Jakobiec FA. A critical analysis of eleven periocular lobular capillary hemangiomas in adults. American Journal of Ophthalmology. 2016;**165**:164-173. DOI: 10.1016/j.ajo.2016.03.010

[33] Krol A, MacArthur CJ. Congenital hemangiomas: Rapidly involuting and noninvoluting congenital hemangiomas. Archives of Facial Plastic Surgery. 2005;**7**(5):307-311

[34] Low CM, Stokken JK. Typical orbital pathologies: Hemangioma. Journal of Neurological Surgery Part B: Skull Base. 2021;**82**(1):20-26. DOI: 10.1055/s-0040-1722633

[35] George A, Mani V, Noufal A. Update on the classification of hemangioma. Journal of Oral and Maxillofacial Pathology. 2014;**18**(Suppl 1):S117-S120. DOI: 10.4103/0973-029X.141321

[36] Darrow DH, Greene AK, Mancini AJ, Nopper AJ; Section on dermatology, section on otolaryngology–Head and neck surgery, and section on plastic surgery. Diagnosis and management of infantile hemangioma. Pediatrics. 2015;**136**(4):e1060-e1104. DOI: 10.1542/peds.2015-2485

[37] Tavakoli M, Yadegari S, Mosallaei M, Aletaha M, Salour H, Lee WW. Infantile periocular hemangioma. Journal of Ophthalmic and Vision Research. 2017;**12**(2):205-211. DOI: 10.4103/jovr.jovr_66_17

[38] Maguiness S, Guenther L. Kasabach-merritt syndrome. Journal of Cutaneous Medicine and Surgery. 2002;**6**(4):335-339. DOI: 10.1177/120347540200600405. Epub 2002 April 15

[39] Hartemink DA, Chiu YE, Drolet BA, Kerschner JE. PHACES syndrome: A review. International Journal of Pediatric Otorhinolaryngology. 2009;**73**(2):181-187. DOI: 10.1016/j.ijporl.2008.10.017

[40] Hernandez JA, Chia A, Quah BL, Seah LL. Periocular capillary hemangioma: Management practices in recent years. Clinical Ophthalmology. 2013;**7**:1227-1232

[41] Sterker I, Gräfe G. Periocular hemangiomas in childhood--Functional and esthetic results. Strabismus. 2004;**12**(2):103-110

[42] Tan X, Guo S, Wang C. Propranolol in the treatment of infantile hemangiomas. Clinical, Cosmetic and Investigational Dermatology. 2021;**14**:1155-1163. DOI: 10.2147/CCID.S332625

[43] de Graaf M, Breur J, Raphaël MF, Vos M, Breugem CC, Pasmans S. Adverse effects of propranolol when used in the treatment of hemangiomas: A case series of 28 infants. Journal of the American Academy of Dermatology. 2011;**65**(2):320-327

[44] Chung SH, Park DH, Jung HL, Shim JW, Kim DS, Shim JY, et al. Successful and safe treatment of hemangioma with oral propranolol in a single institution. Korean Journal of Pediatrics. 2012;**55**(5):164-170

[45] Xue K, Hildebrand GD. Deep periocular infantile capillary hemangiomas responding to topical application of timolol maleate, 0.5%, drops. JAMA Ophthalmology. 2013;**131**(9):1246-1248

[46] Ni N, Langer P, Wagner R, Guo S. Topical timolol for periocular hemangioma: Report of further study. Archives of Ophthalmology. 2011;**129**(3):377-379

[47] Muñoz-Garza FZ, Ríos M, Roé-Crespo E, Bernabeu-Wittel J, Montserrat-García MT, Puig L, et al. Efficacy and safety of topical timolol for the treatment of infantile hemangioma in the early proliferative stage: A randomized clinical trial. JAMA Dermatology. 2021;**157**(5):583-587. DOI: 10.1001/jamadermatol.2021.0596

[48] Nagata E, Kashiwagura Y, Okada E, Tanaka S, Sano S, Nishida M, et al. Efficacy and safety of propranolol cream in infantile hemangioma: A prospective pilot study. Journal of Pharmacological Sciences. 2022;**149**(2):60-65

[49] Awadein A, Fakhry MA. Evaluation of intralesional propranolol for periocular capillary hemangioma. Clinical Ophthalmology. 2011;**5**:1135-1140

[50] Greenberger S, Boscolo E, Adini I, Mulliken JB, Bischoff J. Corticosteroid suppression of VEGF-A in infantile hemangioma-derived stem cells. The New England Journal of Medicine. 2010;**362**(11):1005-1013

[51] Gangopadhyay AN, Sinha CK, Gopal SC, Gupta DK, Sahoo SP, Ahmad M. Role of steroid in childhood haemangioma: A 10 years review. International Surgery. 1997;**82**(1):49-51

[52] Heyns AD, Eldor A, Vlodavsky I, et al. The antiproliferative effect of interferon and the mitogenic activity of growth factors are in-dependent cell cycle events studies with vascular smooth muscle cells and endothelial cells. Experimental Cell Research. 1985;**161**:297-306

[53] Tamayo L, Ortiz DM, Orozco-Covarrubias L, et al. Therapeutic efficacy of interferon alpha-2b in infants with life-threatening giant hemangiomas. Archives of Dermatology. 1997;**133**:1567-1571

[54] Jiménez-Hernández E, Dueñas-González MT, Quintero-Curiel JL, Velásquez-Ortega J, Magaña-Pérez JA, Berges-García A, et al. Treatment with interferon-alpha-2b in children with life-threatening hemangiomas. Dermatologic Surgery. 2008;**34**(5):640-647

[55] Sarihan H, Mocan H, Yildiz K, Abes M, Akyazici R. A new treatment with bleomycin for complicated cutaneous hemangioma in children. European Journal of Pediatric Surgery. 1997;7(3):158-162

[56] Deans RM, Harris GJ, Kivlin JD. Surgical dissection of capillary hemangiomas. An alternative to intralesional corticosteroids. Archives of Ophthalmology. 1992;**110**(12):1743-1747

[57] Kono T, Sakurai H, Groff WF, Chan HH, Takeuchi M, Yamaki T, et al. Comparison study of a traditional pulsed dye laser versus a long-pulsed dye laser in the treatment of early childhood hemangiomas. Lasers in Surgery and Medicine. 2006;**38**(2):112-115

[58] Brauer JA, Geronemus RG. Laser treatment in the management of infantile hemangiomas and capillary vascular malformations. Techniques in

Vascular and Interventional Radiology. 2013;**16**(1):51-54

[59] Chinnadurai S, Sathe NA, Surawicz T. Laser treatment of infantile hemangioma: A systematic review. Lasers in Surgery and Medicine. 2016;**48**(3):221-233. DOI: 10.1002/lsm.22455. Epub 2015 December 29

Chapter 7

Infantile Hemangioma

Sevgi Gözdaşoğlu

Abstract

Infantile hemangiomas (IHs) are the most benign vascular tumors of infancy. IHs occur in 10–12% of infants. They often appear within 1–4 weeks of life. Superficial lesions are bright red or "strawberry" in color, sharply demarcated papules, nodules or plaques. Deep lesions are of bluish hue and dome-shaped. IHs are described as localized or focal, segmental, indeterminate or multifocal pattern, depending on the anatomic appearance. Segmental lesions are often associated with complications. High-risk IH groups which have severe complications can be observed in IHs with disfigurement, life-threatening complications, functional impairment, ulceration and associated structural anomalies; PHACE syndrome (Posterior fossa brain malformations and large facial hemangiomas, Hemangiomas of the cervicofacial region, Arterial anomalies, Coarctation of the aorta and cardiac defects, Eye abnormalities, Sternal cleft and supraumbilical raphe) and LUMBAR syndrome (Lower body hemangioma often extending onto a unilateral lower extremity, Urogenital anomalies, ulceration, Myelopathy, Bony deformities, Anorectal malformations, arterial anomalies and Renal anomalies). Early treatment is vital to avoid complications in high-risk IHs. The presence of segmental IH larger than 5 cm on face, scalp or cervical region is the major sign of PHACE syndrome, whereas segmental IHs affecting the lower body are the significant signs of LUMBAR syndrome.

Keywords: infantile hemangioma, HemSCs, HemECs, VEGFR, PHACE syndrome, LUMBAR syndrome

1. Introduction

Infantile hemangiomas (IHs) are vascular birthmarks and represent the most common benign vascular tumors of infancy. Virchow used the term "angioma" to describe all vascular anomalies. The word "hemangioma" is derived from the ancient Greek word "haima" meaning blood [1]. In 1982, the first biological classification of vascular birthmarks was proposed by Mulliken and Glowacki who divided these lesions into two groups: hemangiomas and vascular malformations [2]. The new classification by the International Society for the Study of Vascular Anomalies (ISSVA) was published in 2018, according to which vascular anomalies are separated into two major categories: the first is vascular tumors and the second is vascular malformations. Vascular tumors are associated with proliferative changes of endothelial cells (ECs) and vascular malformations primarily consisted of structural vascular abnormalities [3]. Infantile hemangiomas are the most common benign vascular tumors, rapidly growing during the first year of life and subsequently involuting. In the literature, the articles on the clinical characteristics

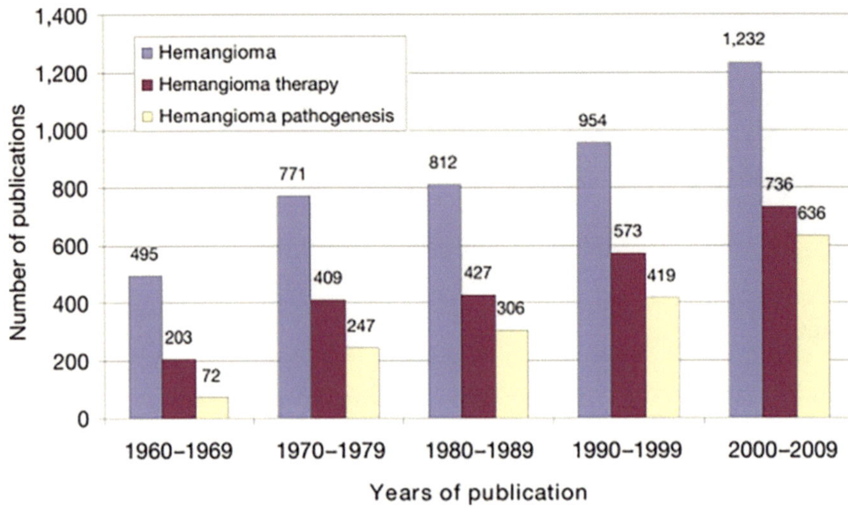

Figure 1.
Results of a PubMed search on August 1, 2011 (used with permission of Frieden).

of IHs, advancement in treatment approaches and the studies on pathogenesis increased remarkably. Frieden published an article detailing the increase of the articles on the issue between 1960 and 2009 in a chronological order (**Figure 1**) [4]. Leung et al. reviewed meta-analyses, randomized controlled trials, clinical trials, observational studies and reviews by PubMed search which were published in the past 20 years and reported the clinical evaluation of IHs, risk factors and congenital abnormalities which are seen with IHs, diagnostic and differential diagnosis criteria and treatment approaches [5]. Lin et al. recently evaluated for the first time the bibliometric analyses specifically focusing on IHs publications. A total of 4333 articles and reviews on IHs were collected from Web of Science (WoS) database from 2000 to 2022. The United States has the highest number of publications, the highest total number of citations and the largest number of scientific research institutions and IH researchers, leading most of the cross-country collaborations. The top five countries with the most publications on IHs are given as follows: USA, China, Italy, United Kingdom and Japan. Although China is ranked as the second country regarding published articles on this issue, the number of citations is low. The top three most influential authors were Frieden, Mulliken and Drolet. The articles published by Léauté-Lebrèze in 2008 had the highest number of citations. A certain research foundation for this field was laid by the articles published by North PE in 2000 and Boye E in 2001 [6].

In this chapter, my main objective is twofold: to review the pathogenesis of IHs and to analyze clinical presentations, risk factors, complications of IHs and hemangioma-related syndromes. The treatment of infantile hemangiomas is excluded in this chapter.

2. Epidemiology and risk factors

The incidence of IHs is estimated to be 1.1–2.6% in neonates and 10–12% in infants by the first year of life [5, 7]. IHs develop more commonly in female infants. The female-to-male ratio is approximately 3:1–5:1 [5, 8]. Ding et al. reported the results of the meta-analysis of the published studies of potential risk factors for IHs. According to this meta-analysis, risk factors, such as preterm birth, low birth weight, female gender, multiple gestation, progesterone therapy and family history, may affect the appearance of IHs [9]. Additionally, twins, white ethnicity, increased maternal age, preeclampsia, placental anomalies (such as placenta previa, placental abruption and abnormal insertion of the umbilical cord), *in vitro* fertilization, maternal vaginal bleeding during the first trimester, gestational diabetes mellitus, gestational hypertension, invasive *antepartum* procedures (such as amniocentesis and chorionic villus sampling), perinatal hypoxia and mechanical stress during delivery may also have an effect on the occurrence of these lesions [5, 8]. On the other hand, Blei et al. identified six kindreds where hemangiomas appear to segregate as an autosomal dominant trait with high penetrance. A linkage to a locus on chromosome 5q31-33 has been identified in genetic mapping of a novel familial form of infantile hemangioma based on recombination breakpoint analyses by the same researchers [10, 11].

3. ISSVA classification

The International Society for the Study of Vascular Anomalies (ISSVA) classification has provided a better understanding of the terminologies, biology and clinical characteristics of vascular tumors and vascular malformations. The ISSVA classification is shown in **Table 1**. Vascular anomalies were classified into two large categories: vascular tumors and vascular malformations [3]. Vascular malformations, which include capillary, lymphatic, venous and arterial vessel formation, are described as congenital developmental disorders [12, 13]. Whereas vascular tumors are characterized by endothelial cell hyperproliferation, typically lesions grow rapidly and most of them are not present at birth [13]. Vascular tumors are classified as benign, locally aggressive or borderline and malignant [3].

4. Pathogenesis

The pathogenesis of IHs is complex and poorly understood. There are many researches that aim to have a better understanding of the pathogenesis of IHs in the literature and several hypotheses have been proposed. Scientists have suggested that IHs are a result of dysregulated vasculogenesis and angiogenesis. Angiogenesis and vasculogenesis are regulated by many important signaling pathways, such as vascular endothelial growth factor (VEGF)/vascular endothelial growth factor receptor (VEGFR) pathway, Notch pathway, β-adrenergic signaling, hypoxia-inducible growth factor-α (HIF-α)-mediated pathway, etc. These pathways have been linked to each other by several interactions in the development of angiogenesis and vasculogenesis [14, 15].

Placental growth factor (PIGF), vascular endothelial growth factor A (VEGF-A), vascular endothelial growth factor B (VEGF-B), vascular endothelial growth factor C (VEGF-C) and vascular endothelial growth factor D (VEGF-D) are members of the human vascular endothelial growth factor (VEGF) family that plays pivotal roles in embryonic development and angiogenesis-dependent disease [15]. The functions of the VEGF family members are defined by their receptors' specificity. Two receptors for VEGF (VEGFR-1 and VEGFR-2) which play the regulation of angiogenesis are located on endothelial cells, bone marrow-derived hematopoietic cells and tumor cells. They are also members of the tyrosine-kinase family. The expression of these receptors is low in normal tissues [15]. Boscolo et al. reported VEGF-A levels in serum samples were found to be significantly higher in proliferating compared to involuting phases [16].

Vascular tumors	Vascular malformations
• Benign vascular tumors *Infantile hemangioma* Congenital hemangiomas *Rapidly involuting (RICH)* *Non-involuting (NICH)* *Partially involuting (PICH)* Tufted angioma Spindle-cell hemangioma Epithelioid hemangioma Pyogenic granuloma (or lobular capillary hemangioma) • Locally aggressive or borderline vascular tumors *Kaposiform hemangioendothelioma* *Other hemangioendotheliomas* *Kaposi sarcoma* • Malignant vascular tumors *Angiosarcoma* *Epithelioid hemangioendotheliomas*	• Simple *Capillary* *Lymphatic* *Venous* *Arteriovenous malformations*[a] *Arteriovenous fistula*[a] • Combined[b] *CVM, CLM* *LVM, CLVM* *CAVM*[a] *CLAVM*[a] *Others* • Major vessels • Associated with other anomalies *Klippel-Trenaunay synd.* *Parkes-Weber synd.* *Servelle-Martorell synd.* *Sturge-Weber synd.* *Limb CM + congenital non-progressive limb hypertrophy* *Maffucci synd.* *Macrocephaly-CM* *Microcephaly-CM* *CLOVES synd.* *Proteus synd.* *Bannayan-Riley-Ruvalcaba synd.*

[a]*High flow lesion.*
[b]*More than one type of vessel (C—capillary, V—venous, L—lymphatic, A—arterial, M—malformation and synd.—syndrome).*

Table 1.
ISSVA classification for vascular tumors and vascular malformations.

The first hypothesis is the somatic mutation of hemangioma stem cells and upregulation of vascular endothelial growth factor receptor (VEGFR) signaling pathway. Hemangioma stem cells (HemSCs) and hemangioma endothelial cells (HemECs) are the two most important cells in the pathogenesis of IHs. Hemangioma stem cells have the ability to undergo self-renewal and can differentiate into HemECs, pericytes and adipocytes (**Figure 2**).

Infantile hemangiomas have three characteristic phases:

1. *Proliferating phase*, it is characterized by the proliferation of a large number of HemECs. Hemangioma stem cells mainly differentiate into HemECs and pericytes to promote angiogenesis.

2. *Involuting phase*, HemSCs mainly differentiate into adipocytes, inhibiting the proliferation of HemECs.

3. *Involuted phase*, the tumor is replaced by fat and/or connective tissues in this phase [14–16].

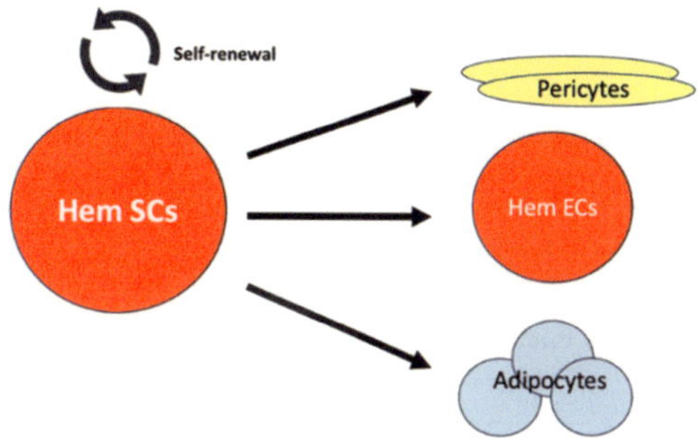

Figure 2.
Multipotent hemangioma-derived stem cells (HemSCs) differentiate into HemECs, pericytes and adipocytes. HemSCs play an important role in the pathogenesis of IHs (adapted from Ref. [16]. Used with permission of Boscolo).

Khan et al. investigated to determine whether HemSCs would form hemangiomas in immunodeficient nu/nu mice. When implanted subcutaneously into nude mice, HemSCs can produce the erythrocyte-type glucose transporter 1 protein (GLUT-1) positive microvessels at 7–14 days. Hemangioma stem cells form hemangioma-like GLUT-1 positive blood vessels in nude mice [17]. This study identified a stem cell as the cellular origin of IHs.

Boscolo and Bischoff recognize that IHs may not only be a disorder of angiogenesis (i.e., the formation of new blood vessels from existing vessels) but also—at least in part—a disorder of vasculogenesis (i.e., the *de novo* formation of new blood vessels from cells) [16].

The second hypothesis is the placental theory which proposes that a fetal placental progenitor cell is the cell type of origin for IHs. North et al. published an article that identified the marker GLUT-1 as a specific feature of IHs during all phases of these lesions. The GLUT-1 is highly expressed in human brain and placenta but not in normal skin or subcutaneous tissue. GLUT-1 immunoreactivity, which is a highly selective and diagnostically useful maker for IHs, was not found in any of the vascular malformations in this research [18]. Placenta-associated antigens, which are Fc gamma receptor II (Fc-gamma-RII), Lewis Y antigen (LeY), merosin and GLUT-1, are expressed in an infantile hemangioma (IH). Infantile hemangioma might also originate from embolized placental tissue [18, 19]. Mihm Jr. et al. suggested that the hemangioma precursor cell comes from the placenta as a "benign metastasis" [20].

The third hypothesis is the tissue hypoxia-induced vascular proliferation theory. Hypoxia is one of the most powerful inducers of angiogenesis and vasculogenesis by stimulating the expression of angiogenic factors, such as VEGF-A and basic fibroblast growth factor (bFGF), on endothelial progenitor cells. Many of the conditions such as preterm birth, low birth weight, preeclampsia and placental anomalies, which predispose an infant to development of IHs, are associated with hypoxia. It is believed that hypoxia stimulates the release of hypoxia-inducible factor-1α (HIF-1α) which promotes the production of VEGF [15, 16].

Hypoxia-inducible factor-1α (HIF-1α) is expressed significantly high in HemECs than normal in endothelial cells (ECs). It is also a significant contributor to the elevated VEGF levels produced in HemECs when it is upregulated. The decreased expression of HIF-1α reduces the proliferation of these cells [15].

MicroRNA (miRNA) and long noncoding RNAs (IncRNAs) also affect the profileration, migration and apoptosis of HemECs. The chromosome 19 miRNA cluster (C19MC) are expressed both in the placenta and in IH endothelial cells, but are not in other vascular anomalies and in the control group of healthy infants. A correlation with the tumor size and clinical response to treatment is demonstrated by circulating C19MC microRNA levels. This is the first potential biomarker for IHs [14].

The fourth hypothesis is the renin-angiotensin system theory. Itinteang et al. reported that IH endothelial cells in the proliferative phase express angiotensin-converting enzyme (ACE) and angiotensin II-receptor-2 (ATII-receptor-2), both integral components of the renin-angiotensin system. According to their hypothesis, the high serum levels of renin lead to a high concentration of angiotensin II [21]. Both angiotensin II and angiotensin II-receptor-2 upregulate VEGF that activates the proliferation of IHs-derived blast cells. The expression of ACE and ATII-receptor-2 on the endothelium of proliferating IH supports this theory [21]. Tan et al. reported that β-adrenergic blockers may be associated with the blocking of β1-adrenergic receptors in the kidney, leading to the inhibition of renin release in the accelerated involution of IH [21, 22]. The spontaneous involution that occurs in IH may be related to decreasing serum renin levels with age and/or depletion of the endothelial progenitor cells with time [23]. Interactions between proposed theories of infantile hemangioma pathogenesis are shown in **Figure 3**.

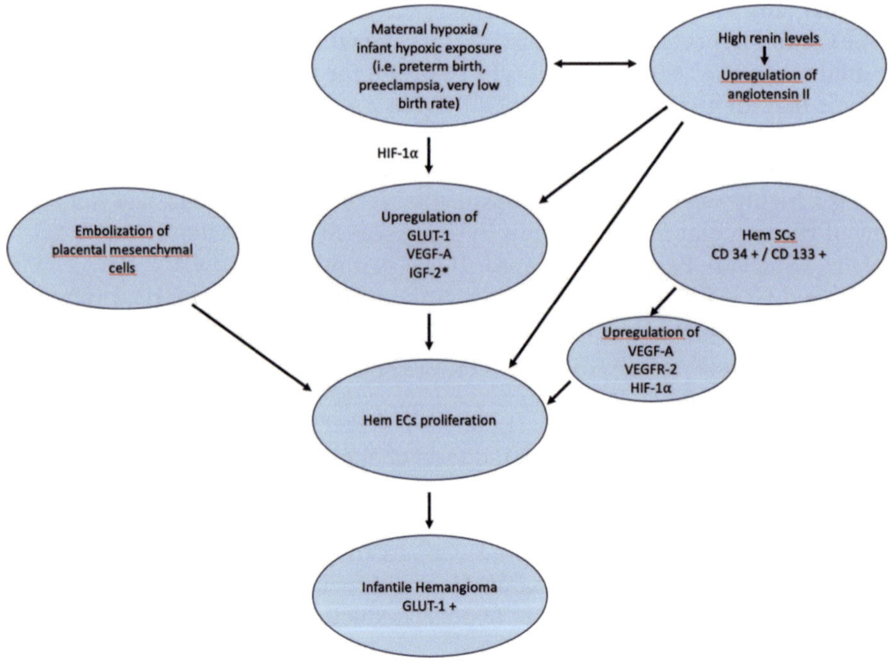

Figure 3.
*Interactions between proposed theories of infantile hemangioma pathogenesis. * IGF-2, insulin-like growth factor (adapted from Ref. [23]. Used with permission of Forbess Smith).*

5. Histopathology

Most of the lesions are developed in the skin and subcutaneous tissues. These are hypervascular, multinodular patterns that are composed of hyperplastic endothelial cells, pericytes and prominent basement membranes (**Figures 4** and **5**) [24, 25].

Glowacki et al. reported that hemangiomas in the proliferative phase contained large numbers of mast cells in comparison with hemangiomas in the involution phase. Mast cells may have an important role in the development of IHs [26]. Dilated vascular lumens and flattened endothelial cells are observed in the involution stage [24]. Placenta-associated antigens staining, including FcRII, Lewis Y antigen (LeY), merosin and GLUT-1, is expressed in an IH [19, 20]. Infantile hemangiomas express GLUT-1 during all phases of their development (**Figure 6**).

GLUT-1 immunoreactivity is a highly selective useful marker for diagnosis [18].

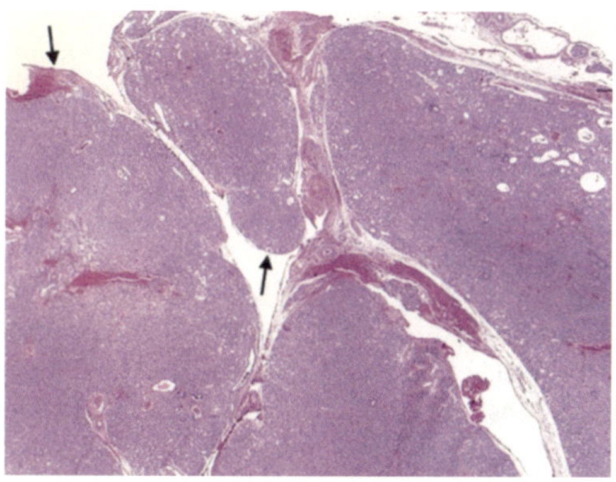

Figure 4.
The image shows lobular growth pattern of infantile hemangioma -a common form of capillary hemangioma (from WebPathology.com).

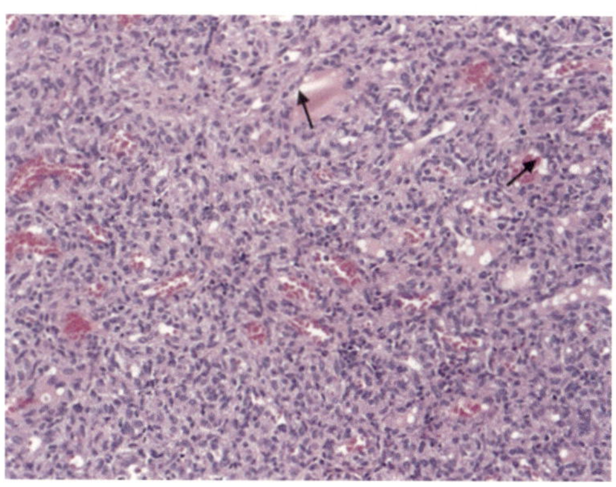

Figure 5.
Plump endothelial cells line with and without lumens in the early phases of the lesions (from WebPathology.com).

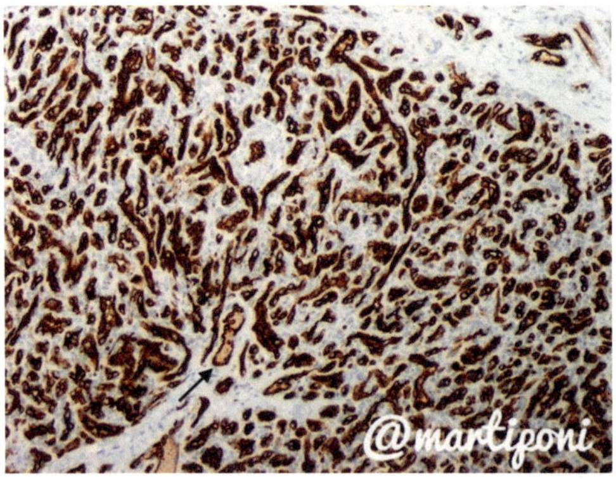

Figure 6.
The endothelial cells of infantile hemangiomas consistently express GLUT-1+, which is a brown colored protein in the endothelial cells, a glucose transport receptor (image courtesy of: Marta Garrido, MD, Barcelona, Spain; from WebPathalogy.com).

6. Clinical manifestations

Infantile hemangiomas are clinically heterogeneous by their appearance in regard to superficially, depth, location and stage of evaluation. Infantile hemangiomas have a triphasic evaluation.

1. *Proliferative phase*: infantile hemangiomas (IHs) grow rapidly in the first 3 months of life but occasionally the proliferative phase may continue up to 12 months of age. The lesion is stable between 6 and 12 months in plateau period.

2. *Involution phase*: this phase begins around 1 year of age and continues for 3–5 years. Approximately 50% of IHs will show complete involution by the time a child reaches age 5.

3. *Involuted phase*: this phase is reached by 5–8 years of age but sometimes up to 10 years of age. The tumor sometimes is replaced by fat and/or connective tissues [14].

In the newborn, hemangiomas may originate as a pale macule with thread-like telangiectases [7]. They often appear within 1–4 weeks of life [8, 27]. Two types of skin lesions, namely "superficial" and "deeper," can be seen in IHs. Bright red or "strawberry" in color, raised, sharply demarcated, firm papules, nodules or plaques are observed as superficial lesions. Deeper lesions may appear as a skin-colored nodule or can have more of a bluish hue [7, 23]. Mixed lesions in which both epidermis and deeper subcutaneous tissues are involved were also reported in some cases [23].

On the other hand, depending on the anatomic appearance IHs are described as localized or focal, segmental, indeterminate or multifocal pattern. Localized or focal IHs are the most common pattern, well-circumscribed focal lesions appearing to rise from a point while segmental IHs are plaque-like extensive IHs measuring 5 cm in diameter. Segmental IHs may be associated with extracutaneous manifestations. Indeterminate IHs are not clearly localized or segmental and are often called partial segmental, whereas multifocal IHs are multiple discrete IHs located at multiple distant sites [28].

Hemangiomas are usually solitary with a size range from a few millimeters to several centimeters in diameter. Approximately 20% of cases have multiple lesions [7]. Approximately 60% of IHs are superficial, 15% deep and 25% mixed—superficial and deep (**Figures** 7 and **8**) [29, 30].

Head and neck are primary regions where IHs are most frequently located. These are followed by the trunk 25% and the extremities 15%. IHs rarely develop in the intestinal organs, such as the liver, gastrointestinal tract, respiratory tract, urinary tract and central nervous system [8]. Hepatic hemangiomas can be identified as focal, multifocal or diffuse types. Kulungowski et al. investigated that cutaneous hemangiomas are associated with multifocal hepatic hemangioma, diffuse hepatic hemangioma and focal hepatic hemangioma. Hypothyroidism was determined in all the patients with diffuse hepatic hemangioma, 21.4% with multifocal hepatic hemangioma but it was not recognized in any of the patients with focal hepatic hemangioma [31]. Hypothyroidism can be observed due to inactivation of the thyroid hormones by type 3 iodothyronine deiodinase (D3) in the tumor tissue [32].

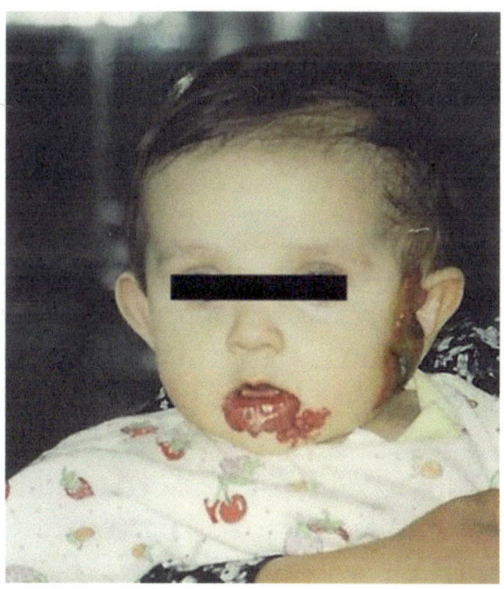

Figure 7.
A 4-month-old girl with a superficial infantile hemangioma on the face.

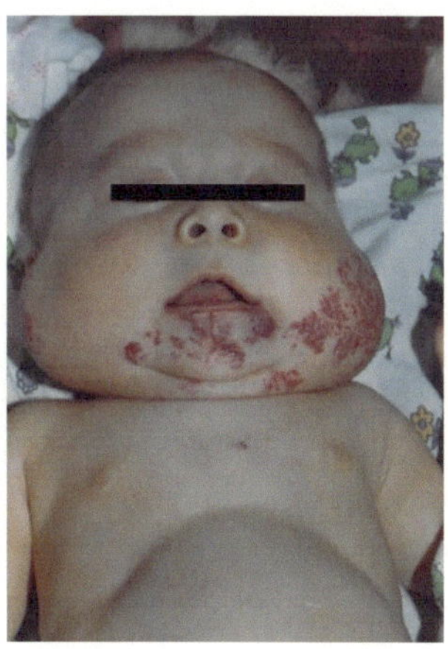

Figure 8.
Infantile hemangioma on the mandibular segment and cardiac failure in a 1-month-old girl.

Infantile hemangioma can be linked to particular congenital organ malformations. Blei et al. reported an infant girl with cutaneous facial and upper trunk hemangioma accompanied supraumbilical midabdominal raphe and sternal atresia. This association is the first report in the dermatologic literature [33]. In 1996, Frieden et al. reported two patients who had large facial hemangioma, congenital cataracts, and structural arterial abnormalities, particularly of the central nervous system vasculature. The authors thought that large >5 cm particularly facial hemangiomas associated with these anomalies are a distinct group and referred to as the "PHACE syndrome" for this association [34].

A 1-month-old infant (**Figure 8**) was admitted to our intensive care unit (ICU) with difficulty in breathing, cyanosis and the large infantile hemangiomas on the mandibular segment. Her eyes were closed and she was unresponsive to painful stimulus. She had all signs of heart failure and massive hepatomegaly. The patient expired due to cardiac failure, despite rapid digitalization. Although the *postmortem* examination could not be realized to make the correct diagnosis, we thought that this patient might have had a PHACE syndrome.

Infantile hemangioma can be linked to particular congenital organ malformations. These dysmorphic features in PHACES syndrome include; *P*osterior fossa brain malformations, *H*emangiomas of the cervicofacial region, *A*rterial anomalies, *C*oarctation of the aorta and cardiac defects, *E*ye abnormalities, *S*ternal cleft and supraumbilical raphe. Sternal defects were added later. Drolet et al. referred to the abnormalities as the PHACES syndrome [7].

Large lumbosacral hemangioma associated with congenital anomalies is LUMBAR syndrome. The LUMBAR syndrome includes: *L*ower body hemangioma often extending onto a unilateral lower extremity, *U*rogenital anomalies, *U*lceration, *M*yelopathy, *B*ony deformities, *A*norectal malformations, *A*rterial anomalies and *R*enal anomalies [7, 32, 35].

The PHACE syndrome is observed in 2–3% of IHs and in these patients cerebrovascular abnormalities 83–91% and cardiac abnormalities 41–67% are the most common manifestations. Higher risk of ocular and central nervous system involvement can be seen when IHs are on the frontotemporal and frontonasal segments, whereas a greater risk of midline and cardiovascular defects is higher when IHs develop on the mandibular segment. Additionally endocrine abnormalities, such as thyroid dysfunction, hypopituitarism with growth hormone deficiency, adrenal insufficiency and neonatal hypoglycemia, have been described [36]. The presence of a large facial segmental often superficial IH is the major sign of PHACE syndrome. In the literature, over 300 patients were reported and it is considered one of the most common neurocutaneous vascular disorders in childhood [36].

6.1 Complications of infantile hemangiomas

Important complications may occur in the patients with IHs according to the size, the anatomic localization, the superficiality and the depth of tumors. High-risk groups of IHs identified by The American Academy of Pediatrics (AAP) published its first clinical practice guideline (CPG) for the management of IHs in 2018.

High-risk IH groups are those with:

1. Disfigurement

2. Life-threatening complications

3. Functional impairment

4. Ulceration

5. Associated structural anomalies:

PHACE syndrome.
LUMBAR syndrome [3].

Segmental lesions are often associated with complications. Pediatricians should identify the high-risk IH group before 3 months of age, ideally at 1 month of age [3]. Risk stratification in these patients is principal for diagnosis and early treatment. Ulceration, infection and bleeding are the most common complications in superficial IHs [32, 37]. Chamlin et al. reported that ulceration occurred in 15.8% of 1096 total patients with IHs and located on the lower lip, neck or anogenital region. Ulceration occurred at a median age of 4 months and bleeding developed in 41%. IHs with ulcerations were large, mixed clinical type and segmental morphologic type [37, 38]. In addition, skin ulceration is causing pain, scarring and unesthetic sequelae [37, 38]. Recurrence occurred in 16% of the treated cases [38]. Infantile hemangiomas with life-threatening complications include obstructive airway hemangiomas and hepatic hemangiomas, heart failure and hypothyroidism. These complications may develop when the IHs localize in the beard area and the patient has multiple >5 cutaneous lesions, respectively [32].

Functional impairment, such as visual disturbances, astigmatism, anisometropia, retrobulbar involvement (**Figures 9** and **10**), tear duct obstruction, proptosis, amblyopia, may occur in periocular IHs, especially in patients of upper eyelid IHs larger than 1 cm.

On the other hand, feeding problems may occur in cases with nasal or lip, oral cavity IHs [3]. Disfigurement develops in IHs localized on noise, ears and perioral area, or large facial area. Segmental and facial IHs show a high risk of unesthetic sequelae, complications and recurrence [38].

Glucocorticosteroids, interferon-alpha-2a and interferon-alpha-2b therapy for high-risk hemangiomas were effective, well-tolerated treatments before

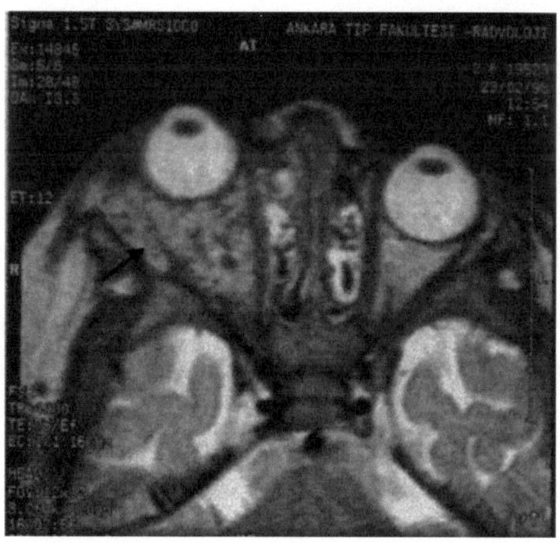

Figure 9.
T2-weighted axial magnetic resonance imaging (MRI) showing retro-orbital infantile hemangioma in a 2-month-old girl.

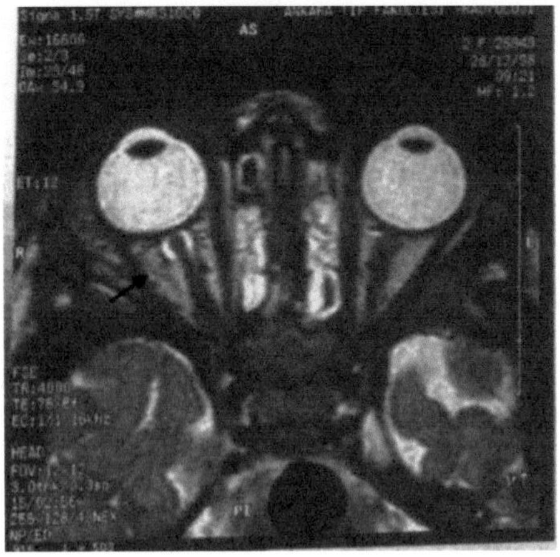

Figure 10.
Significant decrease of the tumor after 11 months of therapy with prednisone + IFN-α-2a.

2008 [39–41]. Léaute-Labrèze et al. discovered the beneficial effects of propranolol for severe IHs and since 2008, propranolol has become the first line of treatment [42].

6.2 Diagnosis and differential diagnosis

The diagnosis is mainly based on clinical appearance. Several factors provide clues for accurate diagnosis, such as the timing of appearance of the lesion, changes in size, color over time and tactile qualities [43]. Dermoscopy, which is useful for evaluating the precise vascular structure, typically shows a polymorphous vascular structure with or without obvious red linear vessels and red dilated vessels in IHs [44, 45]. Biopsy and pathological diagnosis are rarely required when IH is differentiated from congenital hemangiomas (CHs) and vascular abnormalities. Ultrasonography is generally the preferred modality, especially in infants younger than 4 months of age. Doppler ultrasonography and MRI may be helpful in differential diagnosis [46]. Imaging may also be useful in evaluating the extent of complicated hemangioma, evaluating for other potential anomalies such as PHACES syndrome and LUMBAR syndrome or following response to therapy, particularly in the case of hepatic hemangiomas. MRI is the most sensitive technique used for definitive diagnosis of LUMBAR syndrome. In infants with >5 cutaneous lesions, abdominal ultrasonography is recommended [32]. Computed tomography (CT) should be avoided because of the increased susceptibility of children to ionizing radiation [46].

Infantile hemangiomas must be differentiated from other vascular tumors, particularly CHs and vascular malformations. Congenital hemangiomas are fully formed at birth and differ from IHs in their histological and immunohistochemical findings. GLUT-1 immunoreactivity is a diagnostically useful marker that is positive in all the development phases of IHs and negative in CHs and other vascular tumors [18, 25].

Rapidly Involuting Congenital Hemangiomas (RICH) and Non-Involuting Congenital Hemangiomas (NICH) that form *in utero* have no sex predilection, are pink or violet in color and do not grow postnatally (**Figure 11**).

Lesions are usually noted around the elbows and knees and along the mandibular border [44, 47]. Ayturk et al. discovered GNAQ and GNA11 gene mutations in CHs [48], predicting that CHs may represent a distinct clinical entity, caused by

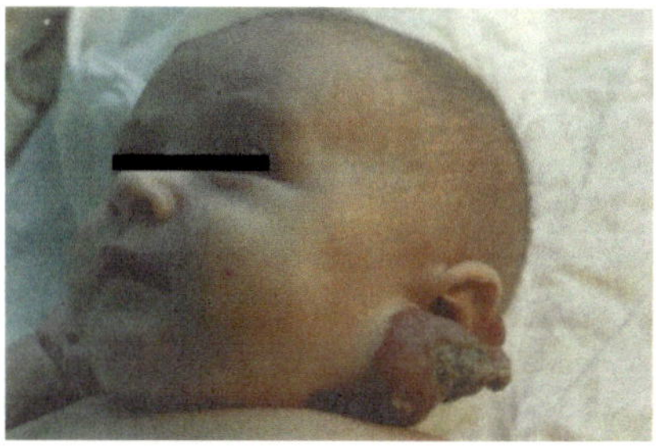

Figure 11.
A 2-month-old boy has congenital hemangioma on the preauricular area.

point mutations in GNAQ and GNA11. It has been suggested that these mutations and alterations affecting related molecular pathways could be a target for future treatment [48, 49].

Melgosa Ramos et al. retrospectively analyzed and compared 34 patients with CHs and 70 patients with IHs. They found that head and neck locations were 42.8% for IHs and the lower limbs/perineum location 32.3% for CHs. Both tumors were more common in girls. The studied risk factors were more common in patients with IHs. The most frequent component in both CHs and IHs was superficial lesions, while deep lesions were more common in CHs (14 vs. 4%). Treatment response was independent of sex, *in vitro* fertilization, lesion depth and location, and type of treatment in this analysis [50]. Other differential diagnoses include tufted angioma, spindle-cell hemangioma, epithelioid hemangioma, pyogenic granuloma, locally aggressive or borderline and malignant vascular tumors.

The International Society for the Study of Vascular Anomalies (ISSVA) classification differentiates lesions with proliferative endothelium from lesions with structural anomalies. Capillary malformations (CMs), which are well-circumscribed pink to purple macular lesions of variable size, typically develop on the head and neck. They are usually unilateral. CMs may develop as an element of Sturge-Weber syndrome (**Figure 12**) and Klippel-Trenaunay-Weber syndrome (**Figure 13**) [3, 51].

6.3 Prognosis

In most cases, the IHs resolve spontaneously during the first few years of life, approximately 30% of IHs have involved by age 4, 50% by age 5 and 75% by age 7. During the involution process, a change in the color from bright red to opaque

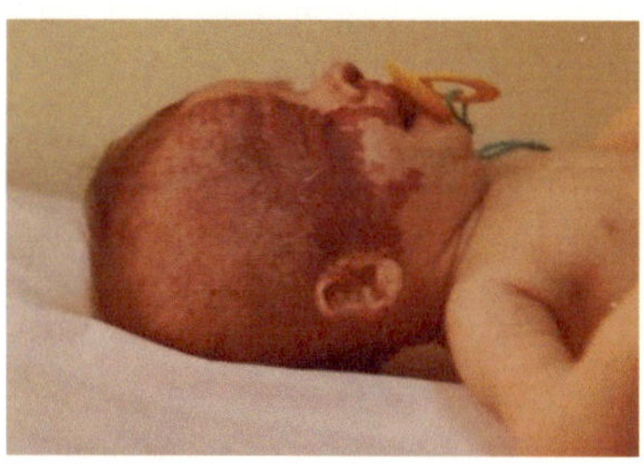

Figure 12.
The picture of a 20-day-old boy with Sturge-Weber syndrome showing port-wine stain on the right upper face and eyelid.

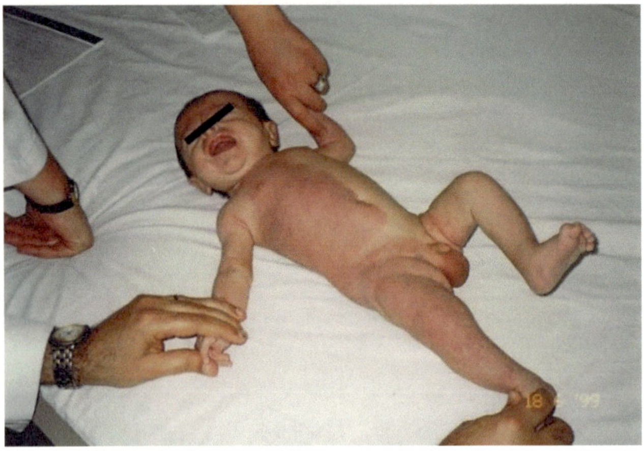

Figure 13.
Klippel-Trenaunay-Weber syndrome consists of port-wine stains of the trunk and the right lower extremities with hemihypertrophy.

pinkish-gray areas is observed in the center of the surface. The affected area may be normal, but more commonly it shows subtle atrophy and telangiectasia, particularly in the lips and eyelids. Areas of previous ulceration frequently leave yellowish scars [29]. Early resolutions are probably not affected by the size of the lesions, by their site or by the number of lesions present. An early onset of resolution is generally associated with a more rapid disappearance and a superior cosmetic result [7].

Infants with multiple (>5) lesions are at risk of extracutaneous involvement, particularly hepatic hemangioma is associated with poor prognosis. A small hemangioma can obstruct the airway or visual pathway with functional impairment and sometimes they can even threaten the patient's life [3]. The vascular and structural anomalies in the brain are the most frequent extracutaneous involvement in the cases with PHACE syndrome. The deficiency of neurological and cognitive functions can be the probable reason for morbidity [36]. Early referral to a specialist, especially patients with high-risk groups, is most important.

7. Conclusion

Infantile hemangioma is the most common benign tumor of infancy, developing in 10 to 12% of infants by the first year of life. Early diagnosis at 1 week to 1 month of age and timely referral of patients with high-risk IHs to a specialist are important in preventing associated morbidity. Segmental IHs may be related to extracutaneous manifestations. Infantile hemagiomas can be rarely associated with multiple congenital structural anomalies, such as PHACE and LUMBAR syndromes. The pediatrician should carefully observe the patient with notable features and should perform the necessary examinations for correct diagnosis and early treatment.

Author details

Sevgi Gözdaşoğlu
Department of Hematology and Oncology, Ankara University Medical School, Ankara, Turkey

*Address all correspondence to: sgozdasoglu@hotmail.com

References

[1] Mendiratta V, Jabeen M. Infantile hemangioma: An update. Indian Journal of Dermatology, Venereology and Leprology. 2010;**76**(5):469-475

[2] Mulliken JB, Glowacki J. Hemangiomas and vascular malformations in infants and children: A classification based on endothelial characteristics. Plastic and Reconstructive Surgery. 1982;**69**(3):412-422

[3] International Society for the Study of Vascular Anomalies (ISSVA). 2018 ISSVA Classification for Vascular Anomalies. Available from: https://www.issva.org/UserFiles/file/ISSVA-Classification-2018.pdf

[4] Frieden IJ. Infantile hemangioma research: Looking backward and forward. The Journal of Investigative Dermatology. 2011;**13**:2345-2348

[5] Leung AKC, Lam JM, Leong KF, Hon KL. Infantile hemangioma: An updated review. Current Pediatric Review. 2021;**17**(1):55-69

[6] Lin Q, Cai B, Shan X, Ni X, Chen X, Ke R, et al. Global research trends of infantile hemangioma: A bibliometric and visualization analysis from 2000 to 2022. Heliyon. 2023;**9**(11):e21300

[7] Drolet BA, Esterly NB, Frieden IJ. Hemangiomas in children. The New England Journal of Medicine. 1999;**341**(3):173-181

[8] Jung HL. Update on infantile hemangioma. Clinical and Experimental Pediatrics. 2021;**64**(11):559-572

[9] Ding Y, Zhang J-Z, Yu S-R, Xiang F, Kang X-J. Risk factors for infantile hemangioma: A meta-analysis. World Journal of Pediatrics. 2020;**16**(4):377-384

[10] Blei F, Walter J, Orlow SJ, Marchuk DA. Familial segregation of hemangiomas and vascular malformations as an autosomal dominant trait. Archives of Dermatology. 1998;**134**(6):718-722

[11] Walter JW, Blei F, Anderson JL, Orlow SJ, Speer MC, Marchuk DA. Genetic mapping of a novel familial form of infantile hemangioma. American Journal of Medical Genetics. 1999;**82**(1):77-83

[12] Park M. Vascular anomaly: An updated review. Clinical Pediatric Hematology Oncology. 2019;**26**:6-11

[13] Steiner JE, Drolet BA. Classification of vascular anomalies: An update. Seminars in Interventional Radiology. 2017;**34**(3):225-232

[14] Sun Y, Qui F, Hu C, Guo Y, Lei S. Hemangioma endothelial cells and hemangioma stem cells in infantile hemangioma. Annals of Plastic Surgery. 2022;**88**(2):244-249

[15] Ji Y, Chen S, Li K, Li L, Xu C, Xiang B. Signaling pathways in the development of infantile hemangioma. Journal of Hematology & Oncology. 2014;7:13

[16] Boscolo E, Bischoff J. Vasculogenesis in infantile hemangioma. Angiogenesis. 2009;**12**(2):197-207

[17] Khan ZA, Boscolo E, Picard A, Psutka S, Melero-Martin JM, Bartch TC, et al. Multipotential stem cells recapitulate human infantile

hemangioma in immunodeficient mice. The Journal of Clinical Investigation. 2008;**118**(7):2592-2599

[18] North PE, Waner M, Mizeracki A, Waner M, Mihm MC Jr. GLUT1: A newly discovered immunohistochemical marker for juvenile hemangiomas. Human Pathology. 2000;**31**(1):11-22

[19] North PE, Waner M, Mizeracki A, Mrak PR, Nicholas R, Kincannon J, et al. A unique microvascular phenotype shared by juvenile hemangiomas and human placenta. Archives of Dermatology. 2001;**137**(5):559-570

[20] Mihm MC Jr, Nelson JS. Hypothesis: The metastatic niche theory can elucidate infantile hemangioma development. Journal of Cutaneous Pathology. 2010;**37**(Suppl 1):83-87

[21] Itinteang T, Brasch HD, Tan ST, Day DJ. Expression of components of the renin-angiotensin system in proliferating infantile haemangioma may account for the propranolol-induced accelerated involution. Journal of Plastic, Reconstructive & Aesthetic Surgery. 2011;**64**(6):759-765

[22] Tan ST, Itinteang T, Day DJ, O'Donnell C, Mathy JA, Leadbitter P. Treatment of infantile haemangioma with captopril. The British Journal of Dermatology. 2012;**167**(3):619-624

[23] Smith CJF, Friedlander SF, Guma M, Kavanaugh A, Chambers CD. Infantile hemangiomas: An updated review on risk factors, pathogenesis, and treatment. Birth Defects Research. 2017;**109**(11):809-815

[24] Tan ST, Velikovic M, Ruger BM, Davis PF. Cellular and extracellular markers of hemangioma. Plastic and Reconstructive Surgery. 2000;**106**(3):529-538

[25] John EF, Davis DM, Tollefson MM, Fritchie K, Gibson LE. Vascular tumors in infants: Case report and review of clinical, histopathologic, and immunohistochemical characteristics of infantile hemangioma, pyogenic granuloma, noninvoluting congenital hemangioma, tufted angioma, and kaposiform hemangioendothelioma. The American Journal of Dermatopathology. 2018;**40**(4):231-239

[26] Glowacki J, Mulliken JB. Mast cells in hemangiomas and vascular malformations. Pediatrics. 1982;**70**(1):48-51

[27] Chamli A, Aggarwal P, Jamil RT, Litaiem N. Hemangioma. Stat-Pearls. Available from: https://www.ncbi.nlm.nih.gov/books/NBK538232/

[28] Atherton DJ. Infantile hemangiomas: A review. Hong Kong Journal of Paediatrics. 1998;**3**(2):89-102

[29] Darrow DH, Greene AK, Mancini AJ, Nopper AJ. Diagnosis and management of infantile hemangioma. Pediatrics. 2015;**136**(4):e1060-e1104

[30] Atherton DJ. Infantile haemangiomas. Early Human Development. 2006;**82**(12):789-795

[31] Kulungowski AM, Alomari AI, Chawla A, Christison-Lagay ER, Fishman SJ. Lessons from a liver hemangioma registry: Subtype classification. Journal of Pediatric Surgery. 2012;**47**(1):165-170

[32] Krowchuk DP, Frieden IJ, Mancini AJ, Darrow DH, Blei F, Greene AK, et al. Clinical practice guideline for the management of infantile hemangiomas. Pediatrics. 2019;**143**(1):e20183475

[33] Blei F, Orlows SJ, Geronemus RG. Supraumbilical midabdominal raphe, sternal atresia, and hemangioma in an

infant: Response of hemangioma to laser and Interferon Alfa-2a. Pediatric Dermatology. 1993;**10**(1):71-76

[34] Frieden IJ, Reese V, Cohen D, PHACE syndrome. The association of posterior fossa brain malformations, hemangiomas, arterial anomalies, coarctation of the aorta and cardiac defects, and eye abnormalities. Archives of Dermatology. 1996;**132**(3):307-311

[35] Iacobas I, Burrows PE, Frieden IJ, Liang MG, Mulliken JB, Mancini AJ, et al. LUMBAR: Association between cutaneous infantile hemangiomas of the lower body and regional congenital anomalies. The Journal of Pediatrics. 2010;**157**(5):795-801

[36] Rotter A, Samorano LP, Rivitti-Machado MC, Oliveira ZNP, Gontijo B. PHACE syndrome: Clinical manifestations, diagnostic criteria, and management. Anais Brasileiros de Dermatologia. 2018;**93**(3):405-411

[37] Chamlin SL, Haggstrom AN, DroletBA,BaselgaE,FriedenIJ,GarzonMC HKA, et al. Multicenter prospective study of ulcerated hemangiomas. The Journal of Pediatrics. 2007;**151**(6):684-689

[38] Mariani LG, Ferreira LM, Rovaris DL, Bonamigo RR, Kiszewski AE. Infantile hemangiomas: Risk factors for complications, recurrence and unaesthetic sequelae. Anais Brasileiros de Dermatologia. 2022;**97**(1):37-44

[39] Ezekowitz RA, Mulliken JB, Folkman J. Interferon-alfa-2a therapy for life-threatening hemangiomas of infancy. The New England Journal of Medicine. 1992;**326**(22):1456-1463

[40] Chang E, Boyd A, Nelson CC, Crowley D, Law T, Keoug KM, et al. Successful treatment on infantile hemangiomas with interferon-alpha-2b. Journal of Pediatric Hematology/ Oncology. 1997;**19**(3):237-244

[41] Gözdaşoğlu S, Uysal Z, Ertem M, Suskan E, Kürekçi E, İleri T, et al. Bebeklik çağı hemanjiomalerında interferon-alfa 2 a tedavisi. Published in IV. Ulusal Pediatrik He-matoloji Kongresi Abstract book, Trabzon. 2003;**125**

[42] Léauté-Labréze C, De la Roque ED, Hubiche T, Boralevi F, Thambo JB, Taieb A. Propranolol for severe hemangiomas of infancy. The New England Journal of Medicine. 2008;**358**(24):2649-2651

[43] Leung AKC, Barankin B, Hon KL. Infantile hemangioma. Pediatrics and Neonatal Nursing Open Journal. 2014;**1**(1):6-11

[44] Oiso N, Kawada A. The dermoscopic features in infantile hemangioma. Pediatric Dermatology. 2011;**28**(5):591-593

[45] Viswan P, Behera B, Sethy M, Dash S, Palit A, Ayyanar P. Dermoscopic analysis of vascular malformations and tumors based upon dominant vascular dermoscopic features: A retrospective analysis from a tertiary care center of East India. Cureus. 2022;**14**(6):e26292

[46] Wildgruber M, Sadick M, Müller-Wille R, Wohlgemuth WA. Vascular tumors in infants and adolescents. Insights Into Imaging. 2019;**10**(1):30

[47] Frieden IJ, Rogers M, Garzon M. Conditions masquerading as infantile hemangioma: Part 1. The Australasian Journal of Dermatology. 2009;**50**(2):77-97

[48] Ayturk UM, Couto JA, Hann S, Mulliken JB, Williams KL, Huang AY,

et al. Somatic activating mutations in GNAQ and GNA11 are associated with congenital hemangioma. American Journal of Human Genetics. 2016;**98**(4):789-795

[49] Olsen GM, Nackers A, Drolet BA. Infantile and congenital hemangiomas. Seminars in Pediatric Surgery. 2020;**29**(5):150969

[50] Melgosa Ramos FJ, Díaz-Corpas T, Santos-Alarcón S, Galarreta Pascual M, Aguado Vázquez A, Mateau PA. Congenital and infantile hemangiomas: Epidemiological, clinical, and treatment characteristics based on 3 years' experience at a tertiary care hospital - A retrospective case comparison and review of the literature. Actas Dermo-sifiliogra. 2023;**114**(7):631-635

[51] George A, Mani V, Noufal A. Update on the classification of hemangioma. Journal of Oral and Maxillofacial Pathology. 2014;**18**(Suppl. 1):S117-S120

Section 6

Common Cancers in Children

Chapter 8

Innovations in Pathophysiology, Diagnosis, Genomic Medicine and State-of-the-Art Treatment Approaches in Pediatric Acute Lymphoblastic Leukemia in the Twenty-First Century

Nawaf AlAnazi, Sarah AlMukhaylid and Zafar Iqbal

Abstract

Innovative advancements in the twenty-first-century technologies have revealed new genetic, immunological, and cellular biological mechanisms that contribute to understanding the biology and pathogenesis of pediatric as well as adulthood diseases. These advancements have sparked a significant revolution in the diagnosis, prognosis, and treatment of different cancers including hematological malignancies, particularly leukemia. Numerous molecular genetic assays have been developed to select optimal drugs and clinical protocols for leukemia patients. This personalized approach to treatment aims to achieve better clinical outcomes with reduced drug side effects. Genomic medicine has made basic genetic testing necessary for every clinic and hospital. This book provides an account of classical and novel developments in pediatric acute lymphoblastic leukemia (ALL) as most common childhood malignancy, that have resulted from state-of-the-art genetic, cell biological, and immunological research during the last three decades. Moreover, it also provides deep insights into the innovation in differential diagnosis, risk stratification, patient-tailored treatment, and accurate therapeutic follow-up for timely therapeutic interventions in the recent era of modern science and technology innovations of the twenty-first century that has fascinatingly improved clinical outcome of this deadly disease of the childhood.

Keywords: pediatric acute lymphoblastic leukemia, childhood cancer, cancer management, genomics, personalized treatment

1. Introduction

Leukemia's origins trace back to the early nineteenth century. In 1811, Peter Cullen first described a case of acute splenitis with the presence of milky-looking blood. Subsequently, Alfred Velpeau described leukemia-like symptoms and noted the appearance of pus within the blood in 1825. Alfred Donné, in 1844, identified the over-production of white blood cells. John Bennett named leucocythemia in 1845 after observing an abnormal increase in white blood cells under the microscope. Rudolf Virchow recognized an imbalance between white and red blood cells, officially naming the medical condition 'leukämie' in 1847 [1].

Leukemia is a broad definition for hematological malignancies characterized by the unregulated proliferation of white blood cells (WBCs) due to the molecular alterations of hematopoietic stem cells (HSCs) [2]. It is marked by the presence of immature leukocytes and blast cells, within both bloodstream and bone marrow. The dysfunction of these cells contributes to the clinical manifestations of the disease. A diagnosis of leukemia is typically confirmed when blast cells constitute equal to or over 20% of the bone marrow composition [3]. Classification of leukemia depends on two key factors: the rapidity of proliferation, resulting in either acute or chronic forms, and the cell of origin, leading to categorization as myeloid or lymphoid lineages [3]. Leukemias of the myeloid lineage include acute myeloid leukemia (AML) and chronic myeloid leukemia (CML), while lymphoid types include acute lymphoblastic leukemia (ALL) and chronic lymphocytic leukemia (CLL).

ALL is a hematologic malignancy marked by both the clonal proliferation and accumulation of lymphoid progenitor cells in the bone marrow and peripheral blood [4]. Multiple genetic abnormalities, such as chromosome translocations, aneuploidies, and mutations, cause ALL initiation [4]. ALL is primarily observed in children, with roughly 75% of cases diagnosed under the age of 6 [4, 5]. Nevertheless, its incidence pattern shows a bimodal distribution, with a second peak occurring in individuals over 60 years old [5, 6]. ALL represents 25% of all childhood cancers and encompasses 72% of childhood leukemia cases, with occurrence estimated to range from two to five cases per 100,000 children [5].

Over the past years, extensive research into the biological mechanisms of ALL has been carried out, particularly through the incorporation of genomic technologies in cancer diagnostics, which has resulted in breakthroughs in prognosis prediction and the development of novel treatments. This chapter presents a detailed overview of the historical development and understanding of pediatric ALL.

2. Pediatric acute lymphoblastic leukemia

Among childhood cancers, pediatric ALL is the most prevalent, which arises from cells called lymphoblasts [7]. Terminology, "acute" indicates the rapid progression onset of leukemia, which, if untreated, could be fatal in a few months [3]. ALL is marked by immature white blood cells that are overpopulated, specifically lymphocytes and blast cells. These blast cells are early-stage lymphoid precursor B or T cells that are halted in their developmental process [8]. The proliferation of blast cells in ALL results in the replacement of normal cells within the bone marrow and bloodstream, leading to neutropenia, anemia, thrombocytopenia, and, rarely, pancytopenia [8]. Moreover, blast cells proliferate extensively in diverse anatomical sites, including the blood, bone marrow, liver, lymph nodes, spleen, and central nervous system (CNS) [9, 10]. Cytogenetic alterations, such as germline and somatic karyotypic abnormalities, translocations, and deletions, form the primary basis for ALL etiology [11].

B-cell acute lymphoblastic leukemia (B-ALL) predominates as the most common subtype of ALL, with T-cell acute lymphoblastic leukemia (T-ALL) comprising only approximately 20% of all cases of ALL [10, 12]. Therapeutic progress in treating pediatric ALL over the past 50 years has resulted in a remarkable increase in survival rates, flourishing from less than 10% in 1962 to approximately 90% today [11]. The development of new agents has marked significant progress in overcoming resistance to traditional chemotherapy, leading to elevated remission rates in patients with relapsed ALL. These emerging therapeutics encompass a diverse range of approaches, including monoclonal antibodies, immunomodulators, chimeric antigen receptor T (CAR-T) cells, and hematopoietic stem cell transplantation [4]. Despite these advancements, relapse still occurs in approximately 20% of pediatric ALL cases. This is often associated with a high rate of chemoresistance development, treatment failure, and mortality [4].

3. Epidemiology of pediatric acute lymphoblastic leukemia

Representing the predominant malignancy in the pediatric population, ALL accounts for approximately 25% of cancer diagnoses among children and 72% of leukemia cases diagnosed in this age group [5]. Its estimated incidence ranges from two to five cases per 100,000 children with a noted predominance among males [5, 13]. The peak occurrence is observed between the ages of two and five years [5]. Nevertheless, the incidence of ALL differs across geographic areas due to multiple factors including ethnicity, infections, and socioeconomic influences. In the USA, according to the Surveillance, Epidemiology, and End Results (SEER) program data, the incidence of ALL was 4.2 cases per 100,000 [14]. An incidence rate of 4.0 per 100,000 children per year has been reported in Nordic countries [15]. The estimated overall incidence in Europe is 1.28 cases per 1,000,000 individuals annually [16].

On the other hand, ALL reports of incidence in Saudi Arabia are lacking. Based on a Saudi study carried out from 2001 to 2014, the overall incidence was found to be 2.35 per 100,000 population in 2014 through the Saudi Cancer Registry (SCR). Detailed depth into the study revealed a rise from 1.58 per 100,000 population to 2.35 per 100,000 population, from 2001 to 2014, respectively. Furthermore, a global trend where ALL is more common in male children than females is a pattern consistent in Saudi Arabia as well. Based on these incidence rates, the study projected that, by 2025, the incidence of ALL in Saudi males is expected to rise to 3.8 cases per 100,000 population, while in Saudi females, it is anticipated to reach 2.9 cases per 100,000 population [17].

4. Etiology of pediatric acute lymphoblastic leukemia

4.1 Proposed hypothesis

Certain etiology of ALL remains unclear, yet numerous hypotheses have been proposed to explain potential pathogenic mechanisms underlying the development of pediatric ALL. In 1990, Gardner et al. hypothesized that parental preconception exposure to irradiation might be the factor [18, 19]. In the same year, Kinlen et al. proposed that childhood leukemia is linked to population mixing in rural or isolated areas. As people from different regions move into these communities, new infections are introduced. The lack of frequent infections in infancy could increase immunological vulnerability when encountering infections later in life [19, 20]. This vulnerability triggers a subsequent molecular event essential for initiating the cancerous process, which explains why ALL peaks between children aged 2 and 7 years [20]. A recent hypothesis "two-hit" emphasizes that the cause of ALL is based on two-step as the name implies.

Predisposing genetic mutation is the first step, and exposure to one or more infections containing *Aspergillus flavus* is the second step [21]. Furthermore, ALL is believed to be initiated in utero through the formation of fusion genes or hyper-diploidy, leading to the development of a pre-leukemic clone. Fusion oncogenes like *BCR-ABL*, *ETV6-RUNX1*, *MLL-AF4*, *SIL-TAL1*, and *TCF3-PBX1* are associated with ALL [21].

4.2 Pathogenesis

Due to a series of gene mutations, oncogenes are activated and tumor suppressor genes are inactivated, leading to increased cell proliferation, resistance to apoptosis, and impaired differentiation of HSCs [21]. This disruption leads to rapid and abnormal proliferation of undifferentiated lymphoid progenitor cells. Chromosomal abnormalities in ALL encompass hyperdiploidy (> 50 chromosomes), hypodiploidy (< 44 chromosomes), as well as translocations involving chromosomes [1, 4, 9, 11, 12, 19, 21, 22], and rearrangements such as *MYC* and *MLL*. These abnormalities lead to the dysregulation of oncogenes or the formation of chimeric fusion genes [22]. Each subtype of ALL is associated with specific genetic alterations. In B-ALL, common alterations include but are not limited to *BCR-ABL1*, *ETV6-RUNX1*, or *TCF3-PBX1* fusions. In T-ALL, alterations in genes such as *TAL1*, *TAL2*, *TLX1*, *TLX2*, or *HOXA* are frequently observed [21, 23]. However, these are not exhaustive, and other alterations may also occur. Further elaboration is discussed in Section 7.

4.3 Risk factors

As with other types of leukemia, various factors act as contribution to the development of ALL. These factors include a range of genetic alternation, environmental, and immunological influences, the interplay of which may contribute to the onset of the disease. Understanding the multifactorial nature of ALL development is crucial for elucidating its etiology and identifying potential targets for prevention and treatment strategies.

- *Environmental exposure:* In line with the two-hit hypothesis, researchers propose that the first genetic change occurs before birth, followed by additional genetic alterations after birth. Elevated exposure to ionizing radiation (IR) is widely recognized as a significant environmental risk factor for childhood cancer [24]. Furthermore, parent exposure to benzene, a known carcinogen present in paint fumes and cigarette smoke, increases the risk of childhood ALL. Benzene undergoes metabolism in either the liver or lungs, producing benzene oxide and hydroquinone. These compounds are subsequently converted to benzoquinone within the bone marrow, leading to cytotoxic effects and DNA damage. A recent report found that minimizing exposure to benzene in both occupational and environmental settings during pregnancy reduces the likelihood of childhood ALL in offspring [23].

- *Infections:* Viral infections can induce leukemogenesis through DNA methylation. Even after viral clearance, abnormal expression of hematopoietic and proliferation genes persists. Abnormal DNA methylation has been observed in patients with ALL who have a history of parvovirus B19 infection [23]. Furthermore, a study observed that newborns infected with adenovirus C were more likely to develop ALL compared to those who did not acquire the infection [25]. Yet, other infections have the potential to modify genes related to cell proliferation and DNA methylation patterns, consequently influencing the progression of ALL [23].

- *Genetic disorders:* Genetic abnormalities, whether primary or secondary, are associated with leukemias and contribute significantly to their development. Such disorders include Down syndrome, Bloom syndrome, Fanconi anemia, Shwachman syndrome, ataxia telangiectasia, and inherited genetic polymorphisms [20]. About one-half to two-thirds of acute leukemia cases in children with Down syndrome are ALL. In approximately 50% of cases where children are diagnosed with both ALL and Down syndrome, common interstitial deletion is found in the pseudoautosomal region (PAR) of chromosomes X and Y. Children with Down syndrome have a more than 60% likelihood of having this deletion, which involves the juxtaposition of CRLF2's first coding region with P2RY8's noncoding exon, resulting in the P2RY8-CRLF2 fusion oncogene. This fusion oncogene is only reported in 10% of non-Down syndrome children [12, 26]. *JAK2* mutations accounted for 18% of Down syndrome patients [26].

- *Birth-weight:* The "Pedersen hypothesis" suggests that maternal hyperglycemia during pregnancy, along with the resulting fetal hyperinsulinemia, contributes to accelerated fetal growth or macrosomia (excessive birth weight) in babies born to diabetic or hyperglycemic mothers. Insulin-like growth factor I (IGF-1) is known to stimulate B-lymphocyte proliferation. There has been speculation about the involvement of IGF-1 in the development of pediatric ALL, suggesting a potential etiological role for IGF-1 in this disease [23].

- *Monozygotic twins:* The first case of concordant childhood leukemia in twins was reported in 1882. Throughout the twentieth century, previously published review papers proposed the prenatal origins of childhood leukemia, citing several case reports that highlighted the occurrence of leukemia in twins. A total of 70 twin pairs with concordant childhood leukemia have been reported to date, 37 of which can be attributed to ALL [27]. The mechanism begins with the initial genetic change emerging in utero, which is then shared among the blood cells of both twins through their shared blood supply, thereby substantiating the two-hit mechanism of leukemogenesis. This model suggests that the primary lesion originates prenatally, followed by the occurrence of secondary somatic mutations during the postnatal period, ultimately leading to the development of acute leukemia [27].

5. Clinical characteristics of pediatric acute lymphoblastic leukemia

5.1 Symptoms

From a symptomatic perspective, ALL diverse and non-specific symptoms are a result of both bone marrow infiltration with lymphoblasts and extramedullary disease. These may include prolonged fever, bone pain, swollen lymph nodes, petechiae, and dyspnea, often attributed to mediastinal enlargement. Additionally, leukemia may be suspected based on imaging findings, including X-rays and/or magnetic resonance imaging (MRI) [18]. Other symptoms like bone pain, limping, and arthritis are observed in 21–59% of children diagnosed with ALL. This occurrence results from leukemic-cell infiltration exerting pressure on the periosteum, while joint pain is mainly due to lesions affecting the periosteum [28]. Additionally, during physical examination, it is noted that more than 40% of patients exhibit lymphadenopathy, hepatomegaly, or splenomegaly [10, 29].

Due to the infiltration of leukemic cells in the thymus, an anterior mediastinal mass often develops, accounting for 10% of newly diagnosed cases of ALL, particularly in T-ALL. Involvement of the central nervous system (CNS) may manifest with symptoms indicative of increased intracranial pressure, such as headache, confusion, vomiting, seizures, and neck stiffness [28]. Thus, cerebrospinal fluid (CSF) analysis is the standard of care at the time of diagnosis to rule out CNS involvement and determine intrathecal chemotherapy administration [30, 31]. Rare extramedullary and endocrinological manifestations are uncommon in ALL patients, typically occurring during relapse or refractory cases. These manifestations may involve various sites, including ocular, bone, renal, hepatic, abdominal, bladder, skin, oral, pericardial, and pancreatic regions [32]. Moreover, as reported by a few studies, superior vena cava syndrome is seen in T-cell ALL patients mainly due to lymphadenopathy [33, 34].

5.2 Clinical diagnosis

Leukemia diagnosis encompasses a variety of procedures, including a complete blood count (CBC), coagulation studies, and a chemistry profile focusing on liver and kidney function tests. Discrimination between different types of leukemia relies significantly on the morphological appearance observed in bone marrow aspiration [29]. The confirmation of pediatric ALL diagnosis relies on detecting 20% or higher lymphoblasts in either bone marrow or peripheral blood as a first step [8]. Upon scientific development for better diagnostic approaches, immunophenotyping was discovered in 1977 by Jonosy and coworkers through the application of monoclonal antibodies. Hybridoma technology has produced monoclonal antibodies to many cell clusters of differentiation (CDs) epitopes [35].

Currently, ALL classification is made through flow cytometric immunophenotyping (FCI), which enables a comprehensive assessment of the surface and intracellular antigens expressed by leukemic cells. Furthermore, FCI assists in the identification and characterization of blast cells, facilitating lineage determination and the assessment of potential therapeutic targets, as well as predicting specific genetic abnormalities. Furthermore, the rapid cell acquisition capabilities of flow cytometers enable the detection of rare abnormal cells post-treatment. Integration of minimal/measurable residual disease (MRD) data into treatment plans permits personalized optimization of therapy, aligning with the objective of personalized medicine [36].

However, despite all the FCI advantages, it has limitations as cells must be fresh and viable. Immunohistochemistry stains serve as an alternative diagnostic tool [37]. Biopsies of bone marrow trephine can provide information on immunophenotypes [37, 38]. Additionally, employing a terminal deoxynucleotidyl transferase (TdT) assay in conjunction with a panel of monoclonal antibodies (MoAbs) targeting antigens associated with T cells and B cells enables the detection of almost all instances of ALL [38].

6. ALL classification

The classification of leukemia relies on cell morphology, immunophenotype, and cytogenetic and molecular genetic features. This comprehensive analysis is crucial for accurately identifying and categorizing different leukemia subtypes, guiding personalized treatment approaches, and prognostic evaluations.

6.1 Cell morphology classification

The primary step in the diagnostic process for both identifying ALL and distinguishing it from acute myeloid leukemia (AML) involves a morphological examination of bone marrow. A crucial discrepancy lies in the characteristics of the blast population. In ALL, lymphoblasts typically exhibit a homogeneous appearance, whereas myeloblasts in AML tend to display heterogeneity [39].

6.1.1 French-American-British classification

In the 1970s and 1980s, the French-American-British (FAB) classification system for acute leukemias was established [40]. This classification primarily utilized morphological features and the examination of standard histologic stains to differentiate between lymphoid and myeloid neoplasms. However, stains' role in distinguishing ALL from AML is mostly historical, as immunophenotyping now offers more objective results, rendering stains less significant [40]. FAB classification categorized ALL into three subgroups, L1 (children), L2 (older children and adults), and L3 (patients with leukemia secondary to Burkitt's lymphoma [40].

- *FAB L1:* Being mostly observed in children, morphological characteristics include small homogenous lymphoblasts with scant blue cytoplasm, regular nuclear morphology, partially condensed chromatin, barely visible nucleoli, and a high nuclear-to-cytoplasmic ratio (N: C) (**Figure 1**) [40].
- *FAB L2:* Mostly seen in adults, lymphoblasts are larger in size with irregular nuclear outlines, heterogeneous lacy chromatin, and moderately plentiful weakly basophilic cytoplasm (**Figure 1**) [40].

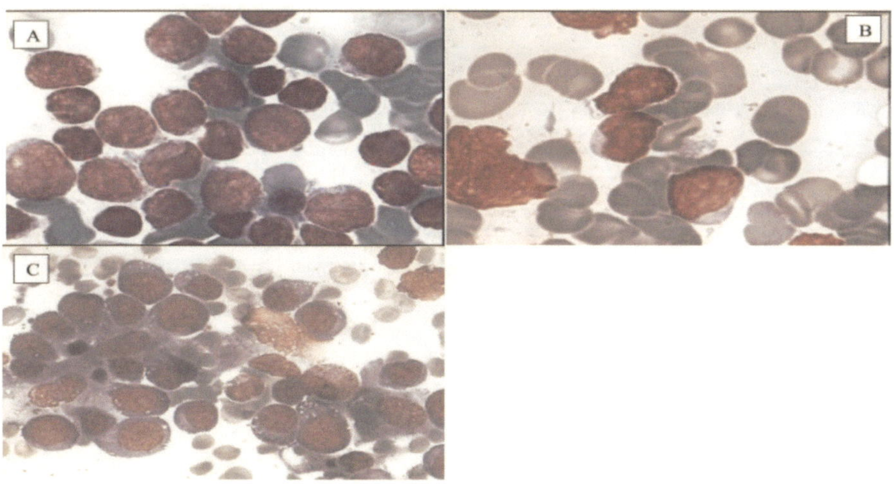

Figure 1.
(A) FAB1 small lymphoblast with little cytoplasm and regularly shaped nuclei. (B) FAB L2 Lymphoblast appears more immature, heterogeneous cell with varying nuclear shape. (C) FAB L3 Larger lymphocyte with abundant cytoplasm which is vacuolated [40].

- *FAB L3 (Burkitt):* Homogeneous lymphoblasts appear large and feature finely granular stippled nuclear chromatin with prominent nucleoli. Their cytoplasm is vacuolated and exhibits **a midnight blue hue (Figure 1)** [40].

Nevertheless, The World Health Organization's (WHO) International Panel on ALL suggests discontinuing the use of the FAB classification, noting its lack of clinical or prognostic relevance. Instead, the panel advocates for adopting the immunophenotypic classification outlined as follows.

6.2 World Health Organization classification

The 2008 classification protocols established by the World Health Organization (WHO) categorize leukemia based on cell morphology, immunophenotype, and genetic/cytogenetic characteristics. Unlike the approach mentioned above advocated by the FAB group, which is now obsolete, the WHO classification system is currently utilized. While the FAB classification was once clinically valuable, particularly in identifying potential cases of Burkitt lymphoma in the leukemic phase, it has been supplanted by the WHO classification. The WHO classified lymphoid neoplasms are categorized into two main groups: those originating from B- and T-lineage lymphoid precursors [41, 42]. In the WHO 2008 classification, seven types of B-ALL were outlined, each characterized by distinct recurring genetic abnormalities, while T-ALL was identified as a singular neoplastic disorder (**Table 1**). The genetic anomalies specified in the WHO 2008 classification were typically detectable through cytogenetic analysis and fluorescence in situ hybridization (FISH).

As the field progresses toward more comprehensive genomic analysis, after the WHO 2008 classification, new editions of the WHO classification have been published. These updated classifications, including the fifth edition (WHO-HAEM5) released in 2022, have integrated newly identified types of B-ALL uncovered through advanced genomic techniques as distinct subtypes of the disease (**Table 2**).

B-lymphoblastic leukemia/lymphoma
B-lymphoblastic leukemia/lymphoma, NOS*
B-lymphoblastic leukemia/lymphoma with recurrent genetic abnormalities
B-lymphoblastic leukemia/lymphoma with t(9;22)(q34;q11.2);*BCR-ABL 1*
B-lymphoblastic leukemia/lymphoma with t(v;11q23);*MLL* rearranged
B-lymphoblastic leukemia/lymphoma with t(12;21)(p13;q22) *TEL-AML1* (*ETV6-RUNX1*)
B-lymphoblastic leukemia/lymphoma with hyperdiploidy
B-lymphoblastic leukemia/lymphoma with hypodiploidy
B-lymphoblastic leukemia/lymphoma with t(5;14)(q31;q32) *IL3-IGH*
B-lymphoblastic leukemia/lymphoma with t(1;19)(q23;p13.3);*TCF3-PBX1*
T lymphoblastic leukemia/lymphoma

**NOS: not otherwise specified, t: translocation.*

Table 1.
WHO 2008 classification [41].

• *B-lymphoblastic leukemias/lymphomas*
B-lymphoblastic leukemia/lymphoma
B-lymphoblastic leukemia/lymphoma with high hyperdiploidy
B-lymphoblastic leukemia/lymphoma with hypodiploidy
B-lymphoblastic leukemia/lymphoma with iAMP21
B-lymphoblastic leukemia/lymphoma with *BCR::ABL1* fusion
B-lymphoblastic leukemia/lymphoma with *BCR::ABL1*-like features
B-lymphoblastic leukemia/lymphoma with *KMT2A* rearrangement
B-lymphoblastic leukemia/lymphoma with *ETV6::RUNX1* fusion
B-lymphoblastic leukemia/lymphoma with *ETV6::RUNX1*-like features
B-lymphoblastic leukemia/lymphoma with *TCF3::PBX1* fusion
B-lymphoblastic leukemia/lymphoma with *IGH::IL3* fusion
B-lymphoblastic leukemia/lymphoma with *TCF3::HLF* fusion
• *B-lymphoblastic leukemia/lymphoma with other defined genetic alterations*
B-lymphoblastic leukemia with *DUX4* rearrangement
B-lymphoblastic leukemia with *MEF2D* rearrangement
B-lymphoblastic leukemia with *ZNF384* rearrangement
B-lymphoblastic leukemia with *PAX5*alt
B-lymphoblastic leukemia with *PAX5* p.P80R
B-lymphoblastic leukemia with *NUTM1* rearrangement
B-lymphoblastic leukemia with *MYC* rearrangement
B-lymphoblastic leukemia/lymphoma, not otherwise specified
• *Precursor T-cell neoplasms*
T-lymphoblastic leukemia/lymphoma
T-lymphoblastic leukemia/lymphoma, not otherwise specified
Early T-precursor lymphoblastic leukemia/lymphoma

Table 2.
WHO-HAEM5 2022 Classification [42].

6.3 Immunophenotyping classification

Immunophenotyping is a crucial method in the classification of ALL, and it is the standard method of diagnosis. It involves the analysis of cell surface markers on leukemia cells to determine their lineage and maturity through multi-channel flow cytometry (MFC) [39]. By identifying specific markers, such as CD19, CD20, and CD3, immunophenotyping helps differentiate between B-cell and T-cell ALL subtypes. Additionally, it provides valuable information about the stage of cell development and can help in predicting treatment response and prognosis which in turn assist in guiding appropriate treatment strategies for patients. Furthermore, the detection and monitoring of minimal residual disease (MRD) through MFC serves as gold standard.

This methodology adheres to the guidelines set forth by the European Group for the Immunological Classification of Leukemias (EGIL). According to the consensus established by the EGIL, blast cells are deemed to have a positive reaction to a specific monoclonal antibody when they reach a threshold of 20% expression. However, exceptions apply to certain markers such as MPO, CD3, CD79a, and TdT, which are considered positive at a lower expression level of 10%. This standardized approach ensures uniformity in the interpretation of immunophenotyping results and aids in the accurate diagnosis and classification of leukemia subtypes [39].

The European Group for the Immunological Classification of Leukemias (EGIL):

6.3.1 Immunophenotype of B-lineage ALL

B-progenitor cells, arising from common lymphoid progenitors within the bone marrow, progress through a specific sequence of three maturation phases to develop

B lineage	CD10	CD19	CD22	CD34	CD79a	Ig
B-I subtype (Pro-B) ALL	–	+	+	+	+	–
B-II subtype (pre-pre-B or common B) ALL	+	+	+	–	+	–
B-III (pre-B) ALL	+		–	–	–	C-mu
B-IV (mature B) ALL	±	+	+	–	+	C-mu

Table 3.
B- linage ALL classification based on the EBIL.

into fully mature B-lymphoid cells. These phases include early/pre-B-I (hematogenous type I), intermediate/pre-B-II (hematogenous type II), and late/transitional B-cells (hematogenous type III) [40]. The intensity of CD45 and CD20 expression increases progressively across these stages, while CD34 and CD10 show a gradual decrease, ultimately being lost at the late stage. CD19 expression is lowest in stage I, significantly increases in stage II, and slightly decreases in mature B cells. Mature B cells do not express CD34, CD10, or TdT, but they are positive for CD20 and CD45 and exhibit surface expression of polytypic immunoglobulins [43].

B-cell lineage in ALL is characterized by its specific markers which include CD19, CD20, CD22, CD24, CD79a, and cytoplasmic or surface expression of IgM heavy chain (mu) protein, cIgμand sig, respectively. EGIL classified B lineage into the following (**Table 3**):

1. *B-I Subtype (Pro-B) ALL:* CD19+, CD34+, CD22+, CD10+ and CD79+

2. *B-II subtype (pre-pre-B or common B) ALL:* CD10+,

3. *B-III (pre-B) ALL:* CD10+,cIg+

4. *B-IV (mature B) ALL:* CD19+,CD22+,CD79a+, CD10+, cIgμ+, sIgμ+, Tdt+

Furthermore, in B-ALL, various markers play crucial roles in subclassification [39]. B-I and B-II ALL often exhibit positivity for CD24 and 4G7 (pro- and pre-B surrogate light chain-specific MoAb). Surface markers like CD20 and CD22 may also variably express beyond the B-I stage [39]. Myeloid/cross-lineage antigens CD13 and CD33, as well as the stem cell antigen CD34, can be present, especially in Ph + ALL (commonly B-II with CD34, CD38, CD25, and CD13/33). However, myeloid-specific CD117 should not be present and can aid in differentiating ALL from rare myeloid leukemias with negative MPO expression. Pro-B ALL with t(4;11)/MLL rearrangements often exhibit myeloid antigen positivity, including CD15 expression [39].

6.3.2 Immunophenotype of T-lineage ALL

T-acute lymphoblastic leukemias (T-ALLs) represent about 15% of pediatric ALL cases. T-cell markers include CD1a, CD2, CD3 (both membrane and cytoplasmic), CD4, CD5, CD7, and CD8. CD2, CD5, and CD7 indicate immature T-cell populations, though not entirely lineage-specific. Thus, definitive diagnosis relies on demonstrating surface or cytoplasmic CD3 expression. In T-ALL, CD10 expression is relatively common (around 25%) but lacks specificity. CD34 and myeloid antigens CD13 and/or CD33 may also be present [42]. EGIL classified T-ALL into the following (**Table 4**):

Marker	Pro-T-ALL	Pre-T-ALL	Cortical T-ALL	Medullary T-ALL
CD1	–	–	+	–
CD2	+	+	+	+
SmCD3	–	–	+	–
CyCD3	+	+	+	+
CD4–/CD8-	+	+	–	–
CD4–/CD8+	–	±	±	±
CD4+/CD8-	–	±	±	+
CD4+/CD8+	–	–	+	±
CD5	–	+	+	+
CD7	+	+	+	+

Table 4.
EGIL classification for T-ALLs.

1. *T-I (Pro-T-ALL):* cCD3+, CD7+, CD1+, CD2+

2. *T-II (Pre-T-ALL):* cCD3+, CD7+ and CD5/CD2+

3. *T-III (Cortical T-ALL):* cCD3+, Cd1a+, sCD3+/–,CD2

4. *T-IV (Medullary T-ALL):* CD2+, CyCD3, CD5+, CD7+

7. ALL genetics and molecular cytogenetics abnormalities and prognostication

Genetic analysis stands out as the foremost method for pinpointing genomic alterations crucial for diagnosing, determining risk, and selecting treatment in ALL. This analysis is divided into two levels: the discovery phase, which investigates the discovery of novel molecular targets to enhance comprehension of ALL's biology, and clinical practice, which focuses on identifying alterations essential for optimal disease management. Before the advent of high-throughput sequencing, extensive genome-wide investigations relied on genomic and transcriptome microarrays (**Table 5**). These studies were instrumental in pinpointing crucial molecular targets and pathways linked to high-risk ALL [4].

Genomic analyses unveiled that ALL patients typically lack significant genomic instability, despite the identification of numerous recurrent copy number alterations (CNAs) [4]. These alterations involve genes pivotal for lymphoid growth or tumorigenesis, such as *PAX5* and *IKZF1* for B-lymphoid development, tumor suppressors like *CDKN2A*/*CDKN2B* and *RB1*, and drug response-related genes such as *NR3C1* for B-ALL and *LMO2*, *MYB*, *PTEN*, and *WT1* for T-ALL. Often, these genes are affected by specific types of alterations—such as focal or broad deletions, translocations, or mutations—functioning in a haploinsufficient or dominant-negative manner. The below context will further discuss each genetic mutation in detail [4].

Technique(s)	Scope/target of test	Abnormality resolution	Sensitivity	Detectable types of abnormality
G-banded cytogenetics	Evaluation of chromosome number and morphology	Low	Low/ medium	Translocations (gene fusions), deletions, amplifications, aneuploidy
Locus specific FISH	Enumeration and localisation of specific DNA target sequences	Medium	Medium/ high	Translocations (gene fusions), deletions, amplifications, aneuploidy
DNA index	Measurement of DNA content	N/A	High	Aneuploidy
Reverse transcription (RT) polymerase chain reaction (PCR)	Qualitative and quantitative assessment of fusion transcripts. Can be multiplexed	N/A	High	Gene fusions (translocations)
Multiplex ligation-dependent probe amplification (MLPA)	Enumeration of multiple specific DNA target sequences	High	Medium	Copy number alterations – deletions and amplifications
Single nucleotide polymorphism (SNP) arrays	Simultaneous evaluation of tens of thousands SNPs across the genome	Very high (depends on distribution of SNPs)	Medium	Copy number alterations (deletions and amplifications), aneuploidy, and copy number neutral (CNN) loss of heterozygosity (LOH)a
Array comparative genome hybridisation (aCGH)	Simultaneous enumeration of tens of thousands of DNA probes across the genome	Very high (depends on distribution of probes)	Medium	Copy number alterations – deletions and amplifications – and aneuploidy
Targeted gene sequencing	Next-generation sequencing of genomic regions using a customized library	Very high	Very high	Originally developed to detect sequence mutations but with appropriate library definition, sophisticated bioinformatic pipelines and long read lengths all types of abnormality can be accurately detected

Table 5.
Overview of the principal genetic techniques used for the diagnosis and classification of ALL [44].

7.1 B-cell ALL

Specific chromosomal abnormalities, like chromosomal rearrangements and aneuploidy, categorize pediatric B-ALL into distinct subtypes. These abnormalities strongly influence therapeutic response and prognosis (**Table 6**). Notably, the distribution of chromosomal abnormalities varies with age, indicating age-dependent leukemogenic mechanisms.

7.1.1 Somatic aneuploidy

Detection of somatic chromosomal gains and losses in leukemia cells is commonly achieved through karyotyping, fluorescence in situ hybridization (FISH), and

Genetic subtype	Genetic alterations	Frequency	Prognosis	Comment
B-ALL				
Abnormalities in Chromosome Number				
High hyperdiploidy (51–67 chromosomes)		25%	Favorable	
Low hyperdiploidy (47–50 chromosomes)		14%	Previously unfavorable, now intermediate	
Hypodiploidy (<44 chromosomes)	Near-haploidy (24–31 chromosomes), low-hypodiploidy (32–39 chromosomes)	1–2%	Unfavorable	Association with *TP53* mutations, *IKZF2* and *IKZF3* deletions, and RAS and PI3K pathway mutations
Recurrent Chromosomal Translocations				
t(12;21)(p13;q22)	*ETV6-RUNX1* (*TEL-AML1*)	20%	Favorable	
t(1;19)(q23;p13.1)	*TCF3-PBX1* (*E2A-PBX1*)	4%	Intermediate	
t(17;19)(q22;p13)	*TCF3-HLF*	<0.5%	Unfavorable	
KMT2A (*MLL*) rearrangements		5–6%	Unfavorable (infants), intermediate (non-infants)	Highest frequency in younger infants (80%); associated with *FLT3* overexpression and epigenetic dysregulation
t(1;11)(q21;q23)	*KMT2A-MLLT11*		Less unfavorable	Rare
t(4;11)(q21;q23)	*KMT2A-AFF1* (*AF4*)		Particularly unfavorable	Comprises 50% of infant *KMT2A*-rearranged ALL
t(9;11)(p22;q23)	*KMT2A-MLLT3* (*AF9*)			Comprises 15% of infant *KMT2A*-rearranged ALL
t(10;11)(p12;q23)	*KMT2A-MLLT10* (*AF10*)			Comprises 5% of infant *KMT2A*-rearranged ALL
t(11;19)(q23;p13.3)	*KMT2A-MLLT1* (*ENL*)			Comprises 20–25% of infant *KMT2A*-rearranged ALL
Other fusion partners				
t(9;22)(q34;q11.2)	*BCR-ABL1*	3–5%	Unfavorable prior to TKI therapy, intermediate with TKI therapy?	Associated with *IKZF1* deletions

Genetic subtype	Genetic alterations	Frequency	Prognosis	Comment
Other				
Ph-like	*IGH-CRLF2*, *P2RY8-CRLF2*	7–8%	Unfavorable	50% of Ph-like; associated with *JAK1* and *JAK2* mutations, *CDKN2A/B* deletions, *IKZF1* deletions; increasing incidence with older age; possibly targetable with TKIs
	ABL1, *ABL2*, *CSF1R*, *PDGFRB* rearrangements	5–6%	Unfavorable	10–20% of Ph-like; potentially targetable with TKIs
	EPOR, *JAK2* rearrangements	2%	Unfavorable	10% of Ph-like; potentially targetable with TKIs
Trisomy 21-associated ALL	*P2RY8-CRLF2*, *JAK2* mutations	50–60% of DS-ALL	Intermediate	
iAMP21	Multiple copies of *RUNX1*	2%	Unfavorable	Rare rob(15;21)(q10;q10)c associated with greatly increased risk of iAMP21 ALL
DUX4 rearrangements	*IGH-DUX4*, *ERG-DUX4*	3–7%	Favorable	Associated with *IKZF1* deletions, *ERG* dysregulation, aberrant CD2 expression
MEF2D rearrangements	*MEF2D-BCL9*, *MEF2D-HNRNPUL1*	3–6%	Unfavorable	Multiple fusion partners, a possible role for epigenetic therapies
ZNF384 rearrangements	*EP300-ZNF384*	4%	Intermediate	Multiple fusion partners, a possible role for JAK inhibitors

Table 6.
Summary of genetic implication in BCP-ALL [12].

chromosomal microarray analysis [45]. These techniques are routinely employed to identify structural aberrations in chromosomes, providing valuable insights into the genetic profile of leukemia.

- *Hyperdiploidy:* High hyperdiploid is characterized by an increased number of chromosomes per leukemia cell (ranging from 51 to 67), predominantly featuring additional copies of chromosomes +4, +6, +10, +14, +17, +18, +21, and + X [46]. It is present in around 25% of childhood ALL cases, particularly among younger children. Patients with high-hyperdiploid B-ALL typically exhibit favorable outcomes and may be suitable candidates for reduced-intensity chemotherapy protocols. These regimens have been shown to effectively reduce treatment-related toxicities while maintaining high survival rates. Nevertheless, the clinical prognosis for low-hyperdiploidy cases, characterized by a chromosome count ranging from 47 to 50, demonstrates enhancement under contemporary treatment approaches [4, 12].

- *Hypodiploidy:* Characterized by 43 or fewer chromosomes, includes near-haploid (24–31 chromosomes), low-hypodiploid (32–39 chromosomes), and high-hypodiploid (40–43 chromosomes) subtypes [47]. These subtypes collectively represent 2–3% of childhood ALL cases and are associated with poor prognosis. Children with low-hypodiploid ALL often exhibit TP53 mutations, with many displaying germline TP53 mutations consistent with Li-Fraumeni syndrome. Hypodiploid B-ALL typically displays a non-random pattern of chromosome losses, affecting chromosomes 3, 7, 13, 15, 16, and 17 [4, 12].

7.1.2 Recurrent chromosomal translocations

The vast majority of childhood B-ALL cases exhibit chromosomal translocations, many of which carry important prognostic implications. These recurrent translocations are often among the earliest events driving leukemogenesis. While routine cytogenetic analyses may not detect certain rearrangements in metaphase chromosomes, techniques such as reverse-transcription polymerase chain reaction (RT-PCR) or fluorescence in situ hybridization (FISH) assays can effectively identify such mutations.

- *ETV6-RUNX1*: Roughly 25% of childhood B-ALL cases classified as standard-risk for t(12;21)(p13;q22), resulting in an ETV6-RUNX1 fusion (formerly known as TEL-AML1) [48]. The detection of ETV6-RUNX1 fusions in preserved blood specimens from children who later develop ALL supports the hypothesis of a possible prenatal origin of leukemia. However, these fusions were also identified in children who did not develop ALL, indicating that *ETV6-RUNX1* translocations require additional mutations to contribute to ALL pathogenesis. Children with *ETV6-RUNX1* fusion generally have highly favorable outcomes with standard therapy. In recent reports, several cases of "ETV6-RUNX1-like" B-ALL have been identified without the typical rearrangement, but instead linked to alternative ETV6 fusion events and deletions affecting IKZF1. Despite incomplete understanding of the clinical outcomes for these rare patients, recurrence does not appear to be frequent [4, 12].

- *TCF3*: The fusion protein *TCF3-PBX1*, resulting from the translocation t(1;19)(q23;p13), is detected in roughly 5% of childhood B-ALL cases [49]. This fusion is associated with a pre-B immunophenotype, where leukemic cells express cytoplasmic immunoglobulin heavy chain. Initially considered high-risk leukemia with tendencies for CNS involvement and increased relapse rates, patients harboring the *TCF3-PBX1* fusion are now classified under good or intermediate risk categories with modern intensive treatment protocols [50]. Conversely, although rare (accounting for less than 0.5% of children with B-ALL), the *TCF3-HLF* fusion resulting from t(17;19)(q22;p13.3) is associated with notably unfavorable outcomes [4, 12].

- *KMT2A (MLL) rearrangement*: Childhood leukemia characterized by *KMT2A*, located on chromosome 11q23 formerly known as *MLL*, presents a distinct subtype with both lymphoid and myeloid characteristics, often associated with a poor prognosis [51]. The onset of this leukemia is typically early, likely occurring in utero for most childhood cases, evidenced by the high prevalence of *KMT2A* translocations in infant ALL cases (under 1 year), accounting for approximately 80% of patients, compared to around 3% in childhood ALL [4, 12].

- *BCR-ABL1*: The occurrence of t(9;22)(q34;q11.1)/*BCR-ABL1* leads to the formation of the Philadelphia chromosome (Ph), and it is detected in approximately 3% of cases in pediatric ALL, with its frequency increasing with age. Positive patients for *BCR-ABL1* fusion are linked to unfavorable prognoses across all age groups, frequently associated with leukocytosis, CNS infiltration, and the early onset of resistance to multiple drugs. *BCR-ABL1* functions as a prognostic biomarker for targeted therapy involving tyrosine kinase inhibitors (TKIs) like imatinib or dasatinib, which specifically block the leukemogenic actions of the BCR-ABL1 oncoprotein [52]. Integration of TKIs with standard chemotherapy has significantly improved the traditionally unfavorable prognosis of *BCR-ABL1*-positive ALL [4, 12].

7.1.3 BCR-ABL1*-like or Philadelphia chromosome-like ALL subtype*

Patients with Ph-like ALL exhibit a gene expression pattern similar to *BCR-ABL1* ALL, despite the absence of the gene fusion. Their genomic profile often includes *IKZF1* deletions, deregulation of *CRLF2*, and mutations in *JAK2* [53]. Ph-like ALL constitutes around 15% of childhood BCP-ALL cases and is associated with unfavorable outcomes. Roughly 50% of Ph-like ALL cases feature *CLRF2* rearrangements. Studies utilizing transcriptome and whole genome sequencing have uncovered that Ph-like ALL lacking CRLF2 rearrangements exhibit diverse genomic changes that activate cytokine receptors and tyrosine kinases. These alterations involve genes such as *ABL1*, *ABL2*, *JAK2*, *EPOR*, and *PDGFRB* and are present in up to 5% of B-ALL cases [4, 12].

7.1.4 CRLF2 *rearrangements and Janus kinase mutations in B-ALL*

The cytokine receptor *CRLF2* mutations are detected in 5% of B-ALL cases while accounting for 50% of Down syndrome ALL (DS-ALL). *CRLF2*-rearranged frequently has activating mutations in the Janus kinase genes, *JAK1* and *JAK2*, which are uncommon in B-ALL [54]. These *JAK* mutations primarily consist of missense mutations located at or near p.Arg683 in the pseudokinase domain of *JAK2*, distinct from the *JAK2* p.Val617Phe mutations observed in myeloproliferative diseases [4, 12].

*7.1.5 Intrachromosomal amplification of chromosome 21 (*iAMP21*)*

iAMP21, detected in 2% of childhood B-ALL cases, presents as a significantly aberrant chromosome 21 formed through breakage-fusion-bridge cycles and chromothripsis. These processes lead to the amplification and loss of multiple segments across the length of chromosome 21. Typically identified as a primary cytogenetic anomaly, *iAMP21* is often observed in patients without other major cytogenetic changes, although there are rare instances where *iAMP21* coexists with *ETV6-RUNX1* and *BCR-ABL1* rearrangements [4, 12].

7.1.6 DUX4 *rearrangement and ERG dysregulation*

In recent findings, recurrent *IGH-DUX4* (double homeobox 4) fusions have been identified in up to 7% of childhood B-ALL cases, leading to *DUX4* overexpression and a distinct gene expression profile [55]. The rearrangement of *DUX4* results in ERG (ETS-related gene) loss of function either through intragenic deletion or by inducing a dominant-negative isoform that hampers wild-type ERG activity. Despite the frequent presence of concomitant *IKZF1* deletions, patients with *DUX4* rearrangements exhibit promising clinical outcomes when treated with standard chemotherapy [4, 12, 44].

7.1.7 MEF2D *and* ZNF384 *rearrangements*

MEF2D and Zinc Finger 384 (*ZNF384*) delineate distinct B-ALL subsets, comprising approximately 6% of pediatric cases. *MEF2D* is part of the MEF2 family of transcription factors, essential for neuronal development and the formation of muscle tissue, and its activity is modulated by class II histone deacetylases [56]. Preclinical studies hint at the potential efficacy of histone deacetylase inhibitors in *MEF2D*-rearranged ALL. Additionally, investigations indicate an elevation in *JAK/STAT* signaling in ZNF384-rearranged ALL, suggesting potential therapeutic benefits with JAK inhibitors (**Figure 2**) [44].

7.2 T-cell ALL

T-ALL cases often exhibit translocation rearrangements of *ABL1*, activating mutations of *NOTCH1*, and various genetic alterations typically involving *CDKN2A/CDKN2B*, *PTEN*, and *MYB*. A brief table is provided below (**Table** 7)

- *T-cell receptor gene rearrangement:* Almost half of cases of childhood T-ALL are positive for chromosomal translocations that fuse T-cell receptor genes with oncogenes or result in interstitial deletions. Through comprehensive expression profiling studies, the genomic and epigenomic landscape of these leukemias has been more thoroughly characterized. These findings have enabled the classification of T-ALL into four primary subtypes: *TLX1* (previously *HOX11*), *LYL1*, *TAL1/LMO2*, and *TLX3* (previously *HOX11L2*). Although the prognostic and therapeutic implications of these T-ALL subsets remain unclear, patients with TLX1 alterations appear to respond more favorably to standard therapy.

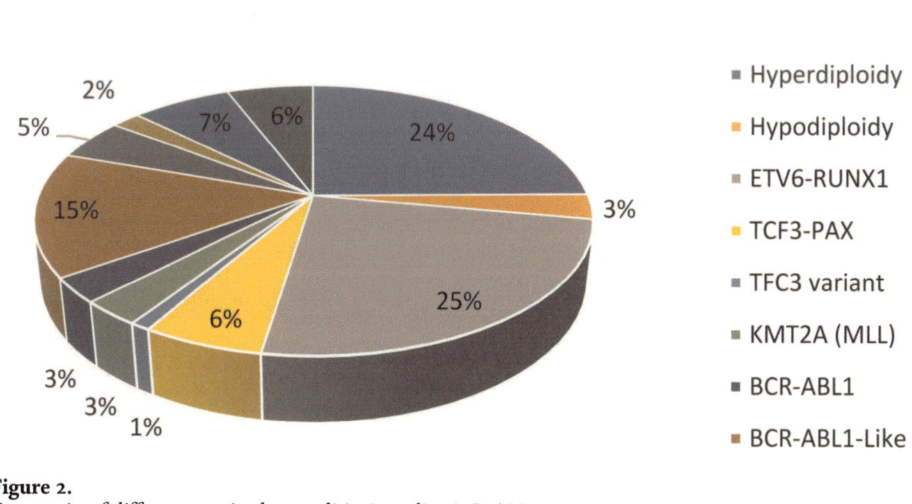

Figure 2.
Frequencies of different genetic abnormalities in pediatric B-ALL.

Genetic subtype	Common alterations	Frequency in ALL	Prognosis	Comment
T-ALL				
Recurrent Chromosomal Translocations				
t(10;14)(q24;q11)	*TLX1 (HOX11)* fusions	5–10% of T-ALL	Favorable	Associated with *PHF6* mutations
t(7;19)(q34;p13)	*LYL1* fusions	10% of T-ALL	Unfavorable	
t(1;14)(p32;q11), t(1;7)(p32;q34), t(11;14)(p15;q11), t(11;14)(p13;q11)	*TAL1, LMO1, LMO2* fusions	50–60% of T-ALL	Unfavorable	Associated with *PHF6* mutations
t(11;14)(p15;q11), t(5;14)(q35;q32)	*TLX3 (HOX11L2)* fusions	20–25% of T-ALL	Unfavorable (some studies), intermediate (some studies), favorable (some studies)	Associated with *PHF6* mutations
t(8;14)(q24;q11)	*TRA-MYC, TRC-MYC*	1% of T-ALL	Probably unfavorable	Associated with MYC activation and aggressive phenotype
7p15 translocations	*HOXA10, HOXA9* overexpression	3% of T-ALL	Unfavorable	
KMT2A (11q23) rearrangements	*KMT2A-AFF1, KMT2A-MLLT1*	5% of T-ALL	Possibly favorable	
t(10;11)(p13;q21)	*PICALM-MLLT10 (CALM-AF10)*	5–10% of T-ALL	Unfavorable (some studies), intermediate (other studies)	Associated with *EZH2* alterations
t(9;14)(q34;q32)	*NUP214-ABL1*	5–15% of T-ALL	Unfavorable (some studies), intermediate (other studies)	Associated with *TLX1* and *TLX3 (HOX11L2)* overexpression
Other				
NOTCH1 mutations		50–60% of T-ALL	Favorable	Associated with *CDKN2A* and *FBXW7* deletions
ETP		10–15% of T-ALL	Unfavorable (some studies), intermediate (other studies)	Associated with Ras pathway mutations; characteristic immunophenotype (CD1a-,CD8-, CD5- or CD5-dim with co-expression of myeloid or stem cell markers)
FBXW7 mutation		15% of T-ALL		Associated with *NOTCH1* activation via impairment of proteasomal degradation of *NOTCH1*

Table 7.
Summary of genetic implication in T-ALL [12].

Rare alterations in T-ALL include t(8;14)(q24;q11), resulting in *TRA-MYC* or *TRD-MYC* fusion [4, 12, 44].

- *PICALM-MLLT10 rearrangement:* The t(10;11)(p13;q21) translocation, leading to the *PICALM-MLLT10* (previously *CALM-AF10*) fusion, is also observed in acute myeloid leukemias and has been linked to unfavorable survival outcomes in pediatric T-ALL [57]. However, recent evidence suggests intermediate outcomes with intensive therapy [4, 12].

- *KMT2A rearrangement:* Like B-ALL, 11q23 translocations leading to *KMT2A* rearrangement occur in 10–15% of T-ALL cases [58]. It remains unclear if *KMT2A-R* T-ALL cases exhibit increased expression of wild-type *FLT3*, resembling infant B-ALL, or if outcomes for these patients could be enhanced by *FLT3* inhibitors [4, 12].

- *ABL1 rearrangement:* The *NUP214-ABL1* fusion resulting from t(5;14) is found in 5–10% of T-ALL cases. Preclinical studies reveal activated ABL1 kinase signaling in *NUP214-ABL1* T-ALL, similar to Ph + and subsets of Ph-like B-ALL [59]. In vitro, inhibition of *ABL1* target phosphoproteins CrkL and *STAT5*, along with increased cell death with dasatinib or nilotinib treatment, has been demonstrated [60]. Clinical reports suggest the potential efficacy of imatinib or dasatinib in refractory *NUP214-ABL1* ALL, although controlled trials are lacking. Additionally, *JAK* inhibition including tofacitinib, momelotinib, and ruxolitinib may hold therapeutic promise in *ABL1*-rearranged and other T-ALL subsets. Common point mutations and indels in *IL7R*, *JAK1*, *JAK3*, and *SH2B3* genes are observed in T-ALL, particularly in the early thymic precursor (ETP) subtype [4, 12].

- *NOTCH mutations:* Up to 50% of T-ALL cases are positive for somatic mutations in *NOTCH1*, which encodes a transmembrane receptor essential for T-cell lineage commitment and survival [61]. This leads to constitutive activation of *PI3K/mTOR* signaling, particularly in leukemias featuring *NOTCH1* mutations or PTEN deletions, a negative regulator of *PI3K* signaling [62]. Additionally, common cooperating deletions of tumor suppressor *CDKN2A* or mutations in ubiquitin-protein ligase FBXW7 can further augment aberrant PI3K signaling by reducing *NOTCH1* protein degradation [4, 12].

7.2.1 Early T-cell precursor ALL

Early T-cell precursor acute lymphoblastic leukemia (ETP-ALL) is a subtype of T-ALL characterized by distinct biological and clinical features classified by the WHO 2016 version [63]. It is recognized as a high-risk subtype due to its aggressive nature and poor response to standard chemotherapy regimens. Prevalence among pediatric EPT-ALL is up to 17% [64]. ETP-ALL arises from immature T-cell precursors that exhibit early developmental arrest, resembling early stages of T-cell differentiation in the thymus. These cells typically lack expression of surface markers that define mature T-cells, such as CD1a, CD8, and CD5, while often expressing myeloid or stem cell markers like CD117 (c-Kit), CD34, and CD13 [65]. This immunophenotypic profile distinguishes ETP-ALL from other T-ALL subtypes and contributes to its aggressive clinical outcomes.

ETP-ALL shares common features with other ALL subtypes, including frequent activating mutations in genes related to the RAS pathway, cytokine receptor signaling, *IL7R* pathway, hematopoietic development, and histone modification [66]. The mutational profile of ETP-ALL resembles myeloid leukemias, suggesting its potential inclusion in a spectrum of leukemias originating from very early hematopoietic progenitor cells or stem cells. Preclinical investigations in childhood T-ALL models, encompassing ETP, indicate the promising therapeutic potential of targeting activated cytokine receptor signaling networks through *FLT3*, *JAK*, or *PI3K/mTOR* inhibitors [4, 12].

8. Treatment of pediatric acute lymphoblastic leukemia

Just half a century ago, ALL was considered incurable. However, the discovery of new drugs and the optimization of treatment protocols have drastically improved the survival rate of children with ALL. Over the last decade, most high-income countries have seen the five-year survival rate for children aged 0–14 years exceed 90% [67]. The marked increase in survival rates is credited to the advancement of novel treatments, derived from insights gleaned through meticulous observation of individual cases by numerous pediatric oncologists, as well as the findings from multiple clinical trials conducted by international cancer cooperative study groups. These groups include the Children's Oncology Group (COG), the Berlin–Frankfurt–Münster (BFM) study group, and the Pediatric Oncology Group (POG) [68].

In standard treatment for ALL, therapy is tailored based on risk assessment. Factors like the child's age at diagnosis, initial white blood cell count, immunophenotypic and cytogenetic characteristics of the blast population, and the speed of response to initial treatment are all taken into consideration. Typically, chemotherapy is administered over 2–3 years.

8.1 Treatment procedure

The treatment of pediatric ALL relies on a multidrug regimen encompassing five distinct phases. These phases are meticulously designed to eradicate cancer cells, prevent relapse, and optimize long-term outcomes for patients. Here's an overview of each phase:

8.1.1 Remission-induction phase

The initial phase aims to induce remission by rapidly reducing the number of leukemia cells in the bone marrow and peripheral blood. Standard induction protocols typically include a three-drug combination consisting of glucocorticoids (prednisone/dexamethasone), vincristine, and L-asparaginase, along with intrathecal therapy BFM protocols, prednisone is administered as a single systemic agent during the initial week of treatment to reduce tumor burden and minimize metabolic complications systematically [69]. There is ongoing debate regarding the selection of glucocorticoids in induction regimens, with prednisone being the more prevalent choice. However, there is a growing preference for dexamethasone due to its potential to reduce rates of bone marrow and central nervous system relapse. This preference is associated with higher levels of the drug in plasma and improved penetration into the CNS [70, 71].

8.1.2 Early intensification

Children in remission, with restored normal hematopoiesis, become eligible for intensification therapy. Intensification therapy is administered to further eradicate residual leukemia cells and prevent the emergence of drug resistance. Specific protocols regarding the optimal treatment regimens and their duration remain elusive. In the BFM protocol, after induction, a course follows comprising 6-mercaptopurine, cyclophosphamide, low-dose cytarabine, and intrathecal methotrexate [70, 71].

8.1.3 Consolidation/CNS preventive therapy

Consolidation therapy aims to eliminate any remaining leukemia cells that may be present in the body, particularly in the bone marrow and central nervous system (CNS). CNS prophylaxis methods vary and include radiation (cranial or craniospinal) and various forms of chemotherapy, either intrathecal or systemic, or combinations thereof [72]. Due to concerns about long-term side effects such as neurologic and neuroendocrine issues, as well as the risk of secondary CNS tumors, cranial irradiation is now reserved for specific high-risk patients. Many modern treatment protocols utilize high-dose systemic methotrexate, typically given in four biweekly doses, along with intrathecal chemotherapy, either methotrexate alone or a combination of methotrexate, cytarabine, and hydrocortisone. The dosage of intrathecal medications is adjusted based on the patient's age. These effective prophylactic strategies have significantly reduced the occurrence of isolated CNS relapse to below 5% [70, 71].

8.1.4 Reinduction therapy

The addition of a delayed intensification (DI) phase post-standard induction/consolidation therapy has enhanced outcomes for pediatric ALL patients. DI's chemotherapy intensity varies by risk group. It predominantly reiterates the initial remission induction and early intensification phases, typically spanning 7 weeks from week 16. To prevent drug resistance, cytotoxic agents like prednisone, doxorubicin, and mercaptopurine were substituted with dexamethasone, daunorubicin, and thioguanine, respectively. This alteration, alongside other medications used, aids in further clearing minimal residual leukemia cells. Studies, including those by the American Children's Cancer Group, incorporating the BFM backbone, validated DI's efficacy, comprising reinduction and reconsolidation, in enhancing treatment success [70, 71].

8.1.5 Maintenance therapy

Maintenance therapy is aimed at preventing leukemia recurrence and maintaining remission over an extended period. Involves lower-dose, long-term chemotherapy regimens administered orally or intravenously. Typically lasts for 2–3 years and includes periodic visits to monitor disease status and adjust treatment as needed.

Throughout the treatment process, patients receive supportive care to manage treatment-related side effects and complications. This multidrug approach, combined with supportive care measures, has significantly improved the outcomes of ALL treatment, with cure rates exceeding 90% in many pediatric oncology centers. However, treatment protocols may vary based on patient age, risk factors, and disease characteristics, highlighting the importance of individualized care in ALL management [73].

8.2 Complete remission (CR)

Pediatric ALL patients, predominantly aged 1–18 years, exhibited a 95% remission rate. Complete remission (CR) was determined by <5% morphologically identified blasts in bone marrow with >20% cellularity and normal maturation [74, 75]. A peripheral blood neutrophil count exceeding 1500/μL, a platelet count surpassing 100,000/μL, and the absence of extramedullary disease were also requisites. This positive response to induction therapy typically occurs within <4–6 weeks of treatment initiation [76]. Additionally, oncologists deem a normal cellular bone marrow with tri-lineage hematopoiesis in leukemia patients as complete remission [76].

8.3 Induction failure

Induction failure, defined as the persistence of >5–25% blast cells in bone marrow, peripheral blood, or an extramedullary site post-induction therapy, occurred in 2.4% of pediatric ALL patients due to the disease's heterogeneity. Patients with T-cell or pre-B-ALL, especially those with high WBC counts or genetic markers like *BCR-ABL/MLL-AF4*, are at high risk. Survival rates up to 10 years are documented in pre-B children aged 1–5 years negative for *BCR-ABL/MLL-AF4*, but not in more than 50% of cases [77].

9. Chimeric antigen receptor T-cell therapy

Chimeric Antigen Receptor T-cell (CAR-T) therapy has emerged as a revolutionary treatment, promising to achieve remission in pediatric patients with relapsed or refractory ALL [78]. A CAR-T-cell therapy trial was conducted simultaneously in pediatric and adult patients, as opposed to the typical development course for oncological therapies, which is often established in adults and extended to children [78, 79]. In recent years, CAR-T cell therapy has seen approvals for clinical use, marking significant milestones in cancer treatment.

The first CAR-T therapy approved by the FDA was tisagenlecleucel (brand name Kymriah), which received approval in August 2017 for the treatment of pediatric and young adult patients up to 25 years of age with B-cell precursor acute lymphoblastic leukemia (ALL) that is refractory or in second or later relapse [80, 81]. Subsequently, in October 2017, another CAR-T therapy, axicabtagene ciloleucel (brand name Yescarta), was approved by the FDA for the treatment of adult patients with relapsed or refractory large B-cell lymphoma, including diffuse large B-cell lymphoma (DLBCL) and high-grade B-cell lymphoma [82]. Brexucabtagene autoleucel (Tecartus), approved in 2020, targets CD19 and is indicated for mantle cell lymphoma [83]. Lisocabtagene maraleucel (Breyanzi) and Abecma (idecabtagene vicleucel), both approved in 2021, target CD19 and are approved for relapsed or refractory large B-cell lymphoma and multiple myeloma, respectively [84, 85]. These approvals have paved the way for personalized medicine approaches and have significantly improved outcomes for patients facing limited treatment options.

9.1 Mechanism of CAR-T therapy

The therapy begins with the collection of the patient's T cells through leukapheresis, which are then engineered to express chimeric antigen receptors

(CARs) on their surface. These CARs are designed to bind to specific antigens present on the surface of cancer cells, such as CD19 in B-cell malignancies [86]. CAR-T-cell infusion is typically preceded by lymphodepleting chemotherapy, which increases T-cell proliferation in vivo by upregulating homeostatic cytokines such as IL-7 and IL-15. Consequently, this in vivo expansion may be more crucial than the dose of T cells as it has been linked to the therapeutic response [87]. Once infused back into the patient, the CAR-T cells proliferate and selectively target cells expressing the targeted antigen, initiating a potent immune response against the cancer. The activation of CAR-T cells leads to the release of cytotoxic molecules and cytokines, inducing apoptosis of cancer cells and stimulating an immune response that enhances tumor clearance [88]. This targeted approach enables CAR-T cell therapy to achieve remarkable clinical responses, particularly in patients with refractory or relapsed hematologic malignancies, ushering in a new era of personalized cancer treatment.

9.2 Impact on overall survival and disease-free survival

The impact of CAR-T cell therapy on overall survival (OS) and disease-free survival (DFS) in pediatric ALL has been profound. Studies have consistently shown that CAR-T cell therapy significantly improves OS rates in children with relapsed or refractory ALL. For example, a study involving 115 pediatric patients demonstrated that those treated with CAR-T cells had an OS rate of over 70% at 12 months post-treatment [89]. Another analysis reported that CAR-T cell therapy led to a DFS rate of approximately 60% at 24 months, indicating long-term remission for many patients [90].

Moreover, compared to traditional therapies such as chemotherapy and hematopoietic stem cell transplantation, CAR-T cell therapy has shown superior results in maintaining remission and extending survival [91]. Studies indicate that CAR-T therapy not only induces higher initial remission rates but also sustains remission longer, significantly reducing the likelihood of relapse [78].

The benefits of CAR-T cell therapy are also reflected in the quality of life improvements for pediatric patients. Reduced relapse rates and prolonged periods of remission mean fewer hospitalizations and less intensive treatments, allowing children to experience a more normal life during and after treatment.

9.3 Is CAR-T cell therapy superior to stem-cell transplantation?

The debate over whether CAR-T cell therapy is superior to stem-cell transplantation in pediatric ALL is ongoing. Recent systematic reviews and research articles provide valuable insights into this comparison. A systematic review by Elsallab et al. [92] compared the efficacy and safety of CAR-T cell therapy with hematopoietic stem cell transplantation (HSCT) in pediatric ALL. The study concluded that CAR-T cell therapy showed superior overall survival and disease-free survival rates compared to HSCT, with fewer late complications.

Additionally, a 2024 research article by Nakayama highlighted that CAR-T cell therapy led to higher remission rates and better quality of life outcomes compared to traditional HSCT. The study emphasized that CAR-T cell therapy could be particularly beneficial for patients who are not candidates for HSCT or who have relapsed after HSCT [90]. Another systematic review by Willyanto et al. [93] found that CAR-T cell therapy had a better safety profile and lower relapse rates compared to HSCT. The review suggested that CAR-T cell therapy should be considered as a first-line treatment for pediatric patients with relapsed or refractory ALL, especially in cases where HSCT is not feasible.

10. Minimal residual disease (MRD)

In pediatric ALL, MRD monitoring is standard practice to assess treatment response and stratify relapse risk. A good prognosis is indicated by undetectable MRD levels post-induction, while persistent MRD suggests a high relapse risk [94]. Classical techniques for MRD detection include flow cytometry and PCR, requiring high sensitivity (≤0.01% or ≤ 10–4) and specific markers like abnormal immunophenotypes, fusion genes, point mutations, and IG or TCR gene rearrangements [4, 95–100].

10.1 Classical methods of MRD monitoring

10.1.1 Flow cytometry (FCM)

Flow cytometry is extensively used for MRD detection due to its ability to identify leukemia-associated immunophenotypes. Traditional FCM methods use 4–5 color panels, but their sensitivity is limited for detecting low levels of residual disease. The technique remains valuable for risk stratification and treatment adjustments based on MRD levels [95].

10.1.2 Ig and TCR PCR

PCR-based methods targeting immunoglobulin (Ig) and T-cell receptor (TCR) gene rearrangements are highly sensitive and specific for MRD detection. These techniques rely on known genetic markers, which can be a limitation as not all leukemias have detectable markers [94, 96].

10.1.3 Fusion oncogene PCR

Fusion oncogene PCR targets specific fusion genes resulting from chromosomal translocations common in ALL. This method is highly specific and sensitive, making it suitable for detecting MRD in patients with known fusion oncogenes, such as BCR-ABL1 and ETV6-RUNX1 [4, 97].

10.2 Novel methods of MRD monitoring

10.2.1 Multicolor flow cytometry

Multicolor flow cytometry (MFC) uses up to 18 colors to analyze multiple parameters simultaneously, increasing the sensitivity and specificity of MRD detection. This method is especially useful in distinguishing between different leukemic clones and normal cells [98].

10.2.2 Next-generation sequencing (NGS)

Next-Generation Sequencing (NGS) offers ultra-deep sequencing of leukemia-specific genetic alterations, enabling the detection of very low levels of residual disease. NGS provides more accurate risk stratification and prediction of relapse compared to traditional methods [99].

10.2.3 Single-cell sequencing

Single-cell sequencing allows for the analysis of individual leukemic cells, providing detailed insights into the heterogeneity of residual disease. This novel method can identify subclonal populations that might be missed by bulk sequencing techniques [100].

10.2.4 Digital PCR (ddPCR)

Digital Droplet PCR (ddPCR) has improved the precision of MRD quantification by partitioning the sample into thousands of droplets, each serving as an individual PCR reaction. This method enhances sensitivity and specificity, making it suitable for routine clinical use in MRD monitoring [101].

10.3 Clinical implications of MRD monitoring

10.3.1 Risk-adapted treatment

MRD monitoring enables risk-adapted treatment strategies in pediatric ALL. High MRD levels post-induction therapy identify high-risk patients who may benefit from intensified treatment, while low or undetectable MRD levels allow for treatment de-escalation, reducing long-term side effects [94, 102].

10.3.2 Early relapse detection

Routine MRD monitoring during and after treatment facilitates early detection of relapse, enabling timely interventions that can improve survival rates. This proactive approach is now a cornerstone in the management of pediatric ALL [4, 103].

10.3.3 Personalized medicine

The integration of advanced MRD monitoring methods supports the move towards personalized medicine. Continuous assessment of MRD status allows clinicians to make informed decisions on treatment modifications, improving patient outcomes and reducing unnecessary exposure to toxic therapies [4, 94, 104].

10.4 Role of MRD detection methods in stem cell transplantation and CAR-T-cell therapy

10.4.1 Stem cell transplantation

MRD monitoring plays a crucial role in assessing the success of stem-cell transplantation in pediatric ALL patients. Detecting MRD before and after transplantation helps in predicting relapse and tailoring post-transplant therapies. Studies have shown that MRD negativity before transplantation is associated with improved outcomes and reduced relapse rates [90, 105]. Pre- and post-transplant MRD status significantly influences the overall survival and event-free survival in pediatric patients undergoing hematopoietic stem cell transplantation (HSCT) [106].

10.4.2 CAR-T-cell therapy

MRD monitoring is vital in evaluating the efficacy of CAR-T-cell therapy. Accurate MRD assessment helps in determining the response to therapy and guiding further treatment decisions. Studies have demonstrated that achieving MRD negativity post-CAR-T-cell therapy is associated with better long-term outcomes and reduced relapse rates [107]. The integration of MRD monitoring in CAR-T-cell therapy protocols has contributed to significant improvements in overall survival and progression-free survival in pediatric ALL patients [108].

10.5 MRD monitoring and improvements in disease outcomes and survival

The advancements in MRD detection methods have greatly improved the outcomes and survival rates of pediatric ALL patients. The integration of MRD monitoring in treatment protocols has allowed for better risk stratification, timely interventions, and personalized treatment plans, leading to improved overall survival and progression towards a cure in this once deadly childhood disease [94, 109].

11. Conclusions

ALL, or acute lymphoblastic leukemia, is the most prevalent form of cancer in children worldwide. Advancements in modern technology in the twenty-first century have resulted in the identification of new genetic, immunological, and cellular pathways that contribute to the biology and parthenogenesis of juvenile acute lymphoblastic leukemia. This has sparked a significant change in the diagnosis, prognosis, and treatment of this disease. The identification of numerous novel molecular genetic anomalies has not only facilitated the selection of suitable pharmaceuticals to meet the specific requirements of individual patients but has also contributed to the development of more efficient clinical procedures with reduced side effects, resulting in personalized treatment for patients. This has led to cure rates of about 95% for pediatric ALL in technologically advanced countries. Advancements in molecular medicine, drug development, and nanotechnology are anticipated to enhance the clinical results for relapsed pediatric ALL and in underdeveloped nations worldwide in the upcoming decades.

Acknowledgements

We acknowledge King Abdullah International Medical Research Center (KAIMRC), our institutional research center, for providing approval of the research project (# RA17/003/A, dated 4th Feb 2019) related to the genetics of pediatric ALL that has paved the way for this article/chapter.

Conflict of interest

The authors declare no conflict of interest.

Notes/thanks/other declarations

Thanks are due to all the authors' dedicated time and compassion for writing this book chapter.

Author details

Nawaf AlAnazi[1,2,3], Sarah AlMukhaylid[3,4,5] and Zafar Iqbal[2,3,4,5]*

1 Department of Pediatrics, King Abdulaziz Hospital, Al-Ahsa, Saudi Arabia

2 King Abdullah International Medical Research Centre (KAIMRC), Al-Ahsa, Saudi Arabia

3 Genomic and Experimental Medicine Group (GEM), Molecular Oncology and Hematology Section (MoOn-Hem); Quality Assurance and Accreditation Unit (QAAA); Clinical Laboratory Sciences Program (CLSP), College of Applied Medical Sciences (COAMS-A), King Saud Bin Abdulaziz University of Health Sciences (KSAU-HS), King Abdulaziz Medical City (KAMC), National Guard Health Affairs, Al-Ahsa, Saudi Arabia

4 Johns Hopkins ARAMCO Healthcare (JHAH), Al-Ahsa, Saudi Arabia

5 Saudi Society for Blood and Bone Marrow Transplantation (SSBMT), King Abdullah International Medical Research Centre (KAIMRC), Al-Ahsa, Saudi Arabia

*Address all correspondence to: iqbalz@ksau-hs.edu.sa; drzafar.medgen1@gmail.com; iqbalza@mngha.med.sa

References

[1] Kampen KR. The discovery and early understanding of leukemia. Leukemia Research. 2012;**36**:6-13. DOI: 10.1016/j.leukres.2011.09.028

[2] Passegué E, Jamieson CHM, Ailles LE, Weissman IL. Normal and leukemic hematopoiesis: Are leukemias a stem cell disorder or a reacquisition of stem cell characteristics? Proceedings of the National Academy of Sciences of the United States of America. 2003;**100**: 11842-11849. DOI: 10.1073/pnas.2034201100

[3] Chennamadhavuni A, Lyengar V, Mukkamalla SKR, Shimanovsky A. Leukemia 2024

[4] Coccaro N, Anelli L, Zagaria A, Specchia G, Albano F. Next-generation sequencing in acute lymphoblastic leukemia. International Journal of Molecular Sciences. 2019;**20**:2929. DOI: 10.3390/ijms20122929

[5] Tuong PN, Kiem Hao T, Kim Hoa NT. Relapsed childhood acute lymphoblastic leukemia: A single-institution experience. Cureus. 2020;**12**. DOI: 10.7759/cureus.9238

[6] DuVall AS, Sheade J, Anderson D, Yates SJ, Stock W. Updates in the management of relapsed and refractory acute lymphoblastic leukemia: An urgent plea for new treatments is being answered! JCO Oncology Practice. 2022; **18**:479-487. DOI: 10.1200/op.21.00843

[7] Huang FL, Chang YM, Lin CY, Yu SJ, Fu JT, Chou TY, et al. Regulating TKT activity inhibits the proliferation of human acute lymphoblastic leukemia cells. American Journal of Cancer Research. 2024;**14**

[8] Terwilliger T, Abdul-Hay M. Acute lymphoblastic leukemia: A comprehensive review and 2017 update. Blood Cancer Journal. 2017;7:e577-e577. DOI: 10.1038/bcj.2017.53

[9] Larson RA, Anastasi J. Acute Lymphoblastic Leukemia: Clinical Presentation, Diagnosis, and Classification. Acute Leukemias, Berlin, Heidelberg: Springer Berlin Heidelberg; 2007. pp. 109-118

[10] Zhu Y, Liu H, Zhang S, Liang Y, Xiao M, Hao Y, et al. A case report of lineage switch from T-cell acute leukemia to B-cell acute leukemia. Medicine (Baltimore). 2020;**99**:e22490. DOI: 10.1097/md.0000000000022490

[11] Zahnreich S, Schmidberger H. Childhood cancer: Occurrence, treatment and risk of second primary malignancies. Cancers (Basel). 2021;**13**: 2607. DOI: 10.3390/cancers13112607

[12] Tasian SK, Hunger SP. Genomic characterization of paediatric acute lymphoblastic leukaemia: An opportunity for precision medicine therapeutics. British Journal of Haematology. 2017;**176**:867-882. DOI: 10.1111/bjh.14474

[13] Singh SK, Lupo PJ, Scheurer ME, Saxena A, Kennedy AE, Ibrahimou B, et al. A childhood acute lymphoblastic leukemia genome-wide association study identifies novel sex-specific risk variants. Medicine (Baltimore). 2016;**95**: e5300. DOI: 10.1097/md.0000000000005300

[14] SEER*Explorer: An Interactive Website for SEER Cancer Statistics [Internet]. Surveillance Research Program, National Cancer Institute. 2023. Available from: https://seer.cancer.gov/statistics-network/explorer/ [Accessed: April 4, 2024]

[15] Garniasih D, Susanah S, Sribudiani Y, Hilmanto D. The incidence and mortality of childhood acute lymphoblastic leukemia in Indonesia: A systematic review and meta-analysis. PLoS One. 2022;**17**:e0269706. DOI: 10.1371/journal.pone.0269706

[16] Hoelzer D, Bassan R, Dombret H, Fielding A, Ribera JM, Buske C. Acute lymphoblastic leukaemia in adult patients: ESMO clinical practice guidelines for diagnosis, treatment and follow-up. Annals of Oncology. 2016;**27**: v69-v82. DOI: 10.1093/annonc/mdw025

[17] Jastaniah W, Essa MF, Ballourah W, Abosoudah I, Al Daama S, Algiraigri AH, et al. Incidence trends of childhood acute lymphoblastic leukemia in Saudi Arabia: Increasing incidence or competing risks? Cancer Epidemiology. 2020;**67**:101764. DOI: 10.1016/j.canep.2020.101764

[18] Kato M, editor. Pediatric Acute Lymphoblastic Leukemia. Springer Singapore: Singapore; 2020

[19] Kristen E, Adrienne M. Does Infection Cause or Prevent Childhood Leukaemia. Children with Leukaemia, London

[20] Belson M, Kingsley B, Holmes A. Risk factors for acute leukemia in children: A review. Environmental Health Perspectives [Internet]. 2007; **115**(1):138-145. DOI: 10.1289/ ehp.9023

[21] Tebbi CK. Etiology of acute leukemia: A review. Cancers (Basel). 2021;**13**:2256. DOI: 10.3390/ cancers13092256

[22] Iacobucci I, Mullighan CG. Genetic basis of acute lymphoblastic leukemia. Journal of Clinical Oncology. 2017;**35**: 975-983. DOI: 10.1200/jco.2016.70.7836

[23] Huang F, Liao E, Li C, Yen C, Yu S. Pathogenesis of pediatric B-cell acute lymphoblastic leukemia: Molecular pathways and disease treatments (review). Oncology Letters. 2020;**20**: 448-454. DOI: 10.3892/ol.2020.11583

[24] Onyije FM, Olsson A, Baaken D, Erdmann F, Stanulla M, Wollschläger D, et al. Environmental risk factors for childhood acute lymphoblastic leukemia: An umbrella review. Cancers (Basel). 2022;**14**:382. DOI: 10.3390/ cancers14020382

[25] Ma X, Urayama K, Chang J, Wiemels JL, Buffler PA. Infection and pediatric acute lymphoblastic leukemia. Blood Cells, Molecules & Diseases. 2009; **42**:117-120. DOI: 10.1016/j. bcmd.2008.10.006

[26] Buitenkamp TD, Izraeli S, Zimmermann M, Forestier E, Heerema NA, van den Heuvel-Eibrink MM, et al. Acute lymphoblastic leukemia in children with down syndrome: A retrospective analysis from the Ponte di Legno study group. Blood. 2014;**123**:70-77. DOI: 10.1182/blood-2013-06-509463

[27] de Smith AJ, Spector LG. In utero origins of acute leukemia in children. Biomedicine. 2024;**12**:236. DOI: 10.3390/ biomedicines12010236

[28] Tragiannidis A, Vasileiou E, Papageorgiou M, Damianidou L, Hatzipantelis E, Gombakis N, et al. Bone involvement at diagnosis as a predictive factor in children with acute lymphoblastic leukemia. Hippokratia. 2016;**20**:227

[29] Brown P, Inaba H, Annesley C, Beck J, Colace S, Dallas M, et al. Pediatric acute lymphoblastic leukemia, version 2.2020, NCCN clinical practice guidelines in oncology. Journal of the National Comprehensive Cancer

Network. 2020;**18**:81-112. DOI: 10.6004/jnccn.2020.0001

[30] Långström S, Huurre A, Kari J, Lohi O, Sievänen H, Palmu S. Bioimpedance spinal needle provides high success and low complication rate in lumbar punctures of pediatric patients with acute lymphoblastic leukemia. Scientific Reports. 2022;**12**:1-8. DOI: 10.1038/s41598-022-10915-4

[31] Ikonomidou C. Cerebrospinal fluid biomarkers in childhood leukemias. Cancers (Basel). 2021;**13**:438. DOI: 10.3390/cancers13030438

[32] Shahriari M, Shakibazad N, Haghpanah S, Ghasemi K. Extramedullary manifestations in acute lymphoblastic leukemia in children: A systematic review and guideline-based approach of treatment. American Journal of Blood Research. 2020;**10**:360

[33] Vemuri KS, Revaiah PC, Bootla D, Chauhan R, Nevali KP, Jandial A, et al. Early T cell precursor leukemia presenting with superior vena cava syndrome and cardiac tamponade. JACC CardioOncology. 2020;**2**:805-809. DOI: 10.1016/j.jaccao.2020.10.009

[34] Özcan A. Vena cava superior syndrome in children with mediastinal Tumors: Single Center experience. Northern Clinics Of Istanbul. 2019;**7**:255. DOI: 10.14744/nci.2019.46354

[35] Tiensiwakul P, Lertlum T, Nuchprayoon I, Seksarn P. Immunophenotyping of acute lymphoblastic leukemia in pediatric patients by three-color flow cytometric analysis. Asian Pacific Journal of Allergy and Immunology. 1999;**17**

[36] DiGiuseppe JA, Wood BL. Applications of flow cytometric immunophenotyping in the diagnosis and posttreatment monitoring of B and T lymphoblastic leukemia/lymphoma. Cytometry. Part B, Clinical Cytometry. 2019;**96**:256-265. DOI: 10.1002/cyto.b.21833

[37] Al Gwaiz LA, Bassioni W. Immunophenotyping of acute lymphoblastic leukemia using immunohistochemistry in bone marrow biopsy specimens. Histology and Histopathology. 2008;**23**. DOI: 10.14670/HH-23.1223

[38] Kalaivani S, Saranya GD, Kar R, Basu D. Role of immunohistochemistry in acute leukemias with myelonecrosis. Indian Journal of Hematology and Blood Transfusion. 2018;**34**:643-647. DOI: 10.1007/s12288-018-0918-0

[39] Chiaretti S, Zini G, Bassan R. Diagnosis and subclassification of acute lymphoblastic leukemia. Mediterranean Journal of Hematology and Infectious Diseases. 2014;**6**:e2014073. DOI: 10.4084/mjhid.2014.073

[40] Keohane E, M, Otto CN, Walenga JM. Rodak's Hematology. Sixth ed. Elsevier; 2020. pp. 466-476, ISBN 9780323530453. DOI: 10.1016/B978-0-323-53045-3.00036-2

[41] Vardiman JW, Thiele J, Arber DA, Brunning RD, Borowitz MJ, Porwit A, et al. The 2008 revision of the World Health Organization (WHO) classification of myeloid neoplasms and acute leukemia: Rationale and important changes. Blood. 2009;**114**:937-951. DOI: 10.1182/blood-2009-03-209262

[42] Alaggio R, Amador C, Anagnostopoulos I, Attygalle AD, de Araujo IBO, Berti E, et al. The 5th edition of the World Health Organization classification of Haematolymphoid tumours: Lymphoid neoplasms.

Leukemia. 2022;**36**:1720-1748. DOI: 10.1038/s41375-022-01620-2

[43] Sharma P, Srinivasan T, Mallik N. Flow cytometry in the diagnostic laboratory workup of acute lymphoblastic leukemias. Indian Journal of Medical and Paediatric Oncology. 2023;**44**:474-481. DOI: 10.1055/s-0043-1772204

[44] Vora A, editor. Childhood Acute Lymphoblastic Leukemia. Switzerland: Springer International Publishing; 2017. DOI: 10.1007/978-3-319-39708-5_1

[45] Ozkan E, Lacerda MP. Genetics, Cytogenetic Testing and Conventional Karyotype. StatPearls Publishing; 2023

[46] Chen Z, Sun Y, Xie W, Wang SA, Hu S, Li S, et al. Is hyperdiploidy a favorable cytogenetics in adults with B-lymphoblastic leukemia? Cancer Medicine. 2019;**8**:4093-4099. DOI: 10.1002/cam4.2255

[47] Carroll AJ, Shago M, Mikhail FM, Raimondi SC, Hirsch BA, Loh ML, et al. Masked hypodiploidy: Hypodiploid acute lymphoblastic leukemia (ALL) mimicking hyperdiploid ALL in children: A report from the Children's oncology group. Cancer Genetics. 2019;**238**:62-68. DOI: 10.1016/j.cancergen.2019.07.009

[48] Zapilko V, Moisio S, Parikka M, Heinäniemi M, Lohi O. Generation of a zebrafish knock-in model recapitulating childhood ETV6::RUNX1-positive B-cell precursor acute lymphoblastic leukemia. Cancers (Basel). 2023;**15**:5821. DOI: 10.3390/cancers15245821

[49] Burmeister T, Gröger D, Gökbuget N, Spriewald B, Starck M, Elmaagacli A, et al. Molecular characterization of TCF3::PBX1 chromosomal breakpoints in acute lymphoblastic leukemia and their use for measurable residual disease assessment. Scientific Reports. 2023;**13**. DOI: 10.1038/s41598-023-42294-9

[50] Zhang H, Wan Y, Wang H, Cai J, Yu J, Hu S, et al. Prognostic factors of childhood acute lymphoblastic leukemia with TCF3::PBX1 in CCCG-ALL-2015: A multicenter study. Cancer. 2023;**129**: 1691-1703. DOI: 10.1002/cncr.34741

[51] Górecki M, Kozioł I, Kopystecka A, Budzyńska J, Zawitkowska J, Lejman M. Updates in KMT2A gene rearrangement in pediatric acute lymphoblastic leukemia. Biomedicine. 2023;**11**:821. DOI: 10.3390/biomedicines11030821

[52] He J, Munir F, Catueno S, Connors JS, Gibson A, Robusto L, et al. Biological markers of high-risk childhood acute lymphoblastic leukemia. Cancers (Basel). 2024;**16**:858. DOI: 10.3390/cancers16050858

[53] Płotka A, Lewandowski K. BCR/ABL1-like acute lymphoblastic leukemia: From diagnostic approaches to molecularly targeted therapy. Acta Haematologica. 2022;**145**:122-131. DOI: 10.1159/000519782

[54] Chang Y, Min J, Jarusiewicz JA, Actis M, Yu-Chen Bradford S, Mayasundari A, et al. Degradation of Janus kinases in CRLF2-rearranged acute lymphoblastic leukemia. Blood. 2021; **138**:2313-2326. DOI: 10.1182/blood.2020006846

[55] Rehn JA, O'Connor MJ, White DL, Yeung DT. DUX hunting—Clinical features and diagnostic challenges associated with DUX4-rearranged leukaemia. Cancers (Basel). 2020;**12**: 2815. DOI: 10.3390/cancers12102815

[56] Ratti S, Lonetti A, Follo MY, Paganelli F, Martelli AM, Chiarini F, et al. B-ALL complexity: Is targeted

therapy still a valuable approach for pediatric patients? Cancers (Basel). 2020;**12**:3498. DOI: 10.3390/cancers12123498

[57] Mark C, Meshinchi S, Joyce B, Gibson B, Harrison C, Bergmann AK, et al. Treatment outcomes of childhood PICALM::MLLT10 acute leukaemias. British Journal of Haematology. 2024; **204**:576-584. DOI: 10.1111/bjh.19067

[58] Peterson JF, Baughn LB, Pearce KE, Williamson CM, Benevides Demasi JC, Olson RM, et al. KMT2A (MLL) rearrangements observed in pediatric/young adult T-lymphoblastic leukemia/lymphoma: A 10-year review from a single cytogenetic laboratory. Genes, Chromosomes & Cancer. 2018;**57**: 541-546. DOI: 10.1002/gcc.22666

[59] Stukaite-Ruibiene E, Norvilas R, Dirse V, Stankeviciene S, Vaitkeviciene GE. Case report: Specific ABL-inhibitor imatinib is an effective targeted agent as the first line therapy to treat B-cell acute lymphoblastic leukemia with a cryptic NUP214::ABL1 gene fusion. Pathology Oncology Research. 2022;**28**. DOI: 10.3389/pore.2022.1610570

[60] Burmeister T, Gökbuget N, Reinhardt R, Rieder H, Hoelzer D, Schwartz S. NUP214-ABL1 in adult T-ALL: The GMALL study group experience. Blood. 2006;**108**:3556-3559. DOI: 10.1182/blood-2006-04-014514

[61] Sanchez-Martin M, Ferrando A. The NOTCH1-MYC highway toward T-cell acute lymphoblastic leukemia. Blood. 2017;**129**:1124-1133. DOI: 10.1182/blood-2016-09-692582

[62] Toribio ML, González-García S. Notch partners in the long journey of T-ALL pathogenesis. International Journal of Molecular Sciences. 2023;**24**:1383. DOI: 10.3390/ijms24021383

[63] Arber DA, Orazi A, Hasserjian R, Thiele J, Borowitz MJ, Le Beau MM, et al. The 2016 revision to the World Health Organization classification of myeloid neoplasms and acute leukemia. Blood. 2016;**127**:2391-2405. DOI: 10.1182/blood-2016-03-643544

[64] Sin C-F, Man P-HM. Early T-cell precursor acute lymphoblastic leukemia: Diagnosis, updates in molecular pathogenesis, management, and novel therapies. Front. Oncologia. 2021;**11**. DOI: 10.3389/fonc.2021.750789

[65] Genescà E, la Starza R. Early T-cell precursor ALL and beyond: Immature and ambiguous lineage T-ALL subsets. Cancers (Basel). 2022;**14**:1873. DOI: 10.3390/cancers14081873

[66] Zhang J, Ding L, Holmfeldt L, Wu G, Heatley SL, Payne-Turner D, et al. The genetic basis of early T-cell precursor acute lymphoblastic leukaemia. Nature. 2012;**481**:157-163. DOI: 10.1038/nature10725

[67] Sasaki K, Jabbour E, Short NJ, Jain N, Ravandi F, Pui C-H, et al. Acute lymphoblastic leukemia: A population-based study of outcome in the United States based on the surveillance, epidemiology, and end results (SEER) database, 1980–2017. American Journal of Hematology. 2021;**96**:650-658. DOI: 10.1002/ajh.26156

[68] Kotecha RS, Gottardo NG, Kees UR, Cole CH. The evolution of clinical trials for infant acute lymphoblastic leukemia. Blood Cancer Journal. 2014;**4**:e200-e200. DOI: 10.1038/bcj.2014.17

[69] Hayashi H, Makimoto A, Yuza Y. Treatment of pediatric acute lymphoblastic leukemia: A historical

perspective. Cancers (Basel). 2024;**16**: 723. DOI: 10.3390/cancers16040723

[70] Ronghe M, Burke GAA, Lowis SP, Estlin EJ. Remission induction therapy for childhood acute lymphoblastic leukaemia: Clinical and cellular pharmacology of vincristine, corticosteroids, L-asparaginase and anthracyclines. Cancer Treatment Reviews. 2001;**27**:327-337. DOI: 10.1053/ctrv.2001.0243

[71] Roganovic J. Acute lymphoblastic leukemia in children. In: Guenova M, Balatzenko G, editors. Leukemia. London, England: InTech; 2013

[72] Cooper SL, Brown PA. Treatment of pediatric acute lymphoblastic leukemia. Pediatric Clinics of North America. 2015; **62**:61-73. DOI: 10.1016/j.pcl.2014.09.006

[73] Toksvang LN, Lee SHR, Yang JJ, Schmiegelow K. Maintenance therapy for acute lymphoblastic leukemia: Basic science and clinical translations. Leukemia. 2022;**36**:1749-1758. DOI: 10.1038/s41375-022-01591-4

[74] Schrappe M, Hunger SP, Pui C-H, Saha V, Gaynon PS, Baruchel A, et al. Outcomes after induction failure in childhood acute lymphoblastic leukemia. The New England Journal of Medicine. 2012;**366**:1371-1381. DOI: 10.1056/nejmoa1110169

[75] Preiss BS, Kerndrup GB, Pedersen RK, Hasle H, Pallisgaard N. Contribution of multiparameter genetic analysis to the detection of genetic alterations in hematologic neoplasia. An evaluation of combining G-band analysis, spectral karyotyping, and multiplex reverse-transcription polymerase chain reaction (multiplex RT-PCR). Cancer Genetics and Cytogenetics. 2006;**165**:1-8

[76] Möricke A, Reiter A, Zimmermann M, Gadner H, Stanulla M, Dördelmann M, et al. Risk-adjusted therapy of acute lymphoblastic leukemia can decrease treatment burden and improve survival: Treatment results of 2169 unselected pediatric and adolescent patients enrolled in the trial ALL-BFM 95. Blood. 2008;**111**:4477-4489. DOI: 10.1182/blood-2007-09-112920

[77] Oudot C, Auclerc M-F, Levy V, Porcher R, Piguet C, Perel Y, et al. Prognostic factors for leukemic induction failure in children with acute lymphoblastic leukemia and outcome after salvage therapy: The FRALLE 93 study. Journal of Clinical Oncology. 2008;**26**:1496-1503. DOI: 10.1200/jco.2007.12.2820

[78] Knight ET, Oluwole O, Kitko C. The implementation of chimeric antigen receptor (CAR) T-cell therapy in pediatric patients: Where did we come from, where are we now, and where are we going? Clinical Hematology International. 2024;**6**:96. DOI: 10.46989/001c.94386

[79] Seng MS, Meierhofer AC, Lim FL, Soh SY, Hwang WYK. A review of CAR-T therapy in pediatric and young adult B-lineage acute leukemia: Clinical perspectives in Singapore. Oncotargets and Therapy. 2023;**16**:165-176. DOI: 10.2147/ott.s271373

[80] Mitra A, Barua A, Huang L, Ganguly S, Feng Q, He B. From bench to bedside: The history and progress of CAR T cell therapy. Frontiers in Immunology. 2023;**14**. DOI: 10.3389/fimmu.2023.1188049

[81] Maude SL, Laetsch TW, Buechner J, Rives S, Boyer M, Bittencourt H, et al. Tisagenlecleucel in children and young adults with B-cell lymphoblastic leukemia. The New England Journal of

Medicine. 2018;**378**:439-448. DOI: 10.1056/nejmoa1709866

[82] Neelapu SS, Locke FL, Bartlett NL, Lekakis LJ, Miklos DB, Jacobson CA, et al. Axicabtagene ciloleucel CAR T-cell therapy in refractory large B-cell lymphoma. The New England Journal of Medicine. 2017;**377**:2531-2544. DOI: 10.1056/nejmoa1707447

[83] Anderson MK, Torosyan A, Halford Z. Brexucabtagene autoleucel: A novel chimeric antigen receptor T-cell therapy for the treatment of mantle cell lymphoma. The Annals of Pharmacotherapy. 2022;**56**:609-619. DOI: 10.1177/10600280211026338

[84] FDA Approves Lisocabtagene Maraleucel for Relapsed or Refractory Mantle Cell Lymphoma. US Food and Drug Administration; Center for Drug Evaluation, Research. 2024. Available from: https://www.fda.gov/drugs/resources-information-approved-drugs/fda-approves-lisocabtagene-maraleucel-relapsed-or-refractory-mantle-cell-lymphoma [Accessed: June 15, 2024]

[85] Sharma P, Kanapuru B, George B, Lin X, Xu Z, Bryan WW, et al. FDA approval summary: Idecabtagene vicleucel for relapsed or refractory multiple myeloma. Clinical Cancer Research. 2022;**28**:1759-1764. DOI: 10.1158/1078-0432.ccr-21-3803

[86] Maude SL, Teachey DT, Porter DL, Grupp SA. CD19-targeted chimeric antigen receptor T-cell therapy for acute lymphoblastic leukemia. Blood. 2015;**125**: 4017-4023. DOI: 10.1182/blood-2014-12-580068

[87] Testa U, Sica S, Pelosi E, Castelli G, Leone G. Car-t cell therapy in b-cell acute lymphoblastic leukemia: CAR-T CELL and B-ALL. Mediterranean Journal of Hematology and Infectious Diseases. 2024;**16**:e2024010. DOI: 10.4084/mjhid.2024.010

[88] Ivanov AV, Alecsa MS, Popescu R, Starcea MI, Mocanu AM, Rusu C, et al. Pediatric acute lymphoblastic leukemia emerging therapies—From pathway to target. International Journal of Molecular Sciences. 2023;**24**:4661. DOI: 10.3390/ijms24054661

[89] Wang Y, Xue Y-J, Zuo Y-X, Jia Y-P, Lu A-D, Zeng H-M, et al. CD19-specific CAR-T cell treatment of 115 children and young adults with acute B lymphoblastic leukemia: Long-term follow-up. Cancer Research and Treatment. 2024. DOI: 10.4143/crt.2023.1205

[90] Nakayama H. Three-year update outcomes of the first chimeric antigen receptor-T therapy for children and young adults with relapsed/refractory acute lymphoblastic leukemia. Translational Pediatrics. 2024;**13**: 535-536. DOI: 10.21037/tp-23-535

[91] Curran KJ, Margossian SP, Kernan NA, Silverman LB, Williams DA, Shukla N, et al. Toxicity and response after CD19-specific CAR T-cell therapy in pediatric/young adult relapsed/refractory B-ALL. Blood. 2019;**134**:2361-2368. DOI: 10.1182/blood.2019001641

[92] Elsallab M, Ellithi M, Hempel S, Abdel-Azim H, Abou-el-Enein M. Long-term response to autologous anti-CD19 chimeric antigen receptor T cells in relapsed or refractory B cell acute lymphoblastic leukemia: A systematic review and meta-analysis. Cancer Gene Therapy. 2023;**30**:845-854. DOI: 10.1038/s41417-023-00593-3

[93] Willyanto SE, Alimsjah YA, Tanjaya K, Tuekprakhon A, Pawestri AR. Comprehensive analysis of the efficacy and safety of CAR T-cell therapy in patients with relapsed or refractory B-

cell acute lymphoblastic leukaemia: A systematic review and meta-analysis. Annals of Medicine. 2024;**56**. DOI: 10.1080/07853890.2024.2349796

[94] Pui C-H, Pei D, Raimondi SC, Coustan-Smith E, Jeha S, Cheng C, et al. Clinical impact of minimal residual disease in children with different subtypes of acute lymphoblastic leukemia treated with response-adapted therapy. Leukemia. 2017;**31**:333-339. DOI: 10.1038/leu.2016.234

[95] Della Starza I, De Novi LA, Elia L, et al. Optimizing molecular minimal residual disease analysis in adult acute lymphoblastic leukemia. Cancers (Basel). 2023;**15**(2):374. DOI: 10.3390/cancers15020374

[96] Mai H, Li Q, Wang G, et al. Clinical application of next-generation sequencing-based monitoring of minimal residual disease in childhood acute lymphoblastic leukemia. Journal of Cancer Research and Clinical Oncology. 2023;**149**(4):1013-1022. DOI: 10.1007/s00432-022-04151-6

[97] Kim IS. Minimal residual disease in acute lymphoblastic leukemia: Technical aspects and implications for clinical interpretation. Blood Research. 2020;**55**(4):244-253. DOI: 10.5045/br.2020.55.4.244

[98] Wu K, Wang Z, Xie Y, et al. One tube 23 color full spectral flow cytometry panel in detecting minimal residual disease in pediatric B-cell acute lymphoblastic leukemia. Blood. 2023. DOI: 10.1016/j.blood.2023.08.002

[99] Ahn WK, Yu K, Kim H, et al. Monitoring measurable residual disease in paediatric acute lymphoblastic leukaemia using immunoglobulin gene clonality based on next-generation sequencing. Cancer Cell International. 2024;**24**:3404. DOI: 10.1186/s12935-024-03404-3

[100] Foltz SM, Loren A, Chen C, et al. Multiomic single-cell tumor evolution models of minimal residual disease in pediatric B-cell acute lymphoblastic leukemia. Cancer Research. 2024. DOI: 10.1158/0008-5472.CAN-23-3952

[101] Schwinghammer C, Koopmann J, Chitadze G, et al. A new view on minimal residual disease quantification in acute lymphoblastic leukemia using droplet digital PCR. The Journal of Molecular Diagnostics. 2022. DOI: 10.1016/j.jmoldx.2022.06.007

[102] Contreras Yametti GP, Ostrow TH, Jasinski S, Raetz EA. Minimal residual disease in acute lymphoblastic leukemia: Current practice and future directions. Cancers (Basel). 2021;**13**(8):1847. DOI: 10.3390/cancers13081847

[103] Ceppi F, Rizzati F, Colombini A, et al. Utilizing the prognostic impact of minimal residual disease in treatment decisions for pediatric acute lymphoblastic leukemia. Expert Review of Hematology. 2021;**14**(10):1001-1012. DOI: 10.1080/17474086.2021.1967137

[104] Senapati J, Kantarjian H, Haddad FG, Short NJ. SOHO state of the art Updates & Next Questions: Acute lymphoblastic Leukemia. Clinical Lymphoma, Myeloma & Leukemia. 2024;**24**(1):e12-e19. DOI: 10.1016/j.clml.2023.10.001

[105] Giarin et al. Pre- and post-transplant minimal residual disease predicts relapse occurrence in children with acute lymphoblastic leukaemia. British Journal of Haematology 2024. DOI: 10.1016/S2468-1245(24)00011-1

[106] Bachanova et al. Unrelated cord blood transplantation in adult and pediatric acute lymphoblastic leukemia: Effect of minimal residual disease on

relapse and survival outcomes. Science Direct. 2023. DOI: 10.1016/S1521-1692 (23)00046-4

[107] Haematologica. Minimal residual disease-guided therapy in childhood acute lymphoblastic leukemia. Haematology. 2023. DOI: 10.3324/ haematol.2023.283848

[108] Tandfonline. Efficacy and Safety of CAR T-cell Therapy for r/r B-ALL: Impact of MRD Status on Outcomes. 2024. DOI: 10.1080/ 07853890.2024.2349796

[109] Nature. CAR T-cell therapy has transformed relapsed/refractory (r/r) B-cell precursor acute lymphoblastic leukaemia (B-ALL) management and outcomes. Nature Reviews. Clinical Oncology. 2024. DOI: 10.1038/ s41408-024-01038-2

Section 7

Common Chest Wall Deformities Cancers in Children

Chapter 9

Chest Wall Defects: An Integrated Multidisciplinary Approach by Assessing Treatment Approaches and Tracking Clinical Progress

Alessandro Maraschi, Erica Cristina Vallocchia and Kunal Bhakhri

Abstract

Chest wall deformities represent a diverse spectrum of conditions encountered frequently in pediatrics' medical practice. They manifest with various phenotypic expressions and, although typically benign, can lead to significant physiological and psychological impacts, some of which pose life-threatening risks. To facilitate systematic understanding, these deformities can be categorized into distinct groups, including: (1) pectus excavatum, (2) pectus carinatum, (3) Poland syndrome, (4) sternal defects, and (5) pectus arcuatum. This chapter aims to comprehensively elucidate these deformities, providing insights into their non-surgical and surgical management, including the latest diagnostic and treatment modalities. Additionally, it delves into the psychological and physiological ramifications experienced by young patients and their families, thereby offering a holistic understanding of the impact of these conditions on their lives.

Keywords: pectus, excavatum, carinatum, vacuum bell, brace

1. Introduction

Chest wall deformities are commonly observed and vary widely in appearance. Although generally benign, they can lead to significant physiological complications. These are categorized into: (1) pectus excavatum, (2) pectus carinatum, (3) Poland syndrome, (4) sternal defects, and (5) pectus arcuatum.

2. Pectus excavatum

Pectus excavatum (PE), also known as "funnel chest," represents the predominant congenital malformation of the anterior chest wall, accounting for 90% of all anterior chest wall deformities. The prevalence of this condition ranges among 1 in every 400 to 1000 live births, and it is three to five times more common in males than in females. While often occurring isolated, pectus excavatum can also be associated with connective tissue disorders, neuromuscular diseases, and genetic syndromes [1, 2].

PE usually becomes noticeable shortly after birth, marked by a posterior indentation of the lower sternum and a curvilinear deformation of the nearby costal cartilages. The deformity primarily affects the lower three to four ribs at their connection to the sternum, while the upper chest including the manubrium, the upper sternum, and the first three ribs remains typically unaffected. Pectus excavatum may also appear asymmetrically, often with the right side more concave, and can include a rotational deviation of the sternum toward the more depressed side.

2.1 Etiology

Although the exact etiology of pectus excavatum remains undetermined, several theories have been proposed. These hypotheses include an imbalance in the growth rates of the ribs compared to the thoracic organs; disproportionate muscular forces exerting unusual stress and strain on the sternum and costal cartilages; anomalies in cartilage structure and growth; irregular rib development; or a combination of these [3].

A significant proportion of pectus excavatum (85–90%) emerge as isolated defect, shortly after birth. Nevertheless, this condition frequently co-occurs with connective tissue disorders, with Marfan syndrome being prevalent. It is also linked to other connective tissue disorders such as Ehlers-Danlos syndrome and osteogenesis imperfecta [4, 5].

In addition to these, there is a substantial link with neuromuscular diseases, for example, spinal muscular atrophy.

Other genetic conditions observed in association with pectus excavatum are Noonan syndrome, Turner syndrome, neurofibromatosis type 1, and multiple endocrine neoplasia type 2b [6].

The higher incidence of pectus excavatum in individuals with connective tissue disorders points to a potential underlying cause rooted in atypical cartilage development like an imbalance in the genetic regulation of cartilage, between genes that promote growth and those that inhibit it [1].

Despite these hypotheses, specific genetic triggers have yet to be identified. Furthermore, histological examinations of cartilage samples from individuals with PE have consistently shown normal tissue structures [7].

The link between congenital diaphragmatic anomalies (diaphragmatic hernia and agenesis) and pectus excavatum is clear because both conditions are often associated [8, 9].

Additionally, there is a significant association between pectus excavatum and scoliosis [10].

There is a pattern of familial aggregation, with approximately one-third of patients reporting at least one family member who has a similar chest wall deformity [11].

2.2 Clinical presentation

2.2.1 Physical findings

On physical examination, is evident the typical depression in the anterior chest wall, primarily affecting the lower half of the sternum and adjacent ribs, and possibly extending laterally up to the mid-clavicular line. The lower costal margins often exhibit an outward flare. Asymmetry, when present, generally shows a deeper indentation on the right side, accompanied by a rotational shift of the sternum from left to right (**Figures 1** and **2**).

Lung sounds are usually normal, but a systolic murmur may be detected, which in some cases is only audible when the patient is in a sitting or standing position.

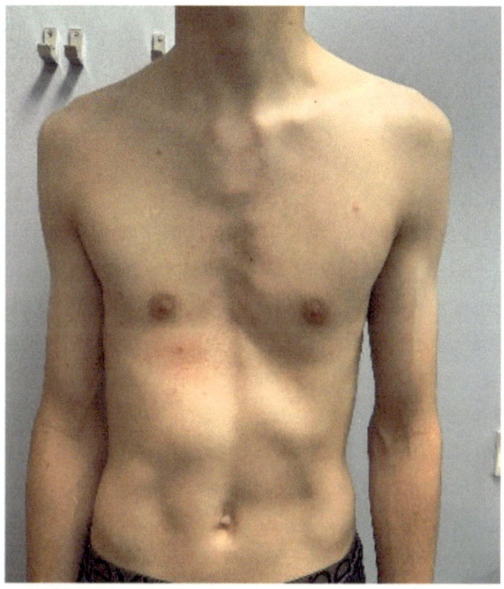

Figure 1.
Frontal view pectus excavatum.

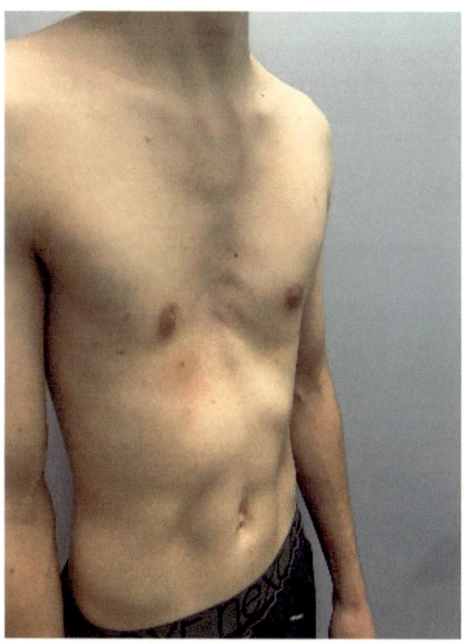

Figure 2.
Lateral view pectus excavatum.

2.2.2 Symptoms

Symptoms can typically be categorized into three main areas: pain, difficulty with exercise, or concerns regarding physical appearance.

In a comprehensive evaluation of patients with severe pectus excavatum, the reported symptoms included [12]:

- Exercise intolerance in 82% of cases,
- Chest pain in 68%,
- Reduced endurance in 67%, and
- Shortness of breath in 42% of the individuals assessed.

The pain is often sharp and brief, localized to the area of the sternal indentation, and can happen sporadically or be triggered by physical activity. Exercise intolerance tends to be of moderate severity. Interestingly, even highly active individuals might find their athletic performance slightly lagging behind their peers.

Concerns about appearance become particularly significant during adolescence, a period often marked by self-consciousness and the desire to fit in. Being perceived as "different" can attract unwanted attention, making the physical manifestations of this condition a source of distress for many young people.

Among patients, females have shown a higher tendency to raise concerns about their physical appearance compared to males (68 vs. 40%). Yet, the level of concern about appearance does not consistently align with the severity of pectus excavatum, indicating a varied perception of the condition's impact among individuals [13].

2.3 Evaluation

Patients with pectus excavatum require an assessment to determine the deformity's severity and identify any coexisting conditions. Those with moderate-to-severe PE, or those exhibiting symptoms indicative of cardiorespiratory compromise, should undergo CT scan.

However, a retrospective study has shown a weak correlation between the physical symptoms and the deformity's severity as seen on chest CT scans [14].

Nevertheless, patients presenting with respiratory symptoms, or those being considered for surgery, should have a pulmonary function test to check for any restrictive respiratory conditions. Exercise tests may be conducted on select patients to assess cardiopulmonary limitations. In cases of significant heart displacement or cardiopulmonary constraints, assessments should include echocardiography and electrocardiography.

For patients not initially recommended for surgery, regular monitoring with focused physical exams is advised, especially during adolescence. This allows for prompt identification and management of any worsening in the deformity or related symptoms, and consideration of non-surgical treatment options.

2.3.1 Physical examination

Thoracic abnormalities—Beyond the hallmark indentation of the sternum, patients with pectus excavatum frequently exhibit a reduced chest wall diameter from front

DOI: http://dx.doi.org/10.5772/intechopen.1006073

to back and possess a chest that appears wide and flat, and commonly exhibits a kyphotic curve. A significant proportion of those with pectus excavatum (10 to 39%) also experience varying degrees of scoliosis. The emergence of scoliosis can occur at any point during the evolution of pectus excavatum, and the impact of corrective pectus surgeries on the evolution of scoliosis remains uncertain [15].

Respiratory symptoms—Up to 98% of patients with pectus excavatum experience resting tachypnoea, which becomes more pronounced during adolescence. Those with more advanced stages of PE often exhibit a diminished aerobic capacity. It is rare to observe significant upper or lower respiratory tract anomalies during physical assessments. Approximately 42% of affected individuals report experiencing shortness of breath [12].

Cardiac assessment—In cases of isolated pectus excavatum, cardiac irregularities are uncommon. However, individuals with PE who also have associated syndromic conditions are more susceptible to cardiovascular issues.

Severe PE may lead to tachycardia, attributed to diminished stroke volume, which in turn is related to the heart's distortion and displacement. A small subset of patients may exhibit functional systolic murmurs, potentially linked to the compression of the left ventricular outflow tract. Additionally, mitral valve prolapse has been observed in a minority of those with PE.

2.3.2 Imaging and index score

Chest X-ray—Standard chest X-rays, including anteroposterior and lateral views, offer limited insight of the deformity but are valuable in identifying accompanying conditions such as kyphoscoliosis or pulmonary disorders.

In certain healthcare settings, conventional radiographs are employed to calculate the Pectus Severity Index (PSI), also known as the Haller Index. However, this method is not as uniformly standardized as CT imaging and may yield less accurate results, particularly for chests with asymmetrical deformities [16].

The PE deformity may present characteristic features on the frontal X-ray, such as opacification in the region of the right middle lobe. This shadowing is often confused with right middle lobe pneumonia or atelectasis but is the result of compression by the anterior chest wall's soft tissues [17].

More than half of the individuals with PE may show a shift of the heart's outline to the left on frontal images [18].

Lateral views show the sternum's posterior displacement, as an opacity that fills the space behind the sternum, with the ribs extending in front of it [17].

Computed tomography scan—CT scans are indicated for patients presenting with moderate to severe pectus excavatum or those experiencing cardiorespiratory difficulties. CT scans are the gold standard to assess the extent of the pectus deformity, including the level of cardiac and pulmonary compression, the displacement of the heart, lung atelectasis, chest wall asymmetry, rotation of the sternum, and the potential development of a compensatory barrel chest.

Magnetic resonance imaging—MRI has also proven effective for these evaluations, offering a significant benefit by avoiding radiation exposure [19].

The Pectus Severity Index—PSI, also known as the *Haller Index*, provides a precise measure of sternal depression severity. It quantifies the depth of the pectus deformity by calculating the ratio of the chest's transverse diameter to its anteroposterior diameter. This measurement is taken from the sternum's posterior surface to the vertebral body's anterior surface at the deepest point of the deformity [20].

A PSI value of ≤2.5 is considered within the normal range, and typically, patients with a PSI of <3.25 are not considered for surgical intervention [21].

These figures, especially when integrated with additional assessments like pulmonary function tests and cardiovascular evaluations, help in identifying candidates for whom surgical intervention is advisable (**Figure 3**) [22, 23].

The Pectus Correction Index (PCI)—has been developed as an alternative to the Haller Index, which might not always capture the true severity of pectus excavatum in cases of atypical chest wall shapes.

The PCI quantifies the proportion of chest depth affected by the pectus deformity.

To calculate the PCI, first imagine the sternum corrected to its ideal position and draw a hypothetical horizontal line across the back at this level. The PCI is calculated by taking the distance from this hypothetical line to the front of the vertebra and subtracting the distance from the deepest point of the sternum's depression to the vertebra. The difference is then divided by the distance from the hypothetical line to the vertebra, and the result is multiplied by 100 to convert it into a percentage.

The PCI is particularly valuable for assessing the severity of pectus deformities in individuals with unusual chest shapes, such as exceptionally wide or narrow chests. A PCI value of 28 per cent or higher, corresponding to a Pectus Severity Index (PSI) of at least 3.25, typically indicates a significant deformity that may warrant surgical intervention [24].

3D body scan—Both the Haller Index (HI) and the Pectus Correction Index (PCI) were initially designed for evaluation through computed tomography. However, the risk associated with ionizing radiation, especially for pediatric patients, raises a significant concern.

As a result, there is a growing interest in, radiation-free, three-dimensional (3D) optical surface imaging as an alternative diagnostic tool.

Given that three-dimensional images concern the external surface, the conventional Haller index, and correction index are not applicable as these are based on internal diameters.

Therefore, external equivalents have been introduced for three-dimensional images. However, cut-off values to help determine surgical candidacy using external indices are not standardized.

A recent paper applied 3D surface imaging to establish the external Haller Index, introducing the external Correction Index.

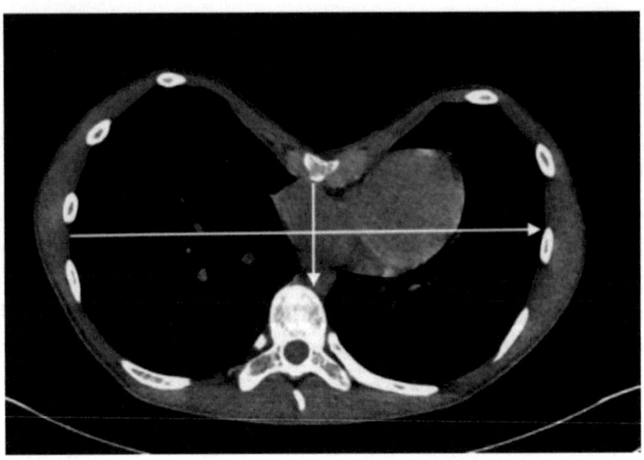

Figure 3.
Haller index on CT scan.

The authors established cut-off values for 3D imaging-derived indices, aligning them with established criteria for surgery: a conventional Haller Index of ≥3.25 and a CT-derived Correction Index of ≥28.0%.

This analysis identified optimal thresholds for surgical consideration: an external Haller Index of ≥1.83 and an external Correction Index of ≥15.2% [25].

In another study, researchers compared the accuracy of optical body surface scanning to conventional CT scans, using a 3D sensor, concluding that this can be effectively used for treatment monitoring [26].

2.3.3 Pulmonary function studies

Pulmonary function testing is recommended for individuals with moderate-to-severe pectus excavatum or those presenting respiratory symptoms. Despite the prevalence of respiratory complaints among PE patients, less than a third exhibit pulmonary function abnormalities, with a weak correlation between subjective symptoms and objective findings [27].

However, normal pulmonary function tests do not rule out the potential cardiopulmonary limitations during physical activity.

Research by Kelly et al. in a cohort of patients seeking surgical correction for PE revealed significant reductions in Forced Vital Capacity (FVC), Forced Expiratory Volume in 1 second (FEV1) and Forced Expiratory Flow at 25–75% (FEF25-75%). These metrics were approximately 10% to 15% lower than the expected averages for the general population [28].

Another study examining lung function before and after the Nuss procedure indicated significant improvements in lung function tests post-surgery, with more pronounced improvements in older patients, showing a trend toward normalization [29].

However, these improvements, while statistically significant, are modest and unlikely to fully account for reported increases in stamina and exercise capacity [30].

2.3.4 Exercise testing

The interest in this topic began with observations by Dr. Sauerbruch, a prominent German thoracic surgeon. He described a case of a 19-year-old, the son of a Swiss watchmaker, who could not sustain a full day's work due to his condition. After surgery to correct his PE, the young man experienced a notable improvement in endurance, able to work longer hours without fatigue. This case inspired numerous studies to objectively evaluate if PE truly affects heart and lung function and to what extent surgical interventions can improve these functions [31].

Exercise testing is advised for individuals with moderate-to-severe PE, or those who show significant respiratory symptoms. This test is more effective at identifying cardiopulmonary abnormalities compared to resting spirometry tests because it evaluates how the cardiac and pulmonary systems interact dynamically under stress.

Small-scale studies have documented diminished maximal exercise capabilities, including lower peak oxygen consumption (VO2max), attributed to decreased stroke volume, alongside a reduced VO2max and an earlier onset of lactate accumulation during physical exertion [21, 32].

Patients with PE may experience an increased metabolic cost of breathing, related to the mechanical inefficiencies of their respiratory system [33].

2.3.5 Cardiac function

Patients with significant displacement of the heart observed on imaging, or those experiencing cardiopulmonary limitations should undergo a cardiology evaluation, including echocardiography and electrocardiography.

Echocardiography might not always confirm cardiac compression; however, it screens potential cardiac manifestations of Marfan syndrome (Mitral valve prolapse and evaluation of the aortic root), and Turner or Noonan syndrome.

In a large series of female patients, 68% showed electrocardiographic evidence of right ventricular strain [7].

Echocardiography has revealed subtle right ventricular outflow obstruction and reduced right ventricular systolic function in severe pectus excavatum cases [34, 35], with improvements noted post-surgery [36, 37].

Studies using intraoperative transoesophageal echocardiography have demonstrated relief of right heart chamber compression and improved cardiac output immediately following surgical repair [38].

2.3.6 Psychological impact

In recent decades, the research literature on anterior congenital chest wall malformations has increasingly focused on the impact on quality of life and psychological well-being.

Pectus excavatum, in particular, exerts a substantial negative psychological impact on patients, leading to significant distress and persistent self-evaluation [39]. Patients often experience embarrassment about their physical appearance, avoiding situations that expose their chest, such as during sports activities or intimate encounters, and report instances of teasing (experienced by 22.8% of patients), primarily from peers [40]. The experience of being teased serves as a strong motivator for seeking help. Psychometric assessments like the Child Behavior Checklist for ages 4 to 18 years (CBCL/4-18) have highlighted psychopathological aspects related to the condition, including withdrawal, anxiety, depression, and social difficulties [41].

Adolescents between 12 and 16 years old with severe malformations appear to be at higher risk of experiencing psychosocial problems, often characterized by low self-esteem, feelings of inferiority, depression, shyness, and social anxiety, which can impact their developmental progress during puberty [42].

While less is known about the experiences of females with these conditions, it is widely acknowledged that they face physiological limitations and esthetic concerns. Female patients with funnel chest deformities often present with asymmetric and underdeveloped chests [43, 44]. Recent research [45] suggests that young female patients with pectus excavatum may have a more challenging experience compared to males, often reporting negative emotions, withdrawal, and poor self-perception. Surveys such as the Modified Pectus Excavatum Evaluation Questionnaire (PEEQ) [46] indicate that patients over 15 years old are significantly more concerned about their appearance, although positive expectations regarding corrective measures remain high in both genders (around 75%). Parents, however, often express uncertainty (67%) or weak support (76%) for surgery, with greater concern for their female children (38.9%). The psychosocial dimension of these conditions extends to the entire family and can influence their expectations regarding treatment options.

While surgery is not recommended for very young patients due to the risk of relapse [47] and potential scarring [48], non-invasive methods such as vacuum bell, bracing, and exercise offer effective alternatives [49].

Studies on the quality of life in patients with pectus excavatum consistently demonstrate improvements in psychological well-being following corrective procedures [50]. Despite increased physical activity post-surgery, adolescents' perceptions of Health-Related Quality of Life (HRQL) are heavily influenced by body image considerations [51].

Comparatively less is known about body image disturbances in patients with pectus carinatum, which often present primarily esthetic concerns rather than cardiopulmonary symptoms. The Pectus Carinatum Body Image Quality of Life (PeCBI-QOL) questionnaire [52], developed to assess psychological repercussions, highlights the importance of treatment motivation and engagement from both patients' and parents' perspectives, with significant improvements observed across all areas following treatment. Non-surgical correction using braces has also shown statistically significant improvements in children's body self-image [53]. Patient compliance is essential for successful non-surgical treatment [54, 55].

2.3.7 Non-surgical approach

Non-surgical options, such as Vacuum bell, are significantly underutilized despite strong evidence supporting their effectiveness, which is comparable to surgery in the majority of cases and do not prevent patients from opting for surgical correction in the future if desired [56].

Treatment decisions should be well-informed and individualized. Considering the results, it is essential to recognize that no patient should be selected for surgery without first attempting a non-operative approach.

The vacuum bell—The most well-known non-surgical treatment for pectus excavatum is the vacuum bell. This device, inspired by suction cup dent pullers used in automobile repairs, was first utilized for treating pectus excavatum in Germany in 1910 [57].

The vacuum bell consists of a silicone ring and a transparent polycarbonate window, creating a vacuum at the chest wall using a hand pump operated by the patient. This vacuum can reach up to 15% below atmospheric pressure. Various sizes of the vacuum bell are available, allowing for selection based on the patient's age and the shape of their chest.

The vacuum bell can significantly lift the ribs and sternum, leading to a permanent correction (**Figure 4**).

Indications—Almost all patients with pectus excavatum are potential candidates for vacuum bell therapy. The best results are typically seen in patients who begin therapy between the ages of 10–12, have a moderate pectus depth ($\leq$ 1.8–1.5 cm), possess sufficient chest wall flexibility, and commit to at least 12 months of treatment [58].

Chest wall flexibility can be assessed by observing sternal elevation when applying the vacuum bell or using the Nuss maneuver:

- Having the patient lie supine with an exposed chest.
- Applying upward pressure on the sternum using a hand or a pectus lifter device, mimicking the surgical bar's effect.
- Visually or instrumentally measuring the sternum's elevation.

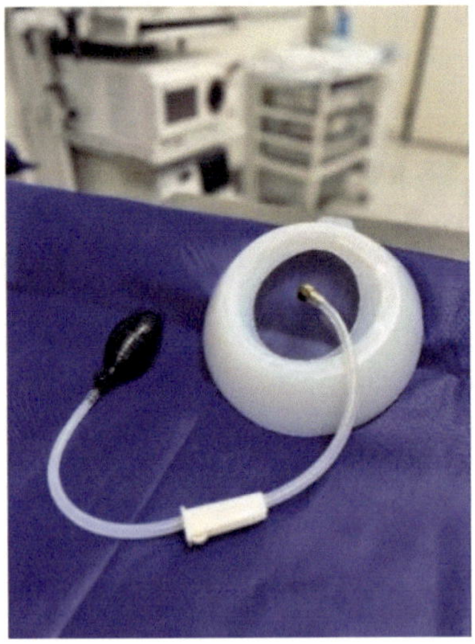

Figure 4.
Vacuum bell.

Older patients, those with more severe deformities, and those with asymmetric pectus excavatum can also benefit from vacuum bell therapy, though they may experience partial correction or require a longer treatment duration. Patients experiencing symptoms like exercise intolerance or chest pain can find relief with vacuum bell therapy.

Contraindications—Cardiac anomalies, skeletal disorders (such as osteogenesis imperfecta and Glisson's disease), vasculopathies (including Marfan syndrome and aortic aneurysms), and coagulopathies are all contraindications for vacuum bell therapy.

Comprehensive history and physical examination should include a detailed family history and an echocardiogram to check for any valvular or aortic diseases. A chest CT may be necessary to calculate the Haller index. Depending on individual circumstances, additional tests such as pulmonary function tests, genetic testing, and photographic documentation of the pectus excavatum may also be required (**Figures** 5 and **6**).

Daily use and treatment length—There is no standardized protocol for the frequency and duration of vacuum bell therapy, as these factors depend on the patient's individual decision and motivation. The initial use of the vacuum bell takes place during an outpatient clinic visit under the supervision of the physician. The correct size and model are chosen based on the patient's age, the shape of the chest wall, and their perception of the deformity. The centre of the device should be aligned with the deepest part of the pectus excavatum.

The general recommendation is to begin using the device twice daily for 30 minutes each session. The ideal daily usage is 4 hours, divided into two sessions, in the morning and in the evening, after a gradual increase [59].

Research indicates that sustained use of the vacuum bell for at least 12–18 months leads to more significant and lasting corrections. Remarkable improvements can be achieved even with shorter daily usage [60–63].

Consistency and adherence over the entire duration of treatment are paramount for achieving optimal results.

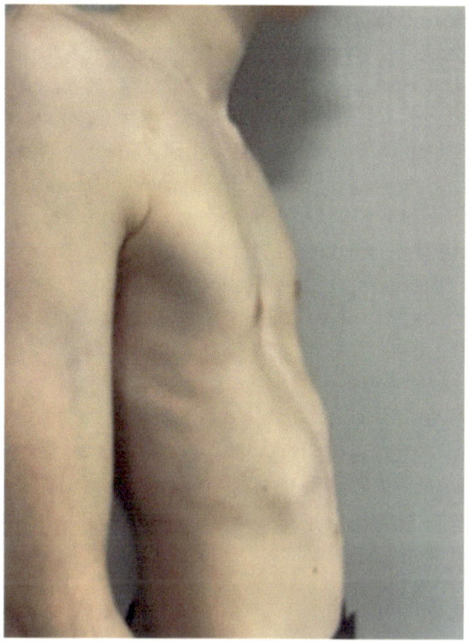

Figure 5.
PE pre-treatment.

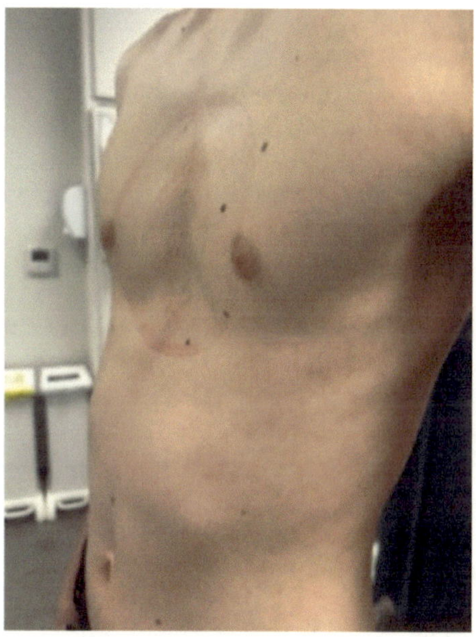

Figure 6.
PE post-treatment with vacuum bell.

The appropriate pressure varies greatly among patients. Patients are encouraged to apply enough pressure to feel their chest rise without causing pain, and they should expect their tolerance to increase as they become more used to the device. It is important for patients to understand that higher pressures do not necessarily correlate with better outcomes.

Outcomes—The vacuum bell has shown to be a highly effective treatment option for certain patients with pectus excavatum. Studies have indicated nearly 100% patient satisfaction, with most patients avoiding surgery. Approximately 20% of patients achieve complete correction, while around 37–80% experience partial correction [59].

The impact of vacuum bell therapy on cardiopulmonary function continues to be debated. The severity of pectus excavatum does not consistently predict symptoms, and clinical improvements following treatment appear to be influenced by multiple factors.

Complications—Generally, patients tolerate the vacuum bell well. Reported complications are mild, including chest wall pain, skin irritation, hematoma, and paraesthesia in the upper extremities. These issues typically resolve on their own once the treatment is discontinued.

Vacuum bell as an adjunct to surgery—Several experts and medical centres are exploring the use of the vacuum bell as a complement to traditional surgical treatments for pectus excavatum. A sterilized vacuum bell can be utilized to elevate the sternum without necessitating additional incisions during the Nuss procedure. It has also been considered for children potentially facing surgery, serving two primary purposes: 1) potentially eliminating the need for surgical intervention and 2) enhancing chest wall flexibility, which could lead to improved surgical outcomes and reduced post-operative discomfort.

Autologous fat grafting—The psychosocial impact of pectus excavatum can be significant, often justifying corrective measures. While even minimally invasive surgical repairs can leave scars, which might cause psychological distress in children, autologous fat grafts offer a less invasive alternative. Suitable for patients with sufficient fat reserves, this method can be used on its own or as a supplement to surgical approaches to enhance cosmetic outcomes.

Hyaluronic acid injections—Hyaluronic acid, widely used in esthetic treatments, presents a non-surgical option for enhancing the appearance of pectus excavatum. Applied as a filler, it aims to improve the visual aspect of the deformity without altering the sternal position. Its effectiveness remains a subject of debate.

2.3.8 Surgical repair

Surgical correction of pectus excavatum often enhances physical appearance and can improve cardiorespiratory function for some patients.

For patients with moderate-to-severe pectus excavatum, a CT scan is recommended to calculate the Pectus Severity Index (PSI).

Surgical intervention is typically considered for patients meeting two or more of the following criteria:

- A PSI greater than 3.25, as measured by CT scan.
- Evidence of cardiac compression, displacement, mitral valve prolapses, murmurs, or conduction abnormalities.
- Pulmonary function tests indicating restrictive respiratory disease.
- History of unsuccessful previous pectus excavatum repair
- Progression of the deformity, with either worsening physiological symptoms or significant patient concern regarding appearance.

There is evidence suggesting that children who undergo early surgical interventions may face a higher risk of recurrence during their adolescent years. Additionally, extensive resection of costal cartilage in young children has sometimes been found to inhibit chest wall growth [60, 62].

The ideal time for corrective surgery for a pectus defect is no earlier than 8 years of age, extending up to the end of adolescence. Children within this age range typically have sufficiently flexible costal cartilage for effective remodeling, while also being old enough to minimize the risk of recurrence during the puberty.

Nuss procedure—This minimally invasive approach developed in the 1990s by Nuss and his team involves correcting the chest deformity without removing any cartilage [61, 63].

The technique uses a custom-shaped metal bar, known as the Nuss bar, which is inserted into the pleural space, positioned behind the sternum at its most inward point, then rotated 180 degrees and secured to the ribs' outer sides.

Modifications to the original Nuss procedure include making small cuts in the cartilage to relieve sternal pressure and better secure the bar, using lateral stabilizers, and employing multiple bars for more complex or extensive deformities.

The bar is typically removed after 2 to 3 years.

Postoperative pain—Patients who undergo the Nuss procedure often experience more postoperative pain compared to those who undergo Ravitch procedure. However, studies involving large patient groups have demonstrated that perioperative pain management is effectively maintained with both procedures, with postoperative pain typically resolving within 1 month.

A significant advancement in managing this postoperative pain is the use of cryoablation of the intercostal nerves in the area of repair. This method temporarily halts the nerves' ability to transmit pain signals without affecting overall nerve function, which allows for the eventual healing and restoration of normal sensation and movement. When combined with intercostal nerve blocks, cryoablation has been shown to significantly enhance pain control post-surgery, reducing or even eliminating the need for opioid pain relievers [64, 65].

Bar displacement—Bar displacement or migration is a serious complication. In some instances, the bar may rotate (90 or 180 degrees posteriorly) or shift laterally. Historically, this issue affected 10 to 20 per cent of patients. However, thanks to increased surgical expertise and technical enhancements in stabilizer designs, the incidence of bar displacement has significantly decreased. Current stabilizing techniques include the use of metal stabilizers, pericostal sutures or wire fixation, and employing two bars when necessary to enhance stability [66].

Cardiac complications—Cardiac perforation can rarely occur during the retrosternal dissection required for placing the Nuss bar in the retrosternal space [67, 68].

Elevating the sternum with an external device can improves visibility and access to the retrosternal area. Additionally, the use of transoesophageal echocardiography has been adopted to ensure safer retrosternal dissection and accurate placement of the Nuss bar.

Pleural effusion—Pleural effusions are a known complication following the Nuss procedure, affecting about 3 per cent of patients. These typically develop around 2 weeks post-operation [69].

Ravitch procedure—The Ravitch procedure, firstly performed in the 1940s [70], has undergone several modifications aimed at enhancing the stability of the sternum internally, optimizing the correction quality, and reducing complications.

Initially, the technique involved extensive resection of the costal cartilages' deformity, removal of the perichondrium, separation of the xiphoid process from the sternum, and a transverse osteotomy of the sternum. The sternum was then positioned anteriorly in an overcorrected position, secured by Kirschner wires or durable silk sutures.

Subsequent revisions by Baronofsky [71] and Welch [72] highlighted the critical role of preserving the perichondrium and its sternal attachments, facilitating rib regeneration. A significant later enhancement involved the incorporation of a support strut, inserted either through or beneath the sternum, to maintain structural integrity while the ribs regenerated.

Typically, these support struts, initially metal, are removed 6- to 12-month post-operation. More recent innovations include the use of bioabsorbable materials or Marlex mesh, though no conclusive evidence favors these newer materials over traditional metal struts in terms of effectiveness.

A key complication of the modified Ravitch procedure is the risk of developing a constricted thorax or secondary thoracic dystrophy, often referred to as acquired Jeune syndrome. This issue can arise from removing too much of the costal cartilage, including the growth centres, or from excessive strain on the perichondrium and damage to the growth centres.

As a result, the chest wall may not grow normally, restricting the development of the lungs and leading to significantly reduced lung capacities.

Risk factors for this condition include surgery before the age of four, removing five or more rib cartilages, disrupting the growth area near the sternum, and improperly aligning the perichondral sheaths.

To lower the risk, it is advisable to delay chest surgery until the child is at least 8 years old and to limit the removal to four or fewer rib cartilages.

Outcomes—There is a lack of extensive prospective studies directly comparing the outcomes of the Nuss and Ravitch procedures.

Patients generally report improved self-esteem and physical appearance following both the modified Ravitch and Nuss procedures. Improvements in exercise tolerance and some cardiopulmonary function metrics have also been observed with both surgical methods.

The outcomes for pulmonary function following the Nuss procedure can vary. Typically, there is an initial dip in lung function after the insertion of the Nuss bar, which then either returns to baseline or improves after the bar's removal.

Additionally, many patients note better exercise capacity post-surgery. For both the Nuss and modified Ravitch procedures, objective measures such as maximum oxygen uptake (VO2 max) tend to remain stable or show modest improvements post-operatively [29, 73].

3. Pectus carinatum

3.1 Evaluation

Pectus carinatum (PC) is the second most prevalent chest wall deformity in children, following pectus excavatum. The name is derived from the Latin term meaning "chest with a keel." This chest wall deformity is also commonly referred to as chicken breast, pigeon chest, pyramidal chest, cuneiform thorax, or sternal kyphosis. It usually does not cause symptoms and is primarily treated for cosmetic reasons.

It affects approximately 1 in 1500 live births and is often found in conjunction with genetic conditions such as Marfan, Noonan, and Poland syndromes. This deformity is more common in males, with a prevalence four times higher than in females, and exhibits a strong genetic link, as up to 25% of patients have a family history of similar chest abnormalities (**Figure 7**) [11, 74, 75].

There are two primary forms of this deformity:

Chondrogladiolar prominence—Commonly referred to as chicken breast or keel chest, this is the most prevalent form of pectus carinatum. It features a forward protrusion of the middle and lower sections of the sternum. The costal cartilages typically show a concave and symmetrically depressed appearance, which emphasizes the sternal prominence. However, the deformity presents asymmetrically in 30 to 50 per cent of cases. Occasionally, patients may exhibit a mixed condition with pectus carinatum on one side and pectus excavatum on the other.

Chondromanubrial prominence—Also known as pectus arcuatum, pouter pigeon breast, or Currarino-Silverman syndrome, this form is a more complex and rarer type of pectus carinatum. In this variation, the upper part of the sternum protrudes forward, while the central section is shorter and leans backward. This creates a distinct Z-shaped appearance of the sternum when viewed from the side. This subtype usually arises from early hardening or the lack of proper segmentation of the sternal joints, resulting in a sternum that is both short and sharply angled. It is often linked with other bone or heart anomalies or with Noonan syndrome. Bracing treatments, unlike with other forms, are generally ineffective for this condition [76].

For many patients evaluated for pectus carinatum, the primary concern is cosmetic, with few physiological complaints reported. However, some patients experience exertional dyspnoea, exercise limitations, frequent respiratory infections, or asthma prior to surgery; these symptoms generally resolve following surgical correction.

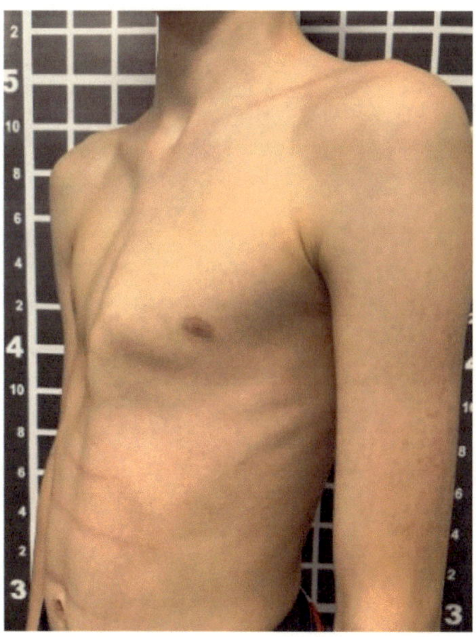

Figure 7.
Pectus carinatum.

The evaluation for pectus carinatum includes a physical examination to assess the severity of the defect. Imaging is typically reserved for those who will undergo surgical treatment as part of their preoperative evaluation.

During the examination, clinicians should document the type of deformity (chondrogladiolar, chondromanubrial, or a mixed carinatum/excavatum), and the degree of asymmetry. It is also important to check if the defect can be manually corrected by applying pressure to the sternum. The presence of scoliosis or other associated abnormalities should be noted.

Photographs are a valuable tool for objective documentation and for comparing changes over time.

Typically, the evaluation includes chest radiographs to document the severity of the deformity and to detect and monitor any scoliosis. Computed tomography scans are used for preoperative planning but are not routinely recommended for patients who are not proceeding to surgery.

For measuring the severity of pectus carinatum, the Pectus Severity Index or Haller index is used. A normal value is 2.54; a lower PSI in patients with pectus carinatum indicates a more severe deformity, which contrasts with pectus excavatum where a higher PSI indicates greater severity.

3.2 Treatment

Pectus carinatum is primarily considered a cosmetic issue, and the decision to treat is based on the severity of the defect and the concerns of the patient and their family. Both bracing and surgery are safe and effective treatment options (**Figures 8** and **9**).

Bracing—This should be the first line of treatment for patients with mild-to-moderate pectus carinatum. It tends to be more successful in patients with flexible chest walls who are committed to following the bracing regimen. Recent advancements in bracing techniques, which use lower pressures, have improved patient compliance and achieved good outcomes.

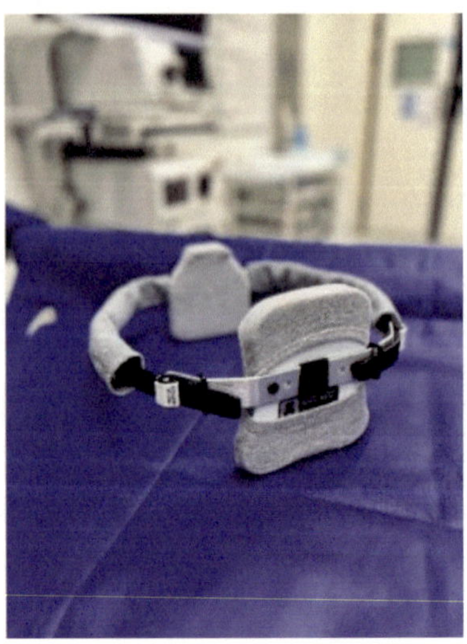

Figure 8.
Brace.

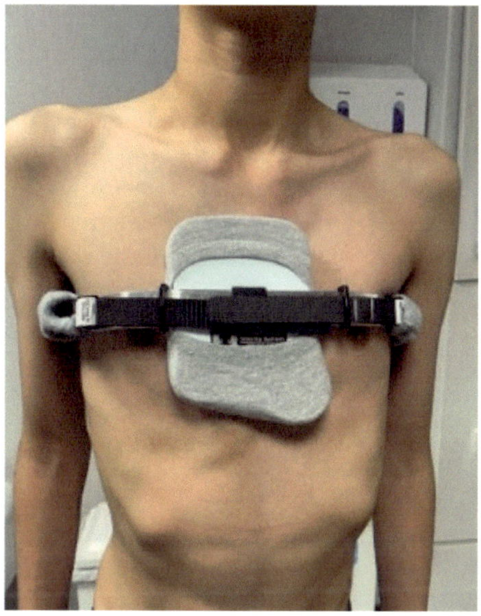

Figure 9.
Brace in place.

Surgery—Surgery may be the preferred option for patients with severe pectus carinatum, those who are skeletally mature, or those suffering from severe pectus arcuatum, as bracing is often less effective in these cases. It is also an option for patients with less severe deformities who are unwilling or unable to comply with a bracing regimen, but only if they have begun their pubertal growth spurt. Surgery should be delayed until after the onset of puberty to minimize the small but significant risk of asphyxiating thoracic dystrophy, particularly following the modified Ravitch repair for pectus carinatum.

4. Poland syndrome

Alfred Poland, a medical student at Guy's Hospital in London, described a patient with a missing anterior chest wall in 1841. This condition, later named "Poland syndrome" (PS) by Clarkson, another physician at the same hospital, involves the absence of chest wall structures on one side (usually the right) and often includes syndactyly of the hand on the same side. Poland syndrome is rare, with an estimated occurrence of 1 in 30,000. It typically presents with a range of abnormalities from underdeveloped chest muscles and ribs to complete absence of the breast and nipple.

While chest deformities are a significant concern, the associated limb abnormalities, such as underdeveloped and fused fingers, are often more disabling. Poland syndrome may also coexist with Mobius' syndrome, characterized by facial and abducens nerve palsies [77, 78].

Hashim et al., in their recent translational analysis, provide a comprehensive overview of the current theories regarding the genesis, evolution, and management of this syndrome [79].

Multiple theories and etiological factors have been proposed to explain the origins of congenital disorders, which result from errors in morphogenesis leading to malformations, deformations, or disruptions. One prominent theory involves embryonic or foetal vascular disruption, which can cause a sequence of developmental disruptions.

The vascular disruption theory is widely accepted as a pathogenic mechanism. It suggests that PS may arise from a disruption in the development of the proximal subclavian artery and its branches that supply the pectoral muscles around the sixth week of gestation. This disruption leads to inadequate blood flow to the distal limb and pectoral region, resulting in tissue loss in these areas. Bavinck and Weaver introduced a pathogenic hypothesis known as the "subclavian artery supply disruption sequence" (SASDS) to describe this vascular disruption during embryonic development [80].

The predictable patterns of defects resulting from SASDS include:

- Absence of the pectoralis major and ipsilateral breast hypoplasia due to interruption of internal thoracic artery flow.

- Terminal transverse limb defects following a disruption of the subclavian artery distal to the origin of the internal thoracic artery.

- Poland syndrome resulting from a disruption of the subclavian artery distal to the origin of the vertebral artery but proximal to the origin of the internal thoracic artery.

Various factors, including mechanical, environmental, and embryologic events, can lead to interruption or reduction of blood flow to the subclavian artery and its branches. Intrinsic factors such as thrombi and emboli, as well as external mechanical influences like cervical ribs, aberrant muscles, and amniotic bands, can cause vascular disruption [81–83].

Other suggested hypotheses include maternal factors, such as smoking and cocaine abuse [84].

Genetic or external factors can disrupt the migration of the pectoralis major muscle and digital separation during the critical period between 6 and 8 weeks of gestation. While most PS cases are sporadic, familial instances have been documented, suggesting a possible autosomal dominant inheritance pattern with variable penetrance. These familial cases exhibit intra-familial variability [85, 86].

Moderate-to-severe PS is typically diagnosed at birth due to visible chest or limb defects. Antenatal diagnosis through foetal ultrasound can detect these abnormalities, and Doppler assessment of the ipsilateral subclavian artery flow is recommended when unilateral skeletal defects are identified. Three-dimensional US enhances the characterization of limb defects [87].

Clinical suspicion of PS arises upon detecting chest defects with or without ipsilateral limb anomalies in newborns or children. The age of diagnosis varies widely due to the spectrum of severity, with some cases presenting later in life for unrelated medical issues, particularly in individuals with milder forms of PS and normal hand development.

Imaging modalities are essential for diagnosing PS and determining the specific location and characteristics of chest wall deformities. Chest X-rays typically reveal hyperlucency in the affected lung field, resembling a "post-radical mastectomy picture." Both CT and MRI are paramount for accurate diagnosis, assessing the extent of musculoskeletal involvement, and guiding surgical reconstruction decisions.

Generally, surgical intervention in Poland Syndrome (PS) may be required for the following indications:

1. Unilateral depression of the chest wall that may worsen with age.

2. Insufficient protection of the lung and heart.

3. Paradoxical movement of the chest wall.

4. Hypoplasia or aplasia of the breast in females.

5. Enhancement of the chest's esthetic appearance in males due to the absence of the pectoralis major muscle and anterior axillary fold.

Surgical correction is tailored to the extent of chest involvement. For simple cases with only breast and muscle deficiencies, the treatment is cosmetic, using myocutaneous flaps, fat transfers, and prosthetics. More complex cases, involving missing ribs, require structural repairs. Generally, surgery is recommended after growth completion to ensure the best outcomes, except in urgent situations like lung herniation that causes breathing difficulties.

5. Conclusion

In conclusion, chest wall deformities in pediatric patients, while typically benign, can have profound physiological and psychological impacts. Emphasizing conservative management strategies is essential, as they are often sufficient in addressing mild-to-moderate cases and can significantly reduce the need for invasive surgical procedures. Early and accurate diagnosis, coupled with regular monitoring, is crucial to promptly address any potential complications and ensure optimal patient outcomes.

A multidisciplinary approach is key in the management of these conditions. Pediatricians, thoracic surgeons, physical therapists, and mental health professionals should work collaboratively to develop comprehensive and individualized care plans. This approach not only addresses the physical aspects of the deformities but also supports the psychological well-being of the young patients and their families.

Non-surgical interventions, such as physical therapy, bracing, and respiratory exercises, can be highly effective in managing symptoms and improving quality of life. When surgical intervention is necessary, it should be carefully considered and tailored to the specific needs of the patient, ensuring that the benefits outweigh the risks.

Ultimately, the goal is to provide holistic care that prioritizes the overall health and well-being of the patient. By focusing on conservative management and fostering a supportive care environment, healthcare providers can help young patients with chest wall deformities lead healthier, more fulfilling lives.

Author details

Alessandro Maraschi[1*], Erica Cristina Vallocchia[2] and Kunal Bhakhri[1]

1 University College London Hospital, London, United Kingdom

2 Psychologist Psychotherapist, Turin, Italy

*Address all correspondence to: alessandro.maraschi@gmail.com

References

[1] Fokin AA, Steuerwald NM, Ahrens WA, Allen KE. Anatomical, histologic, and genetic characteristics of congenital chest wall deformities. Seminars in Thoracic and Cardiovascular Surgery. 2009;**21**(1):44-57. DOI: 10.1053/j.semtcvs.2009.03.001

[2] Fonkalsrud EW. 912 open pectus excavatum repairs: Changing trends, lessons learned: One surgeon's experience. World Journal of Surgery. 2009;**33**(2):180-190. DOI: 10.1007/s00268-008-9793-4

[3] Park CH, Kim TH, Haam SJ, Lee S. Rib overgrowth may be a contributing factor for pectus excavatum: Evaluation of prepubertal patients younger than 10years old. Journal of Pediatric Surgery. 2015;**50**(11):1945-1948. DOI: 10.1016/j.jpedsurg.2015.07.010. Epub 2015 Jul 17

[4] Williams AM, Crabbe DC. Pectus deformities of the anterior chest wall. Paediatric Respiratory Reviews. 2003;**4**(3):237-242. DOI: 10.1016/s1526-0542(03)00053-8

[5] Behr CA, Denning NL, Kallis MP, Maloney C, Soffer SZ, Romano-Adesman A, et al. The incidence of Marfan syndrome and cardiac anomalies in patients presenting with pectus deformities. Journal of Pediatric Surgery. 2019;**54**(9):1926-1928. DOI: 10.1016/j.jpedsurg.2018.11.017. Epub 2018 Dec 27

[6] Billar RJ, Manoubi W, Kant SG, Wijnen RMH, Demirdas S, Schnater JM. Association between pectus excavatum and congenital genetic disorders: A systematic review and practical guide for the treating physician. Journal of Pediatric Surgery. 2021;**56**(12):2239-2252. DOI: 10.1016/j.jpedsurg.2021.04.016. Epub 2021 Apr 24

[7] Kelly RE Jr. Pectus excavatum: Historical background, clinical picture, preoperative evaluation and criteria for operation. Seminars in Pediatric Surgery. 2008;**17**(3):181-193. DOI: 10.1053/j.sempedsurg.2008.03.002

[8] Greig JD, Azmy AF. Thoracic cage deformity: A late complication following repair of an agenesis of diaphragm. Journal of Pediatric Surgery. 1990;**25**:1234-1235

[9] Vanamo K, Peltonem J, Rintala R, et al. Chest wall and spinal deformities in adults with congenital diaphragmatic defects. Journal of Pediatric Surgery. 1996;**31**:851-854

[10] Wang Y, Chen G, Xie L, et al. Mechanical factors play an important role in pectus excavatum with thoracic scoliosis. Journal of Cardiothoracic Surgery. 2012;**7**:118-120

[11] Shamberger RC, Welch KJ. Surgical repair of pectus excavatum. Journal of Pediatric Surgery. 1988;**23**:615-622

[12] Nuss D, Kelly RE Jr. Minimally invasive surgical correction of chest wall deformities in children (Nuss procedure). Advances in Pediatrics. 2008;**55**:395-410. DOI: 10.1016/j.yapd.2008.07.012

[13] Kelly RE Jr, Cash TF, Shamberger RC, Mitchell KK, Mellins RB, Lawson ML, et al. Surgical repair of pectus excavatum markedly improves body image and perceived ability for physical activity: Multicenter study. Pediatrics. 2008;**122**(6):1218-1222. DOI: 10.1542/peds.2007-2723

[14] Ewert F, Syed J, Kern S, Besendörfer M, Carbon RT, Schulz-Drost S. Symptoms in pectus

deformities: A scoring system for subjective physical complaints. The Thoracic and Cardiovascular Surgeon. 2017;**65**(1):43-49. DOI: 10.1055/s-0036-1584355. Epub 2016 Jun 24

[15] Waters P, Welch K, Micheli LJ, Shamberger R, Hall JE. Scoliosis in children with pectus excavatum and pectus carinatum. Journal of Pediatric Orthopedics. 1989;**9**(5):551-556. DOI: 10.1097/01241398-198909010-00009

[16] Poston PM, McHugh MA, Rossi NO, Patel SS, Rajput M, Turek JW. The case for using the correction index obtained from chest radiography for evaluation of pectus excavatum. Journal of Pediatric Surgery. 2015;**50**(11):1940-1944. DOI: 10.1016/j.jpedsurg.2015.06.017. Epub 2015 Jun 30

[17] Mullett R, Jain A, Kotugodella S, Curtis J. Lobar collapse demystified: The chest radiograph with CT correlation. Postgraduate Medical Journal. Jun 2012;**88**(1040):335-347. DOI: 10.1136/postgradmedj-2011-130213. Epub 2012 Jan 25. PMID: 22282740

[18] Orshuis WJ et al. Chest radiography in pectus excavatum: Recognition of pectus excavatum-related signs and assessment of severity before and after surgical correction. European Radiology. 1994;**4**(3):197-202

[19] Marcovici PA, LoSasso BE, Kruk P, Dwek JR. MRI for the evaluation of pectus excavatum. Pediatric Radiology. 2011;**41**(6):757-758. DOI: 10.1007/s00247-011-2031-5. Epub 2011 Mar 8

[20] Haller JA Jr, Kramer SS, Lietman SA. Use of CT scans in selection of patients for pectus excavatum surgery: A preliminary report. Journal of Pediatric Surgery. 1987;**22**(10):904-906. DOI: 10.1016/s0022-3468(87)80585-7

[21] Malek MH, Fonkalsrud EW, Cooper CB. Ventilatory and cardiovascular responses to exercise in patients with pectus excavatum. Chest. 2003;**124**(3):870-882. DOI: 10.1378/chest.124.3.870

[22] Frantz FW. Indications and guidelines for pectus excavatum repair. Current Opinion in Pediatrics. 2011;**23**:486-491

[23] Blanco FC, Elliott ST, Sandler AD. Chest wall reconstruction. Seminars in Plastic Surgery. 2011;**25**:107-116

[24] Poston PM, Patel SS, Rajput M, Rossi NO, Ghanamah MS, Davis JE, et al. The correction index: Setting the standard for recommending operative repair of pectus excavatum. The Annals of Thoracic Surgery. 2014;**97**(4):1176-1179; discussion 1179-80. DOI: 10.1016/j.athoracsur.2013.12.050. Epub 2014 Feb 26

[25] Daemen JHT, Coorens NA, Hulsewé KWE, Maal TJJ, Maessen JG, Vissers YLJ, et al. Three-dimensional surface imaging for clinical decision making in pectus excavatum. Seminars in Thoracic and Cardiovascular Surgery. Winter 2022;**34**(4):1364-1373. DOI: 10.1053/j.semtcvs.2021.08.002. Epub 2021 Aug 8. PMID: 34380079

[26] Deng X, Huang P, Luo J, Wang J, Yi L, Yang G, et al. Journal of Pediatric Surgery. 2020;**55**(8):1448-1452

[27] Redding GJ, Kuo W, Swanson JO, Phillips GS, Emerson J, Yung D, et al. Upper thoracic shape in children with pectus excavatum: Impact on lung function. Pediatric Pulmonology. 2013;**48**(8):817-823. DOI: 10.1002/ppul.22660. Epub 2012 Aug 21

[28] Kelly RE, Shamberger RC, Mellins RB, Mitchell KK, Lawson LM, Oldham K, et al. Prospective multicenter

study of surgical correction of pectus excavatum: Design, perioperative complications, pain, and baseline pulmonary function facilitated by internet-based data collection. Journal of the American College of Surgeons. Aug 2007;**205**(2):205-216. DOI: 10.1016/j.jamcollsurg.2007.03.027

[29] Lawson ML, Mellins RB, Tabangin M, Kelly RE Jr, Croitoru DP, Goretsky MJ, et al. Impact of pectus excavatum on pulmonary function before and after repair with the Nuss procedure. Journal of Pediatric Surgery. 2005;**40**(1):174-180. DOI: 10.1016/j.jpedsurg.2004.09.040

[30] Kelly RE, Mellins RB, Shamberger RC, et al. Multicenter study of pectus excavatum, final report: Complications, static/exercise pulmonary function, and anatomic outcomes. Journal of the American College of Surgeons. 2013;**217**:1080-1089

[31] Ferdinand NS, der Brustorgane DC. 1. Band: Die Erkrankungen der Lunge. Deutsche Zeitschrift f. Chirurgie. 1921;**165**:289-292. DOI: 10.1007/BF02799461

[32] Tardy MM, Filaire M, Patoir A, Gautier-Pignonblanc P, Galvaing G, Kwiatkowski F, et al. Exercise cardiac output limitation in pectus Excavatum. Journal of the American College of Cardiology. 2015;**66**(8):976-977. DOI: 10.1016/j.jacc.2015.06.1087. Erratum in: J Am Coll Cardiol. 2015 Oct 20;66(16):1850. Tardy-Médous, Marie M [corrected to Tardy, Marie M]; Ruddy, Richard [corrected to Richard, Ruddy]

[33] Borowitz D, Cerny F, Zallen G, Sharp J, Burke M, Gross K, et al. Pulmonary function and exercise response in patients with pectus excavatum after Nuss repair. Journal of Pediatric Surgery. 2003;**38**(4):544-547. DOI: 10.1053/jpsu.2003.50118

[34] Mocchegiani R, Badano L, Lestuzzi C, Nicolosi GL, Zanuttini D. Relation of right ventricular morphology and function in pectus excavatum to the severity of the chest wall deformity. The American Journal of Cardiology. 1995;**76**(12):941-946. DOI: 10.1016/s0002-9149(99)80266-5

[35] Kowalewski J, Brocki M, Dryjanski T, Zolyński K, Koktysz R. Pectus excavatum: Increase of right ventricular systolic, diastolic, and stroke volumes after surgical repair. The Journal of Thoracic and Cardiovascular Surgery. 1999;**118**(1):87-92; discussion 92-3. DOI: 10.1016/S0022-5223(99)70145-5

[36] Krueger T, Chassot PG, Christodoulou M, Cheng C, Ris HB, Magnusson L. Cardiac function assessed by transesophageal echocardiography during pectus excavatum repair. The Annals of Thoracic Surgery. 2010;**89**(1):240-243. DOI: 10.1016/j.athoracsur.2009.06.126

[37] Sigalet DL, Montgomery M, Harder J. Cardiopulmonary effects of closed repair of pectus excavatum. Journal of Pediatric Surgery. 2003;**38**(3):380-385; discussion 380-5. DOI: 10.1053/jpsu.2003.50112

[38] Chao CJ, Jaroszewski DE, Kumar PN, Ewais MM, Appleton CP, Mookadam F, et al. Surgical repair of pectus excavatum relieves right heart chamber compression and improves cardiac output in adult patients–An intraoperative transesophageal echocardiographic study. American Journal of Surgery. 2015;**210**(6):1118-1124; discussion 1124-5. DOI: 10.1016/j.amjsurg.2015.07.006. Epub 2015 Sep 24

[39] Kolvekar SK, Simon NL, Kolvekar T. Patient experience before and after

treatment: Psychological effects and patients' personal experience. In: Kolvekar SK, Pilegaard HK, editors. Chest Wall Deformities and Corrective Procedures. Switzerland: Springer; 2016. pp. 161-167. DOI: 10.10007/978-3-319-23968-2

[40] Ji Y, Liu W, Chen S, Xu B, Tang Y, Wang X, et al. Assessment of psychosocial functioning and its risk factors in children with pectus excavatum. Health and Quality of Life Outcomes. 2011;**9**:28. DOI: 10.1186/1477-7525-9-28

[41] Achenbach TM. Manual for the Revised Child Behavior Checklist/4-18 and 1991 Profile. Burlington: University of Vermont Department of Psychiatry; 1991

[42] Habelt S, Korn S, Berger A, Bielek J. Psychological distress in patients with pectus excavatum as an indication for therapy. International Journal of Clinical Medicine. 2011;**2**:295-300. DOI: 10.4236/ijcm.2011.23050

[43] Fonkalsrud EW. Management of pectus chest deformities in female patients. The American Journal of Surgery. 2004;**187**:192-197. DOI: 10.1016/j.amjsurg.2003.11.010

[44] Beier JP, Weber PG, Reingruber B, Huemmer HP, Kesser U, Dragu A, et al. Aesthetic and functional correction of female, asymmetric funnel chest. A combined approach. The Breast. 2009;**18**:60-65. DOI: 10.1016/j.breast.2008.12.001

[45] Kostic M, Sretenović A, Radulović D, Milačić Vidaković I, Savić M, Popović M, et al. Influence of psychosocial characteristics of patients and opinions of their relatives on indication for surgical treatment of pectus excavatum. ANZ Journal of Surgery. 2023;**93**:2974-2980. DOI: 10.1111/ans.18746

[46] Lawson ML, Cash TF, Akers R, Vasser E, Burke B, Tabangin M, et al. A pilot study of the impact of surgical repair on disease-specific quality of life among patients with pectus excavatum. Journal of Pediatric Surgery. 2003;**38**:916-918. DOI: 10.1016/S0022-3468(03)00123-

[47] Nuss D, Obermeyer RJ, Kelly RE Jr. Pectus excavatum form a pediatric surgeon's perspective. Annals of Cardiothoracic Surgery. 2016;**5**:493-500. DOI: 10.21037/acs.2016.06.04

[48] Kwong JZ, Gulack BCH. Non-surgical approaches to the management of chest wall deformities. Seminars in Pediatric Surgery. 2024;**33**:1511388. DOI: 10.1016/j.sempedsurg.2024.151388

[49] Haje DP, Haje SA, Volpon JB, Silva ACO, Lima LFB, Huang W. Localized pectus excavatum treated with brace and exercise: Long term results of a Brazilian technique. Acta Ortopedica Brasileira. 2021;**29**:143-148. DOI: 10.1590/1413-785220212903241550

[50] Walsh J, Walsh R, Redmond K. Systematic review of physiological and psychological outcomes of surgery for pectus excavatum supporting commissioning of service in the UK. BMJ Open Respiratory Research. 2023;**10**:8. DOI: 10.1136/bmjresp-2023-001665

[51] Lam MWC, Klassen AF, Montgomery CJ, LeBlanc JG, Skarsgard ED. Quality-of-life after surgical correction of pectus excavatum: A comparison of the Ravitch and Nuss procedures. Journal of Pediatric Surgery. 2008;**43**:819-825. DOI: 10.1016/j.jpedsurg.2007.12.020

[52] Paulson JF, Ellis KE, Obermeyer RJ, Kuhn MA, Frantz FW, McGuire MM, et al. Development and validation of the pectus carinatum body image quality of life (PeCBI-QOL) questionnaire. Journal of Pediatric Surgery. 2019;**54**:2257-2260. DOI: 10.1016/j.jpedsurg.2019.03.019

[53] Orrick BA, Pierce AL, McElroy SF. Changes in self-image after pectus carinatum brace treatment. Journal of Pediatric Surgery. 2022;**57**:1579-1583. DOI: 10.1016/j.jpedsurg.2021.12.002

[54] Fraser S, Harling L, Patel A, Richards T, Hunt I. External compressive bracing with initial reduction of pectus carinatum: Compliance is the key. The Annals of Thoracic Surgery. 2020;**109**:413-419. DOI: 10.1016/j.athoracsur.2019.08.026

[55] Frediani S, Zarfati A, Pardi V, Aloi I, Bertocchini A, Accinni A, et al. A new custom-made bivalve brace for pectus carinatum in children and adolescents: Preliminary promising experience of 140 patients from a tertiary center. Frontiers in Pediatrics. 2024;**12**:1321633. DOI: 10.3389/fped.2024.1321633

[56] Jung Y, Yi E, Lee K, Chung JH, Cho S, Lee S. Surgical versus vacuum bell therapy for the correction of pectus excavatum: A comparison of 1-year treatment outcomes. Journal of Chest Surgery. 2021;**54**(6):473-479. DOI: 10.5090/jcs.21.073

[57] Lange F. Thoraxdeformitäten. In: Pfaundler M, Schlossmann A, editors. Handbuch der Kinderheilkunde, Chirurgie und Orthopädie im Kindesalter. Vol. V. Leipzig: FCW Vogel; 1910. p. 157

[58] Toselli L, Chinni E, Nazar-Peirano M, et al. Determinants of success associated with vacuum bell treatment of pectus excavatum. Journal of Pediatric Surgery. 2022;**57**:550-554

[59] Obermeyer RJ, Cohen NS, Kelly RE, et al. Nonoperative management of pectus excavatum with vacuum bell therapy: A single center study. Journal of Pediatric Surgery. 2018;**53**:1221-1225

[60] Haecker FM, Sesia S. Vacuum bell therapy. Annals of Cardiothoracic Surgery. 2016;**5**:440-449

[61] Prada Arias M, Gómez Veiras J, Rodríguez Iglesias P, et al. Treatment of pectus excavatum with vacuum bell during puberty. Cirugía Pediátrica. 2023;**36**:116-121

[62] Haller JA Jr, Colombani PM, Humphries CT, Azizkhan RG, Loughlin GM. Chest wall constriction after too extensive and too early operations for pectus excavatum. The Annals of Thoracic Surgery. 1996;**61**(6):1618-1624; discussion 1625. DOI: 10.1016/0003-4975(96)00179-8

[63] Nuss D, Kelly RE, Croitoru DP, et al. A 10-year review of a minimally invasive technique for the correction of pectus excavatum. Journal of Pediatric Surgery. 1998;**33**:545-552

[64] Kelly RE Jr, Shamberger RC, Mellins RB, Mitchell KK, Lawson ML, Oldham K, et al. Prospective multicenter study of surgical correction of pectus excavatum: Design, perioperative complications, pain, and baseline pulmonary function facilitated by internet-based data collection. Journal of the American College of Surgeons. 2007;**205**(2):205-216. DOI: 10.1016/j.jamcollsurg.2007.03.027. Epub 2007 Jun 21

[65] DiFiore JW, Robertson JO, Chhabada S, DeRoss AL, Hossain MS, Rincon-Cruz L, et al. Next day discharge after the Nuss procedure using intercostal nerve cryoablation, intercostal nerve blocks, and a perioperative ERAS pain protocol. Journal of Pediatric Surgery.

2022;**57**(2):213-218. DOI: 10.1016/j.jpedsurg.2021.10.034. Epub 2021 Oct 30

[66] Fallon SC, Slater BJ, Nuchtern JG, Cass DL, Kim ES, Lopez ME, et al. Complications related to the Nuss procedure: Minimizing risk with operative technique. Journal of Pediatric Surgery. 2013;**48**(5):1044-1048. DOI: 10.1016/j.jpedsurg.2013.02.025

[67] Belcher E, Arora S, Samancilar O, Goldstraw P. Reducing cardiac injury during minimally invasive repair of pectus excavatum. European Journal of Cardio-Thoracic Surgery. 2008;**33**(5):931-933. DOI: 10.1016/j.ejcts.2008.01.030. Epub 2008 Mar 4

[68] Park HJ, Lee SY, Lee CS. Complications associated with the Nuss procedure: Analysis of risk factors and suggested measures for prevention of complications. Journal of Pediatric Surgery. 2004;**39**(3):391-395; discussion 391-5. DOI: 10.1016/j.jpedsurg.2003.11.012

[69] Cheng YL, Lin CT, Wang HB, Chang H. Pleural effusion complicating after Nuss procedure for pectus excavatum. Annals of Thoracic and Cardiovascular Surgery. 2014;**20**(1):6-11. DOI: 10.5761/atcs.oa.12.02067. Epub 2013 Feb 15

[70] Ravitch MM. The operative treatment of pectus excavatum. Annals of Surgery. 1949;**129**:429-444

[71] Baronofsky ID. Technique for the correction of pectus excavatum. Surgery. 1957;**42**:884-890

[72] Welch KJ. Satisfactory surgical correction of pectus excavatum deformity in childhood: A limited opportunity. The Journal of Thoracic Surgery. 1958;**36**:697-713

[73] Johnson JN, Hartman TK, Pianosi PT, Driscoll DJ. Cardiorespiratory function after operation for pectus excavatum. The Journal of Pediatrics. 2008;**153**:359

[74] Yuksel M, Lacin T, Ermerak NO, Sirzai EY, Sayan B. Minimally invasive repair of pectus carinatum. The Annals of Thoracic Surgery. 2018;**105**(3):915-923. DOI: 10.1016/j.athoracsur.2017.10.003. Epub 2018 Jan 9

[75] Cobben JM, Oostra R-J, van Dijk FL. Pectus excavatum and carinatum. European Journal of Medical Genetics. 2014;**67**:414-417

[76] Abdellaoui S, Scalabre A, Piolat C, Lavrand F, Lachkar AA, Lehn A, et al. Pectus arcuatum: A pectus unlike any other. Journal of Pediatric Surgery. 2023;**58**(9):1679-1685. DOI: 10.1016/j.jpedsurg.2023.03.013. Epub 2023 Mar 23

[77] Bavinck JN, Weaver DD. Subclavian artery supply disruption sequence: Hypothesis of a vascular etiology for Poland, Klippel-Feil, and Möbius anomalies. American Journal of Medical Genetics. Apr 1986;**23**(4):903-918. DOI: 10.1002/ajmg.1320230405. PMID: 3008556

[78] Froriep R. Beobachtung eines Falles Von Mangel der Brustdruse. Notizen Gebiete Natur Helkunde. 1839;**10**:9-14

[79] Hashim EAA, Quek BH, Chandran S. A narrative review of Poland's syndrome: Theories of its genesis, evolution and its diagnosis and treatment. Translational Pediatrics. 2021;**10**(4):1008-1019. DOI: 10.21037/tp-20-320

[80] Bavinck JNB, Weaver DD. Subclavian artery supply disruption sequence: Hypothesis of a vascular etiology for Poland, Klippel-Feil, and Mobius anomalies. American Journal of Medical Genetics. 1986;**23**:903

[81] Van Allen MI. Fetal vascular disruptions: Mechanisms and some resulting birth defects. Pediatric Annals. 1981;**10**:219-233

[82] Hoyme HE, Jone KL, Van Allen MI, et al. Vascular pathogenesis of transverse limb reduction defects. The Journal of Pediatrics. 1982;**101**:839-843

[83] Cingel V, Bohac M, Mestanova V, et al. Poland syndrome: From embryological basis to plastic surgery. Surgical and Radiologic Anatomy. 2013;**35**:639-646

[84] Puvabanditsin S, Garrow E, Augustin G, et al. Poland-Möebius syndrome and cocaine abuse: A relook at vascular etiology. Pediatric Neurology. 2005;**32**:285-287

[85] Bamforth JS, Fabian C, Machin G, et al. Poland anomaly with a limb body wall disruption defect: Case report and review. American Journal of Medical Genetics. 1992;**43**:780-784

[86] Fraser FC, Ronen GM, O'Leary E. Pectoralis major defect and Poland sequence in second cousins: Extension of the Poland sequence spectrum. American Journal of Medical Genetics. 1989;**33**:468-470

[87] Berdel AL, Henrich W. Antenatal sonographic features of Poland syndrome on 2- and 3-dimensional sonography. Journal of Ultrasound in Medicine. 2010;**29**:679-680